NUTRITION FUNDAMENTALS AND MEDICAL NUTRITION THERAPY

THIRD EDITION

NUTRITION FUNDAMENTALS AND MEDICAL NUTRITION THERAPY

THIRD EDITION

Julie Zikmund, MPH, RDN, LRD

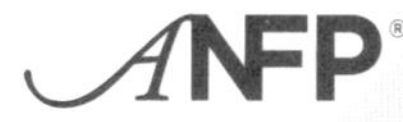

Association of Nutrition & Foodservice Professionals

Association of Nutrition & Foodservice Professionals
PO Box 3610
St. Charles, IL 60174
800.323.1908
www.ANFPonline.org

ISBN: 978-0-578-78016-0

Printed in the United States of America

Dedication

I dedicate this book to those dietitians on whose shoulders I firmly stand and from whom I have had the privilege of learning, for without your gift of shared knowledge, I would not be who I am today.

To my University of North Dakota Nutrition Sherpas: Becky Rude, Jean Hartl, Lynette Borth, Mary Russell, and Brenda Rubash—thank you for always keeping me grounded and yet reaching for new heights.

To the future Certified Dietary Manager,® Certified Food Protection Professional® (CDM®, CFPP®) who does not yet realize the potential and importance of the career they have chosen, and to those CDM, CFPPs who work every day at making their career a success and our world a much better place in which to live, I extend my gratitude.

Finally, and most of all, I dedicate this book to my family (Kevin, Zach, Andrew, Mom, Dad, and Augie) and friends, with all my love and appreciation. I could not have done it without you. I am truly blessed!

—Julie Zikmund, MPH, RDN, LRD

Table of Contents

The chapters are color coded based on CDM, CFPP professional competencies. This book includes two areas. The first six chapters include fundamentals of nutrition. The next 11 chapters include nutrition fundamentals related to the daily practice of the CDM, CFPP.

CHAPTER

Preface

Nutrition is a science that has been studied for centuries and continuously evolves related to new evidence. Research results may often change or modify practice applications. Food and nutrition are critical to human beings across the lifespan. From prenatal care through death, the Certified Dietary Manager®, Certified Food Protection Professional® (CDM®, CFPP®) plays an important role in providing proper nutrition and nutrition care.

The CDM, CFPP faces many opportunities and challenges in providing clinical nutrition care. At one time, health care involved just the physician and the client; however, times have changed. Health care includes many allied health professionals. How many different types of healthcare professionals will the CDM, CFPP work with daily? That list will likely include a/an: Registered Dietitian Nutritionist; Dietetic Technician, Registered; Nutrition and Dietetic Technician, Registered; Registered Nurse; Licensed Practical Nurse; Pharmacist; Licensed Social Worker; Medical Technologist; Respiratory Therapist; Physical Therapist; Occupational Therapist; Speech-Language Pathologist; and Activities Director. All are members of the healthcare team. A healthcare or interdisciplinary team is a group of specialists, in their respective areas, that work together to provide client care.

One component of the healthcare team is the nutrition care team. This may be comprised of some combination of the following: Registered Dietitian Nutritionist (RD/RDN); Nutrition and Dietetics Technician, Registered (NDTR); Certified Dietary Manager, Certified Food Protection Professional (CDM, CFPP); and foodservice staff. These members work together to provide optimal nutrition services to patients or residents. These leaders also recognize the importance and value of the entire department as additional team members.

Nutrition care for the client will include the selection and recommendation of foods based on nutrition science, application of food guides and tools to assess nutritional adequacy, planning menus based on nutrition needs of clients or populations, implementation and service of menus that meet guidelines, management of food allergies, and participation in the nutrition care process including: nutrition screening, documenting in the electronic health record, implementing medical nutrition therapy, and providing feedback and evaluation to the healthcare team as well as to other regulatory agencies.

The author's roadmap in writing this textbook is based on the Professional Standards of Practice for the CDM, CFPP and the role of nutrition care as a critical component of client care. These tasks represent current practice in the United States. Evidence-based nutrition science is the foundation of nutrition care and practice for the future CDM, CFPP. This textbook is intended for students learning to become a CDM, CFPP and as a reference for CDM, CFPPs working in the industry. In addition, this textbook integrates the 2021 Detailed Content Outline.

An additional online resource, *Nutrition Supplemental Materials,* is included for the student. This supplement offers documents, articles, and other information to assist in the learning and practice to become a CDM, CFPP.

Acknowledgments

We want to recognize the contribution of the review team who generously invested their professional expertise and valuable time:

Jill Braten, RD

Jolene Campbell, MEd, RD, LDN

Sona Donayan, MS, RDN

Catherine Kling Nourse, MPH, RDN, LD

Barbara Thomsen, CDM, CFPP, RAC, QCP

We would like to express our appreciation to the individuals who contributed as content editors of this textbook throughout the past few years:

Content Editors:

Melissa Baron, MS, RDN

Dorothy Chen-Maynard, PhD, RDN, FAND

Casey Colin, MS, RDN

Dr. Terri Lisagor, EdD, MS, RDN

Lauri Wright, PhD, RDN

Technical Editor: Diane Everett

ANFP Staff: Cindy Zemko, BS, CDM, CFPP

Art Direction/Graphic Design: Mercy Ehrler

A Personal Invitation

As a student enrolled in the Nutrition & Foodservice Professional Training Program, we invite you to join the Association of Nutrition & Foodservice Professionals (ANFP) as a Pre-Professional member.

ANFP is the premier resource for foodservice managers, directors, and those aspiring towards careers in foodservice management, with more than 14,000 professionals dedicated to the mission of providing optimum nutritional care through foodservice management and food safety.

Pre-Professional membership is a stepping stone for professional growth. Network and connect with members in all practice areas, understand the profession, and gain valuable tools and resources at your fingertips.

Enjoy benefits such as:

- 24/7 Members-only access to website, online community, and social media
- An electronic version of *Nutrition & Foodservice Edge* magazine
- Scholarship opportunities
- eNews monthly online newsletter
- Special discounted member pricing for ANFP products and services
- Network nationally, locally, and even globally with peers

You are the future of our profession. Take the first step in nourishing your career. Join ANFP today! For more information, visit www.ANFPonline.org or call 800-323-1908.

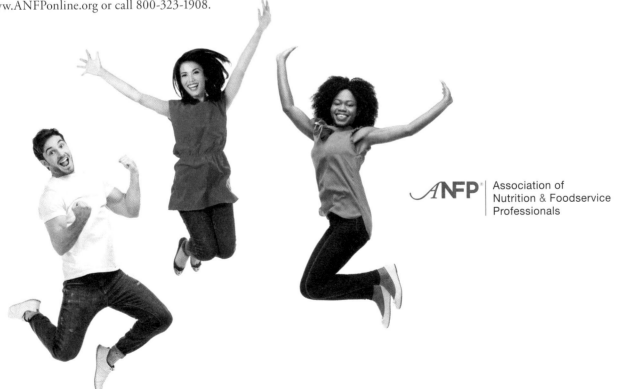

ANFP® Association of Nutrition & Foodservice Professionals

Translate Nutrition Science into Food Intake

Overview and Objectives

A Certified Dietary Manager®, Certified Food Protection Professional® (CDM®, CFPP®) needs to select and recommend food according to established science-based nutrition guidelines. In addition, a CDM, CFPP needs to be able to use guides to assess nutritional adequacy. After completing this chapter, you should be able to:

- Discuss the importance of good nutrition and physical activity for a healthy lifestyle
- Discuss dietary recommendations for simple carbohydrates (sugars) and complex carbohydrates (fiber)
- Discuss dietary recommendations for fats (total fat, saturated fat, and cholesterol)
- Explore health effects of protein
- Distinguish between vitamins and minerals
- Identify the role of water as a nutrient
- Define phytochemicals and functional foods
- Select the best food sources of specific vitamins and minerals
- Define daily fluid requirement
- Differentiate between different food guides
- Analyze dietary intake compared to MyPlate

1

This chapter will help you understand the relationship between overall dietary intake and nutrition status. Nutrition status and "total diet" have to do with consuming food and the body utilizing that food for growth, regulation, and maintenance. The Dietary Guidelines Advisory Committee (DGAC) defines "total diet" as "the combination of foods and beverages that provide energy and nutrients and constitute an individual's complete dietary intake, on average, over time. This encompasses various foods and food groups, their recommended amounts and frequency (to be eaten) and the resulting eating pattern." With so many foods to choose from, what is the best combination of foods that provide a balance of nutrients?

Sound nutrition advice combined with food consumption advice is available from both government and private agencies.

This chapter will explore:

- Healthy People Initiative
- Dietary Reference Intakes (DRIs)
- Dietary Guidelines for Americans
- USDA Food Plans
- MyPlate

Nutrition as a Science

Nutrition is based in science—biology, chemistry, anatomy, physiology, psychology, anthropology—just to name a few. Nutrition has been observed and studied since ancient times, with early observations written by Aristotle and Socrates. Nutrition investigation and scientific discovery continued until the late 1700-1800s when the ability to identify nutrients in food became possible. In those years of "rapid discovery," early nutrition research focused on identifying essential nutrients. During the last century, the 1900s, nutrition advice centered on encouraging intake of certain foods to prevent deficiencies and enhance growth. In recent years, however, the focus has changed, as nutrition scientists devote a great deal of research to the opposite problem: nutritional excess and imbalance. The first Surgeon General's Report on Nutrition and Health in 1988 was a turning point for nutritional planning. The report concluded that over-consumption of certain nutrients—not deficiency—should be the primary nutritional concern for Americans. Generally, the over-consumed nutrients are macronutrients, like fats (certain types), protein and carbohydrates, as well as overall caloric-intake.

The Health Status of the United States

In the early 1990s, the United States Department of Agriculture (USDA) and the U.S. Department of Health and Human Services (HHS) focused attention on the issue of nutrition excess and imbalance. The USDA and HHS were charged with tracking what Americans eat, the nutritional content of the food, and the related health concerns connected with consumption of these foods. These two agencies and the Centers for Disease Control and Prevention (CDC) conduct ongoing national food surveys: USDA's Continuing Survey of Food Intakes by Individuals (CSFII) and CDC's National Health and Nutrition Examination Survey (NHANES). The results of these two surveys give us insight into the eating patterns of Americans.

The NHANES survey results showed that Americans eat excess calories, fats, added sugars, refined grains, and sodium. Conversely, Americans do not consume enough dietary fiber, vitamin D, calcium, potassium, unsaturated fatty acids (specifically omega-3s), and other important nutrients. Many of these nutrients are found in vegetables, fruits, whole grains, low-fat milk and dairy products, and seafood.

Obesity is a major public health challenge, not only in the United States, but worldwide. According to the Surgeon General's Report in 2010, "obesity contributes to an estimated 112,000 preventable deaths in the U.S. annually." Figure 1.1 shows obesity trends for individuals aged 18 and older. This obesity trend is a concern not just for adults, but also youth of all ages. Due to the dramatic increase in childhood obesity, the White House convened a Task Force on Childhood Obesity (including 12 federal agencies) in 2010 to make recommendations to address childhood obesity.

Overweight is calculated by figuring **body mass index (BMI)**. BMI is used to express weight adjusted for height. BMI is calculated as weight in kilograms divided by height in meters squared. There are many charts available where one can just enter height in inches and weight in pounds to pinpoint BMI. **Overweight** is defined as being at a BMI of 25-29.9. **Obesity** is defined as being at a BMI of 30 or greater.

According to the Dietary Guidelines Advisory Committee Report on Energy Balance and Weight Management, 2010, the conditions listed in Figure 1.2 are health risks associated with overweight and obesity and with a sedentary lifestyle. Note the health risks that are the same.

Obesity is influenced by many factors. For each individual, body weight is the result of a combination of genetic, metabolic, behavioral, environmental, cultural, and socioeconomic influences. However, based on a growing amount of evidence provided by the Dietary Guidelines Advisory Committee, there are two factors that have a significant impact on the obesity epidemic:

- The food environment
- Amount of physical activity

GLOSSARY

Body Mass Index (BMI)
A proportion of weight to height

Overweight
Having a BMI of 25.0-29.9 Kg/m^2

Obesity
Having a BMI of 30.0 Kg/m^2 or greater

Figure 1.1
2018: Percent of Adults Aged 18 Years and Older Who Have Obesity

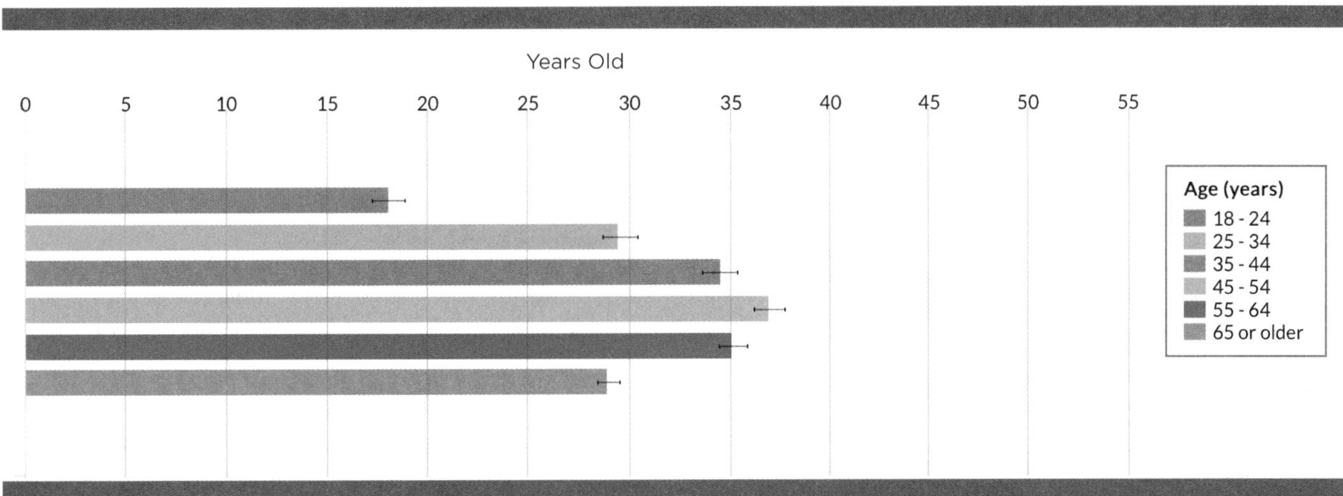

Source: Centers for Disease Control and Prevention

Figure 1.2

Health Risks Associated with Overweight, Obesity, and Sedentary Lifestyles

Overweight and Obesity Associated Health Risks	Sedentary Lifestyle Associated Health Risks
• Type 2 Diabetes • Hypertension • Cardiovascular Disease (CVD) • Stroke • Certain Kinds of Cancer • Osteoarthritis • Gallbladder Disease • Sleep Apnea • Dyslipidemia	• Type 2 Diabetes • Hypertension • Coronary Artery Disease • Stroke • Certain Kinds of Cancer • Osteoporosis • Depression • Decreased Health-Related Quality of Life • Overweight and Obesity • Decreased Overall Fitness

Note that some of the health risks are the same in both categories.
Source: Centers for Disease Control and Prevention and Healthy People 2020

The food environment is associated with a lower intake of fruits and vegetables and an increased body weight. Food environment includes the distance from a supermarket that offers a large variety of fruits and vegetables, and the density of fast food restaurants in the area where a person lives. The strongest documented relationship between fast food and obesity is when one or more fast food meals are consumed in a week. There is also a direct relationship between portion size and body weight. Discussions of food environment must also include "screen time" (amount of time spent on watching TV, the computer, or video games) for both adults and children. The strongest association with overweight and obesity is with television screen time.

Research indicates that there is an imbalance with excess energy intake when compared to energy expenditure at the current level of physical activity. While food alone does not cause, cure, or control obesity, weight control is an important nutrition issue. When consuming more than what is expended, weight gain can be seen. Exercise is a key component in disease prevention and weight management. Regular (daily) exercise helps a person:

- Balance energy intake and energy expenditure (see Figure 1.3)
- Prevent heart disease by strengthening the heart and cardiovascular system
- Achieve a healthy weight and reduce the risk of developing certain types of cancer (breast, colon, and other forms linked to obesity)

It is obvious from the information above that both dietary intervention and regular physical activity are needed in order to reach goals of maintaining energy balance and preventing disease. Figure 1.4 provides physical activity goals and facts on inactivity.

1. What would BMI be for an individual who is 5'6" tall and weighs 175 lbs.?

Figure 1.3
Energy Balance

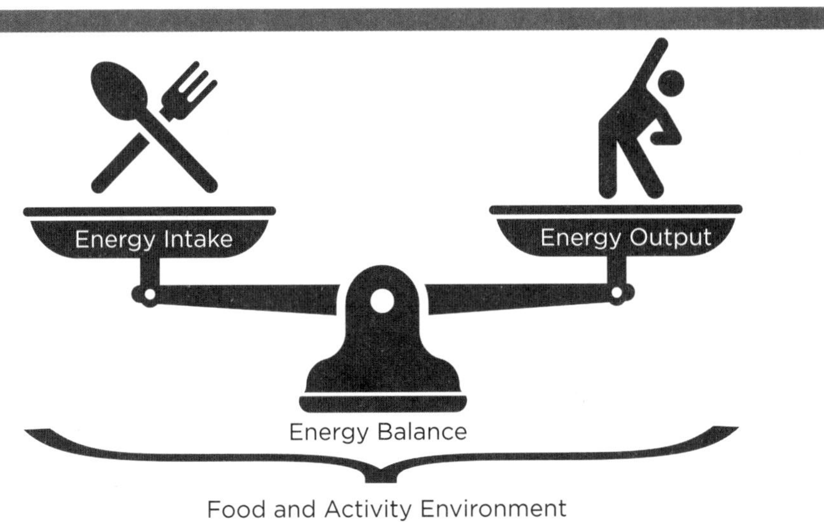

Figure 1.4
Physical Activity Goals and Facts on Inactivity

- It is recommended that Americans accumulate at least 30 minutes (adults) or 60 minutes (children) of moderate physical activity most days of the week. More may be needed to prevent weight gain, to lose weight, or to maintain weight loss.
- Less than 1/3 of adults engage in the recommended amounts of physical activity.
- Many people live sedentary lives; in fact, 40 percent of adults in the United States do not participate in any leisure time physical activity.
- 43 percent of adolescents watch more than 2 hours of television each day.
- Physical activity is extremely helpful in maintaining weight loss, especially when combined with healthy eating.

Source: US Surgeon General and American Cancer Society

Healthy People Initiative

For the past three decades, the U.S. Department of Health and Human Services (HHS) has set science-based, 10-year national objectives for promoting health and preventing disease. Healthy People 2020 is the current edition. Healthy People Initiatives have established benchmarks for the United States population and monitor progress made towards achieving these goals. Healthy People 2020 national objectives are aimed at improving the health of all Americans. The focus of Healthy People 2020 is to encourage collaborations across communities and sectors, empower individuals toward making informed health decisions, and to measure the impact of prevention activities.

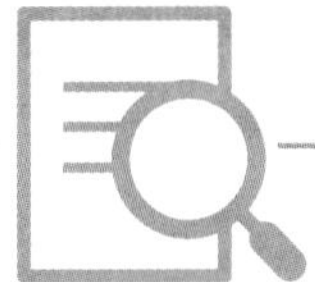

View the Supplemental Material to see the latest Healthy People 2030.

Healthy People 2020 was launched in December 2010. It is an ambitious, yet achievable, 10-year agenda for improving the nation's health. Healthy People 2020 is the result of a multiyear process that reflects input from a diverse group of individuals and organizations. The vision of Healthy People 2020 is stated as "A society in which all people live long, healthy lives."

Here is a bit more background information on the overarching activities to support the vision of Healthy People 2020:

- Identify nationwide health improvement priorities.
- Increase public awareness and understanding of the determinants of health, disease and disability, and the opportunities for progress.
- Provide measurable objectives and goals that are applicable at the national, state, and local levels.
- Engage multiple sectors to take actions to strengthen policies and improve practices that are driven by the best available evidence and knowledge.
- Identify critical research, evaluation, and data collection needs.

Overarching Goals: Healthy People 2020 is working to:

- Attain high-quality, longer lives free of preventable disease, disability, injury, and premature death.
- Achieve health equity, eliminate disparities, and improve the health of all groups.
- Create social and physical environments that promote good health for all.
- Promote quality of life, healthy development, and healthy behaviors across all life stages.

There are 38 categories of objectives that range from A (Access to Health Services) to V (Vision). Many categories have a tie to nutrition and the role of nutrition in disease prevention. Figure 1.5 shows the objectives for the Nutrition and Weight Status category.

The purpose of these objectives is to provide direction for diverse groups of people to combine their efforts and work as a team. All parts of health care should address these objectives, and as an organization work towards improving health, as set forth in Healthy People 2020. Remember, the Healthy People Initiative is a population-based approach to improve the health status of all Americans.

Dietary Reference Intakes (DRIs)

Since 1941, the Food and Nutrition Board of the National Academy of Sciences has been preparing recommendations on nutrient intakes for Americans. Contemporary studies address topics ranging from the prevention of classical nutritional deficiency diseases to the reduction of risk of chronic diseases such as osteoporosis, cancer, and cardiovascular disease. In partnership with Health Canada, the Food and Nutrition Board has responded to these developments by making fundamental changes in its approach to setting nutrient reference values. This partnership issued the first of its new standards in 1997, replacing Recommended Dietary Allowances (RDAs). Dietary Reference Intakes is the inclusive name given to the new approach.

Dietary Reference Intakes (DRIs) is a generic term used to refer to four types of reference values: **Estimated Average Requirement, Recommended Dietary Allowance, Adequate Intake,** and **Tolerable Upper Intake Level**. Dietary reference intakes are designed for various age and gender groups, because nutrient needs vary from childhood through adulthood and some vary between males and females.

Estimated Average Requirement

The Estimated Average Requirement (EAR) is the intake value that is estimated to meet the requirement defined by a specified indicator of adequacy in 50 percent of a specific group (age and gender group). A requirement is how much is needed in the

GLOSSARY

Dietary Reference Intakes (DRIs)
A generic term that encompasses four types of reference values: Estimated Average Requirement, Recommended Dietary Allowance, Adequate Intake, and Tolerable Upper Intake Level

Estimated Average Requirement (EAR)
Intake value that is estimated to meet the requirements defined by a specific indicator of adequacy in 50 percent of a specific group (age/gender)

Recommended Dietary Allowance (RDA)
The amount of a nutrient adequate to meet the known nutrient needs of practically all healthy persons

Adequate Intake (AI)
A specific judgment or the amount of some nutrients for which a specific RDA is not known

Tolerable Upper Intake Level (UL)
The maximum level of a daily nutrient that is considered safe

Figure 1.5
Healthy People 2020 Nutrition and Weight Status Objectives

- Increase the proportion of adults who are at a healthy weight.
- Reduce the proportion of adults who are obese.
- Reduce iron deficiency among young children and females of childbearing age.
- Reduce iron deficiency among pregnant females.
- Reduce the proportion of children and adolescents who are overweight or obese.
- Increase the contribution of fruits to the diets of the population aged 2 years and older.
- Increase the variety and contribution of vegetables to the diets of the population aged 2 years and older.
- Increase the contribution of whole grains to the diets of the population aged 2 years and older.
- Reduce consumption of saturated fat in the population aged 2 years and older.
- Reduce consumption of sodium in the population aged 2 years and older.
- Increase consumption of calcium in the population aged 2 years and older.
- (Developmental) Increase the proportion of worksites that offer nutrition or weight management classes or counseling.
- Increase the proportion of physician office visits that include counseling or education related to nutrition or body weight.
- Eliminate very low food security among children in U.S. households.
- (Developmental) Prevent inappropriate weight gain in youth and adults.
- Increase the proportion of primary care physicians who regularly measure the body mass index of their patients.
- Reduce consumption of calories from solid fats and added sugars in the population aged 2 years and older.
- Increase the number of States that have State-level policies that incentivize food retail outlets to provide foods that are encouraged by the Dietary Guidelines.
- Increase the number of States with nutrition standards for foods and beverages provided to preschool-aged children in childcare.
- Increase the percentage of schools that offer nutritious foods and beverages outside of school meals.

Source: Centers for Disease Control and Prevention and Healthy People 2020

diet to prevent symptoms of deficiency. A deficiency is the illness that occurs over time when a nutrient is not present in adequate amounts. For example, not eating enough vitamin C causes the deficiency disease scurvy. Not having enough vitamin D causes the deficiency disease rickets. Scurvy and rickets are examples of nutrient deficiency illnesses. At the EAR level of intake, 50 percent of the specified group would not have its needs met. In other words, if everyone consumed exactly the EAR levels of nutrients, some people would actually develop nutrient deficiencies. Thus, the EAR is designed only for setting a benchmark for baseline nutrient requirements. An EAR is not intended for use in evaluating an individual's dietary intake.

Recommended Dietary Allowance

A Recommended Dietary Allowance (RDA) is the amount of a nutrient that is adequate to meet the known nutrient needs of practically all healthy persons. Contrary to popular belief, an RDA is not a minimum daily requirement. It is a dietary recommendation. To develop RDAs, scientists first review research studies that indicate what minimum levels of nutrients might be required to prevent nutrient deficiencies. Then, they adjust the requirements to account for additional factors that might affect requirements. They also consider the numbers to account for the difference between the amount of a nutrient consumed and the amount the body can actually use. The scientists use statistics to calculate individual variations in nutrient needs and project figures that address the needs of most healthy people. Thus, an RDA is truly a recommendation about how much of a nutrient to consume through food. If everyone consumed exactly the RDA levels of nutrients, very few people in that group would develop nutrient deficiencies. Also, RDAs are for healthy individuals. RDAs do not always apply to someone who is suffering from a chronic illness or who has special medical conditions. Unlike the EAR, an RDA is a goal for groups of individuals.

Adequate Intake

For some nutrients, there is simply not enough science to set a meaningful RDA. Currently, the scientific research that backs up the calculation of requirements has not been done. When this is the case, an Adequate Intake (AI) value is issued. For example, there is no information about the physiological requirements for choline. Instead of setting an RDA, experts have designated an AI for choline. An AI represents a scientific judgment. An AI covers the nutrient needs of groups or individuals, but the AI value seems to be a reasonable point of reference based on what is currently available in the research. When the only standard available for a nutrient is an AI, it is fine to apply the AI to both groups and individuals.

Tolerable Upper Intake Level

The Tolerable Upper Intake Level (UL) is the maximum level of daily nutrient intake that is unlikely to pose risks of adverse health effects. ULs have been developed for some nutrients as safety guidelines. For example, these points of reference are helpful in determining whether the doses of nutrients contained in nutritional supplements represent safe intakes.

Setting dietary reference intakes is a complex task. Scientists are working to develop figures that can be referred to when assessing individuals' diets and planning menus. Due to the enormity of this undertaking, the Dietary Reference Intake project has been divided into seven nutrient groups, which are updated intermittently based on the latest scientific findings.

How Should the Dietary Reference Intakes be Used?

The RDAs were developed to assess the diets of groups of people rather than individuals. Be sure to use the DRIs to plan and evaluate the diets of clients. Because the body stores nutrients for later use, it is not necessary to eat the RDAs every day. The USDA has a website that lists the current DRI tables (http://fnic.nal.usda.gov/interactiveDRI/). Log on to use the interactive tool to calculate daily nutrient recommendations for a client and for dietary planning based on the Dietary Reference Intakes (DRIs).

2. Which would be a more appropriate DRI for someone planning a menu in a facility: EAR or RDA?

Nutrition Guidance for Americans

With so much nutrition information, so many recommendations, and plenty of health and nutrition goals, how can a person make sense of it all? How can one evaluate diets, plan adequate menus, or advise others about how to choose the "right" foods?

The Center for Nutrition Policy and Promotion, under the umbrella of the United States Department of Agriculture, was established in 1994 to improve the nutrition and wellbeing of Americans. The Center has two primary objectives:

1. Advance and promote dietary guidance for all Americans, and
2. Conduct applied research and analyses in nutrition and consumer economics.

The Center has six core initiatives to reach its objectives: (those starred below will be addressed in this chapter)

1. Dietary Guidelines for Americans*
2. USDA Food Patterns
3. MyPlate*
4. Healthy Eating Index
5. Nutrient Content of the U.S. Food Supply
6. Expenditures on Children by Families

Dietary Guidelines for Americans

The *2015-20 Dietary Guidelines for Americans* (*Dietary Guidelines* for short) support a total diet approach to achieving dietary goals. The *Dietary Guidelines* are issued jointly by the U.S. Department of Agriculture (USDA) and the U.S. Department of Health and Human Services (HHS). According to the USDA, "The *Dietary Guidelines* is designed for professionals to help all individuals ages 2 years and older and their families consume a healthy, nutritionally adequate diet. The information in the *Dietary Guidelines* is used in developing Federal food, nutrition, and health policies and programs. It also is the basis for Federal nutrition education materials designed for the public and for the nutrition education components of HHS and USDA food programs."

According to the USDA and HHS, the *2015-20 Dietary Guidelines for Americans (8th Edition)* focuses on healthy eating patterns and regular physical activity to help people achieve and maintain good health and reduce the risk of chronic disease throughout all stages of the lifespan. The 2015-20 Dietary Guidelines encourages healthy eating patterns and healthy food and beverage choices focusing on variety, nutrient density, and amount, and supports healthy eating patterns.

Helping Americans incorporate these Guidelines into their everyday lives is important to improving the overall health of the American people. The *2015-20 Dietary Guidelines for Americans* includes 5 general guidelines that encourage healthy eating patterns for the general population and additional Key Recommendations for specific population groups, such as women who are pregnant. Key Recommendations are the most important messages within the Guidelines in terms of their implications for improving public health and reducing development of chronic diseases. The recommendations are intended as advice to achieve an overall healthy eating pattern. To get the full benefit, all Americans should achieve all of the Dietary Guidelines' recommendations in their entirety. Find it at: https://www.dietaryguidelines.gov/current-dietary-guidelines/2015-2020-dietary-guidelines.

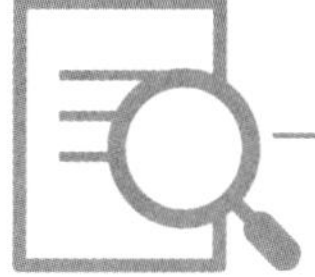

View supplemental material for more information on Dietary Guidelines

The USDA solicits the foremost nutrition experts in the country to serve on the Dietary Guidelines Advisory Committee. These experts convene to examine the most current research surrounding nutrition outcomes, and use this updated research to revise and publish the newest Dietary Guidelines every five years. The Dietary Guidelines Advisory Committee also takes into account feedback from professionals and consumers when formulating the newest guidelines. The latest *Dietary Guidelines* can be found in the Supplemental Material.

The USDA and HHS also developed more consumer-friendly advice and tools, such as MyPlate. Below is a preview of some of the tips to help consumers translate the Dietary Guidelines into their everyday lives:

Balance the Energy Intake

- Enjoy your food, but eat less.
- Avoid oversized portions.

Foods to Increase

- Make half your plate fruits and vegetables.
- Switch to fat-free or low-fat (1%) milk.
- Make at least half your grains whole grains.

Foods to Reduce

- Compare sodium in foods like soup, bread, and frozen meals—and choose the foods with lower numbers.
- Drink water instead of sugary drinks.

The *Dietary Guidelines* "summarize and synthesize knowledge regarding individual nutrients and food recommendations into a pattern of eating that can be adopted by the public." They are updated every five years based on new scientific information.

Dietary Guidelines generally categorize and make recommendations under topic areas/groups. Each topic area or group contains a series of key recommendations, including some for specific population groups. The *Dietary Guidelines* are full of the science, recommendations, and goals for healthy eating. Even with all of that information, it seems an average American is not any closer to understanding what foods need to be eaten to attain good health.

Healthy Eating Plans

An **eating plan** or **eating pattern** translates dietary recommendations and current research into a healthy way of eating for most individuals. The plans or patterns are examples of how to eat in accordance with the Dietary Guidelines. Three eating plans based on the Dietary Guidelines are:

- USDA Food Patterns
- MyPlate
- DASH Diet (covered in Chapter 6)

GLOSSARY

Eating Plan or Eating Pattern
Translation of the dietary recommendations and research into a healthy way of eating for most individuals

USDA Food Patterns

The USDA Food Patterns, based on the *Dietary Guidelines*, were developed to translate the science into a workable form for individuals to make food choices. They identify daily amounts of foods from each food group. Individuals need to eat from five major food groups, as well as specific amounts of foods from subgroups from the major food groups. In addition, the patterns also include an allowance for oils and limits on the maximum number of calories that should be consumed from solid fats and added sugars (empty calories or low nutrient density food).

Recommended amounts and limits in the USDA Food Patterns at 12 calorie levels, ranging from 1,000 calories to 3,200 calories, are shown in Figure 1.7 USDA Food Patterns. Food Patterns at 1,000, 1,200 and 1,400 calorie levels meet the nutritional needs of children ages 2 to 8 years. Patterns at 1,600 calories and above meet the needs for adults and children ages 9 years and older. Individuals should follow a pattern that meets their estimated calorie needs—shown in the "Estimated Calorie Needs per Day" table.

The USDA Food Patterns (see Figure 1.7a and 1.7b) are the recommended daily intake amounts from each food group or subgroup at all calorie levels. Recommended intakes from vegetable subgroups are per week. This food pattern can be used to plan menus for school foodservice, correctional facilities, and healthcare facilities. Additional food patterns are available online at: www.fns.usda.gov/cnd/menu/menu_planning.doc

The USDA Food Patterns help simplify the *Dietary Guidelines* for Americans into a form that can be quantified or measured daily or weekly. For most, this is still a complex system to ensure that our bodies get the nutrition we need. Let's look at MyPlate, which helps clarify what should be eaten at each meal.

MyPlate

For the past 100 years or so, the United States Department of Agriculture (USDA) has been providing food guidance to the public. The USDA has had many different food guidance systems based on the nutrition science of the time. There have been as few as 4 food groups. There have also been as many as 9 different food groups. The basis for all of these food guidance systems is to attempt to help people *visualize* what should be on our plates and ultimately in the body to help it grow and be healthy.

In addition to the food guidance systems, there have been many attempts by USDA to help us understand "how much" food should be eaten (portion sizes). Many figures discuss how to select foods, what protection or health benefits they may have, and to focus primarily on eating foods rather than eating "nutrients." Some of the other key messages include variety, consistency ("eat this way every day" for example), moderation, and nutrition adequacy.

When taking a look at the history of the food guidance systems, many focus on the reduction of certain foods to make Americans aware of dietary excesses. This is true when focusing on the concepts of eating fats, oils, and sweets less often to maintain energy balance. When looking at the messages over time, the shift in attention to the rise in obesity in the United States is quite evident. As America has become heavier, the messages found in the food guidance system also reflect a similar message. More recently, an increase in the physical activity messages and its role in maintaining health have been added. Glimpses of this message appeared in the 1940s through the 1970s, then it reappeared with a strong emphasis in 2005.

Fast forward to the newest Food Guidance from USDA: MyPlate. In the summer of 2011, MyPlate became the newest in a long line of Food Guidance Systems that helps people visualize what should be put on the plate at each meal. Here are some features about 2011 MyPlate:

- Introduced along with updated USDA food patterns for the 2020 *Dietary Guidelines for Americans*
- Different shape to help grab consumers' attention with a new visual cue
- Icon that serves as a reminder for healthy eating, not intended to provide specific messages

Figure 1.6

MyPlate—Estimated Calorie Needs per Day by Age, Gender, and Activity Level

Estimated amounts of calories[a] needed to maintain calorie balance for various gender and age groups at three different levels of physical activity. The estimates are rounded to the nearest 200 calories for assignment to a USDA Food Pattern. An individual's calorie needs may be higher or lower than these average estimates. *(Source: USDA)*

	MALE			FEMALE[c]		
ACTIVITY LEVEL[b]	Sedentary	Moderately Active	Active	Sedentary	Moderately Active	Active
2	1,000	1,000	1,000	1,000	1,000	1,000
3	1,200	1,400	1,400	1,000	1,200	1,400
4	1,200	1,400	1,600	1,200	1,400	1,400
5	1,200	1,400	1,600	1,200	1,400	1,600
6	1,400	1,600	1,800	1,200	1,400	1,600
7	1,400	1,600	1,800	1,200	1,600	1,800
8	1,400	1,600	2,000	1,400	1,600	1,800
9	1,600	1,800	2,000	1,400	1,600	1,800
10	1,600	1,800	2,200	1,400	1,800	2,000
11	1,800	2,000	2,200	1,600	1,800	2,000
12	1,800	2,200	2,400	1,600	2,000	2,200
13	2,000	2,200	2,600	1,600	2,000	2,200
14	2,000	2,400	2,800	1,800	2,000	2,400
15	2,200	2,600	3,000	1,800	2,000	2,400
16	2,400	2,800	3,200	1,800	2,000	2,400
17	2,400	2,800	3,200	1,800	2,000	2,400
18	2,400	2,800	3,200	1,800	2,000	2,400
19-20	2,600	2,800	3,000	2,000	2.200	2,400
21-25	2,400	2,800	3,000	2,000	2,200	2,400
26-30	2,400	2,600	3,000	1,800	2,000	2,400
31-35	2,400	2,600	3,000	1,800	2,000	2,200
36-40	2,400	2,600	2,800	1,800	2,000	2,200
41-45	2,200	2,600	2,800	1,800	2,000	2,200
46-50	2,200	2,400	2,800	1,800	2,000	2,200
51-55	2,200	2,400	2,800	1,600	1,800	2,200
56-60	2,200	2,400	2,600	1,600	1,800	2,200
61-65	2,000	2,400	2,600	1,600	1,800	2,000
66-70	2,000	2,200	2,600	1,600	1,800	2,000
71-75	2,000	2,200	2,600	1,600	1,800	2,000
76+	2,000	2,200	2,400	1,600	1,800	2,000

a. Based on Estimated Energy Requirements (EER) equations, using reference heights (average) and reference weights (healthy) for each age-gender group. For children and adolescents, reference height and weight vary. For adults, the reference man is 5 feet 10 inches tall and weighs 154 pounds. The reference woman is 5 feet 4 inches tall and weighs 126 pounds. EER equations are from the Institute of Medicine. Dietary Reference Intakes for Energy, Carbohydrate, Fiber, Fat, Fatty Acids, Cholesterol, Protein and Amino Acids. Washington (DC): The National Academies Press; 2002.

b. Sedentary means a lifestyle that includes only the light physical activity associated with typical day-to-day life. Moderately active means a lifestyle that includes physical activity equivalent to walking about 1.5 to 3 miles per day at 3 to 4 miles per hour, in addition to the light physical activity associated with typical day-to-day life. Active means a lifestyle that includes physical activity equivalent to walking more than 3 miles per day at 3 to 4 miles per hour, in addition to the light physical activity associated with typical day-to-day life.

c. Estimates for females do not include women who are pregnant or breastfeeding.

Source: U.S. Department of Agriculture, Center for Nutrition Policy and Promotion

Figure 1.7a

USDA Food Patterns

The Food Patterns suggest amounts of food to consume from the basic food groups, subgroups, and oils to meet recommended nutrient intakes at 12 different calorie levels. Nutrient and energy contributions from each group are calculated according to the nutrient-dense forms of foods in each group (e.g., lean meats and fat-free milk). The table also shows the number of calories from solid fats and added sugars (SoFAS) that can be accommodated within each calorie level, in addition to the suggested amounts of nutrient-dense forms of foods in each group.

Daily Amount of Food from Each Group

Calorie Level[1]	1,000	1,200	1,400	1,600	1,800	2,000	2,200	2,400	2,600	2,800	3,000	3,200
Fruits[2]	1 cup	1 cup	1-1/2 cups	1-1/2 cups	1-1/2 cups	2 cups	2 cups	2 cups	2 cups	2-1/2 cups	2-1/2 cups	2-1/2 cups
Vegetables[3]	1 cup	1-1/2 cups	1-1/2 cups	2 cups	2-1/2 cups	2-1/2 cups	3 cups	3 cups	3-1/2 cups	3-1/2 cups	4 cups	4 cups
Grains[4]	3 oz.-eq.	4 oz-eq.	5 oz-eq.	5 oz-eq.	6 oz-eq.	6 oz-eq.	7 oz-eq.	8 oz-eq.	9 oz-eq.	10 oz-eq.	10 oz-eq.	10 oz-eq.
Protein Foods[5]	2 oz-eq.	3 oz-eq.	4 oz-eq.	5 oz-eq.	5 oz-eq.	5-1/2 oz-eq.	6 oz-eq.	6-1/2 oz-eq.	6-1/2 oz-eq.	7 oz-eq.	7 oz-eq.	7 oz-eq.
Dairy[6]	2 cups	2-1/2 cups	2-1/2 cups	3 cups	3 cups	3 cups	3 cups	3 cups	3 cups	3 cups	3 cups	3 cups
Oils[7]	15 g	17 g	17 g	22 g	24 g	27 g	29 g	31 g	34 g	36 g	44 g	51 g
Limit on calories from SoFAS[8]	137	121	121	121	161	258	266	330	362	395	459	596

Vegetable Subgroup Amounts Per Week

Calorie Level	1,000	1,200	1,400	1,600	1,800	2,000	2,200	2,400	2,600	2,800	3,000	3,200
Dark-green Vegetables	1/2 c./wk.	1 c./wk.	1 c./wk.	1-1/2 c./wk.	1-1/2 c./wk.	1-1/2 c./wk.	2 c./wk.	2 c./wk.	2-1/2 c./wk.	2-1/2 c./wk.	2-1/2 c./wk.	2-1/2 c./wk.
Red and Orange Vegetables	2-1/2 c./wk.	3 c./wk.	3 c./wk.	4 c./wk.	5-1/2 c./wk.	5-1/2 c./wk.	6 c./wk.	6 c./wk.	7 c./wk.	7 c./wk.	7-1/2 c./wk.	7-1/2 c./wk.
Beans and Peas (e.g. pintos, lentils, split peas)	1/2 c./wk.	1/2 c./wk.	1/2 c./wk.	1 c./wk.	1-1/2 c./wk.	1-1/2 c./wk.	2 c./wk.	2 c./wk.	2-1/2 c./wk.	2-1/2 c./wk.	3 c./wk.	3 c./wk.
Starchy Vegetables	2 c./wk.	3-1/2 c./wk.	3-1/2 c./wk.	4 c./wk.	5 c./wk.	5 c./wk.	6 c./wk.	6 c./wk.	7 c./wk.	7 c./wk.	8 c./wk.	8 c./wk.
Other Vegetables	1-1/2 c./wk.	2-1/2 c./wk.	2-1/2 c./wk.	3-1/2 c./wk.	4 c./wk.	4 c./wk.	5 c./wk.	5 c./wk.	5-1/2 c./wk.	5-1/2 c./wk.	7 c./wk.	7 c./wk.

Protein Foods Subgroup Amounts Per Week

Calorie Level	1,000	1,200	1,400	1,600	1,800	2,000	2,200	2,400	2,600	2,800	3,000	3,200
Seafood	3 oz./wk.	5 oz./wk.	6 oz./wk.	8 oz./wk.	8 oz./wk.	8 oz./wk.	9 oz./wk.	10 oz./wk.	10 oz./wk.	11 oz./wk.	11 oz./wk.	11 oz./wk.
Meats, Poultry, Eggs	10 oz./wk.	14 oz./wk.	19 oz./wk.	24 oz./wk.	24 oz./wk.	26 oz./wk.	29 oz./wk.	31 oz./wk.	31 oz./wk.	34 oz./wk.	34 oz./wk.	34 oz./wk.
Nuts, Seeds, Soy	1 oz./wk.	2 oz./wk.	3 oz./wk.	4 oz./wk.	4 oz./wk.	4 oz./wk.	4 oz./wk.	5 oz./wk.	5 oz./wk.	5 oz./wk.	5 oz./wk.	5 oz./wk.

1 **Calorie Levels** are set across a wide range to accommodate the needs of different individuals. The table "Estimated Daily Calorie Needs" can be used to help assign individuals to the food pattern at a particular calorie level.

2 **Fruit Group** includes all fresh, frozen, canned and dried fruits and fruit juices. In general, 1 cup of fruit or 100% fruit juice, or ½ cup of dried fruit can be considered as 1 cup from the fruit group.

3 **Vegetable Group** includes all fresh, frozen, canned and dried vegetables and vegetable juices. In general, 1 cup of raw or cooked vegetables or vegetable juice, or 2 cups of raw leafy greens can be considered as 1 cup from the vegetable group.

4 **Grains Group** includes all foods made from wheat, rice, oats, cornmeal, barley, such as bread, pasta, oatmeal, breakfast cereals, tortillas and grits. In general, 1 slice of bread, 1 cup of ready-to-eat cereal, or ½ cup of cooked rice, pasta, or cooked cereal can be considered as 1 ounce-equivalent from the grains group. At least half of all grains consumed should be whole grains.

5 **Proteins Group** includes meat, poultry, seafood, eggs, processed soy products and nuts and seeds. In general, 1 ounce of lean meat, poultry, or seafood, 1 egg, 1 Tbsp. peanut butter, or 1/2 ounce of nuts or seeds can be considered as 1 ounce equivalent from the protein group. Also, 1/4 cup of beans or peas may be counted as a 1 ounce equivalent in this group.

6 **Dairy Group** includes all milks, including lactose-free products and fortified soy milk (soy beverage) and foods made from milk that retain their calcium content, such as yogurt and cheese. Foods made from milk that have little to no calcium, such as cream cheese, cream and butter, are not part of the group. Most dairy group choices should be fat-free or low-fat. In general, 1 cup of milk or yogurt, 1½ ounces of natural cheese, or 2 ounces of processed cheese can be considered as 1 cup from the dairy group.

7 **Oils** include fats from many different plants and from fats that are liquid at room temperature, such as canola, corn, olive, soybean and sunflower oil. Some foods are naturally high in oils, like nuts, olives, some fish and avocados. Foods that are mainly oil include mayonnaise, certain salad dressings and soft margarine.

8 **SoFAs** are solid fats and added sugars. The limits for calories from SoFAS are the remaining amount of calories in each food pattern after selecting the specified amounts in each food group in nutrient-dense forms (forms that are fat-free or low-fat and with no added sugars).

Source: U.S. Department of Agriculture, Center for Nutrition Policy and Promotion

Figure 1.7b
USDA Food Patterns

Estimated Daily Calorie Needs

To determine which food intake pattern to use for an individual, the following chart gives an estimate of individual calorie needs. The calorie range for each age/sex group is based on physical activity level, from sedentary to active.

	CALORIE RANGE	
Children	**Sedentary**	**Active**
2-3 years	1,000	1,400
Females	**Sedentary**	**Active**
4-8 years	1,200	1,800
9-13	1,600	2,200
14-18	1,800	2,400
19-30	2,000	2,400
31-50	1,800	2,200
51+	1,600	2,200
Males	**Sedentary**	**Active**
4-8 years	1,400	2,000
9-13	1,800	2,600
14-18	2,200	3,200
19-30	2,400	3,000
31-50	2,400	3,000
51+	2,200	2,800

Sedentary means a lifestyle that includes only the light physical activity associated with typical day-to-day life.

Active means a lifestyle that includes physical activity equivalent to walking more than 3 miles per day at 3 to 4 miles per hour, in addition to light physical activity associated with typical day-to-day life.

Source: U.S. Department of Agriculture, Center for Nutrition Policy and Promotion

- Visual is linked to food and is a familiar mealtime symbol in consumers' minds, as identified through testing
- "My" continues the personalization approach from USDA

Upon the announcement of the 2015-20 Dietary Guidelines for Americans, the United States Department of Agriculture (USDA) and the Department of Health and Human Services (HHS) said, "The *2015-20 Dietary Guidelines* provides guidance for choosing a healthy diet and focuses on preventing the diet-related chronic diseases that continue to affect our population. Its recommendations are ultimately intended to help individuals improve and maintain overall health and reduce the risk of chronic disease. Its focus is disease prevention, not treatment."

Because more than one-third of children and more than two-thirds of adults in the United States are overweight or obese, the 2015-2020 version of the *Dietary Guidelines* placed stronger emphasis on the overall eating pattern and increasing physical activity.

When the *2015-20 Dietary Guidelines for Americans* were released, the majority of adults were overweight. In addition, one in three children were also overweight or obese. This was a crisis that could no longer be ignored. These new and improved dietary recommendations give individuals the information to make thoughtful choices of healthier foods in the right portions and to complement those choices with physical activity. The bottom line is that most Americans need to trim our waistlines to reduce the risk of developing diet-related chronic disease. Improving our eating habits is not only good for every individual and family, but also for our country.

MyPlate was developed to provide a visual and practical guidance about how to eat at each meal. It is a concrete example of how the plate should look, in spite of gender, age or caloric requirements. It offers a way of making dietary choices, based on sound nutrition principles. For the general healthy public over the age of two, it represents solid "basic nutrition" advice that can help individuals choose healthy foods that will contribute to health, balance calorie intake with physical activity and provide nutrient-dense food choices.

MyPlate can be found at www.ChooseMyPlate.gov. The site is an interactive nutrition resource to explore and design a personal eating plan.

Ten Tips—MyPlate

The MyPlate plan illustrates 10 recommendations/categories as follows:

1. **Balance Calories**—Find out how many calories *you* need for a day as a first step in managing your weight. Go to www.ChooseMyPlate.gov to find your calorie level. Being physically active also helps you balance calories.
2. **Enjoy Your Food, But Eat Less**—Take the time to fully enjoy your food as you eat it. Eating too fast or when your attention is elsewhere may lead to eating too many calories. Pay attention to hunger and fullness cues before, during, and after meals. Use them to recognize when to eat and when you've had enough.
3. **Avoid Oversized Meals**—Use a smaller plate, bowl, and glass. Portion out foods before you eat. When eating out, choose a smaller size option, share a dish, or take home part of your meal.
4. **Foods to Eat More Often**—Eat more vegetables, fruits, whole grains, and fat-free or 1% milk and dairy products. These foods have the nutrients you need for health, including potassium, calcium, vitamin D, and fiber. Make them the basis for meals and snacks.
5. **Make Half Your Plate Fruits and Vegetables**—Choose red, orange, and dark-green vegetables like tomatoes, sweet potatoes, and broccoli, along with other vegetables for your meals. Add fruit to meals as part of main or side dishes or as dessert.
6. **Switch to Fat-Free or Low-Fat (1%) Milk**—They have the same amount of calcium and other essential nutrients as whole milk, but fewer calories and less saturated fat.
7. **Make Half Your Grains Whole Grains**—To eat more whole grains, substitute a whole-grain product for a refined product—such as eating whole wheat bread instead of white bread or brown rice instead of white rice.

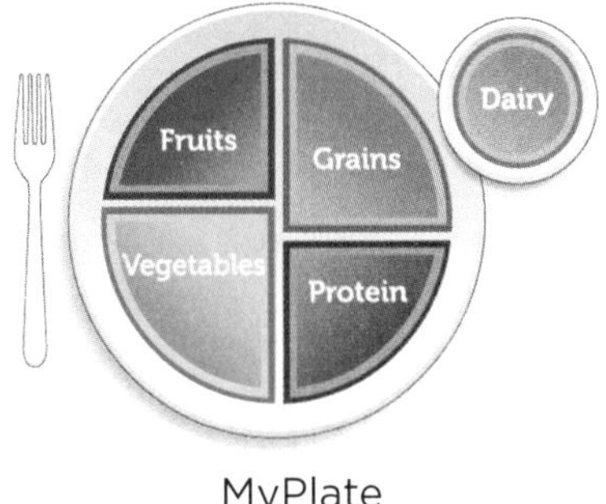

MyPlate

Figure 1.8

MyPlate Overview of Messages

Food Group	MyPlate Message	What Foods Are Included	Amounts Measured In...	Other Messages
Fruit	Focus on fruit	Any fruit or 100% fruit juice counts as part of the fruit group. Fruits may be fresh, canned, frozen, or dried and may be whole, cut-up, or puréed.	Cups per day	Limit juice to 6 ounces or less per day.
Vegetables	Vary your veggies	Any vegetable or 100% vegetable juice counts as a member of the vegetable group. Vegetables may be raw, cooked, fresh, frozen, canned, dried, or dehydrated and may be whole, cut-up, or mashed.	Cups per day	Based on their nutrient content, vegetables are organized into 5 subgroups: dark green vegetables, red and orange vegetables, starchy vegetables, beans and peas, and other vegetables.
Protein	Go lean with protein	All foods made from meat, poultry, seafood, beans, peas, eggs, processed soy products, nuts, and seeds are considered part of the protein foods group.	Ounces per day	Select a variety of protein foods to improve nutrient intake and health benefits, including at least 8 ounces of cooked seafood per week.
Grains	Make half your grains whole	Any food made from wheat, rice, oats, cornmeal, barley, or another cereal grain is a grain product. Bread, pasta, oatmeal, breakfast cereals, tortillas, and grits are examples of grain products.	Ounces per day	Grains are divided into 2 subgroups: whole grains and refined grains. Whole grains contain the entire grain kernel—the bran, germ, and endosperm.
Dairy	Get your calcium-rich foods	All fluid milk products and many foods made from milk are considered part of the dairy food group. Most dairy group choices should be fat-free or low-fat. Foods made from milk that retain their calcium content are part of the group. Foods made from milk that have little to no calcium, such as cream cheese, cream, and butter, are not. Calcium-fortified soymilk (soy beverage) is also part of the dairy group.	Cups per day	

Source: U.S. Department of Agriculture, Center for Nutrition Policy and Promotion

8. **Foods to Eat Less Often**—Cut back on foods high in solid fats, added sugars, and salt. They include cakes, cookies, ice cream, candies, sweetened drinks, pizza, and fatty meats like ribs, sausages, bacon, and hot dogs. Use these foods as occasional treats, not everyday foods.
9. **Compare Sodium in Foods**—Use the Nutrition Facts label to choose lower sodium versions of foods like soup, bread, and frozen meals. Select canned foods labeled "low sodium," "reduced sodium," or "no salt added."
10. **Drink Water Instead of Sugary Drinks**—Cut calories by drinking water or unsweetened beverages. Soda, energy drinks, and sports drinks are a major source of added sugar and calories in American diets.

Ounce or Ounce Equivalent for Grains and Protein Groups

What is an **ounce** or ounce equivalent? An ounce is a measurement of weight. The weight of one ounce is 28 grams. But still, what does that mean?

GLOSSARY

Ounce
A measurement of weight. One ounce = 28 grams

In general, 1 ounce of meat, poultry or fish, ¼ cup cooked beans, 1 egg, 1 tablespoon of peanut butter, or ½ ounce of nuts or seeds can be considered as 1 ounce equivalent from the Protein Foods Group. In general, 1 slice of bread, ½ bun, 1 cup of ready-to-eat cereal, or ½ cup of cooked rice, cooked pasta, or cooked cereal can be considered as 1 ounce equivalent from the Grains Group. Let's look at an example: consider the MyPlate guide for a person targeting 2,200 calories per day. The suggested intake from the Grains group is 7 ounces. To meet that total, a person may choose many different combinations and amounts of grain foods, such as:

- 1/2 cup oatmeal at breakfast (1 ounce), plus
- 2 slices of rye bread at lunch in a sandwich (2 ounces), plus
- 1 small bag of corn tortilla chips (1 ounce) for a snack, plus
- 1-1/2 cups of rice or pasta at dinner (3 ounces)

This would provide a total of seven ounces from this group for a day.

For mixed foods, estimate food groups based on the main ingredients. For example, a generous serving of pizza would count in the Grains group (crust), the Dairy group (cheese), and the Vegetable group (tomato). A serving of beef stew would count in the Protein and the Vegetable groups. Figure 1.9 provides examples of counting mixed dishes with MyPlate.

The MyPlate approach provides a simple tool that is readily understood. Most people can select their own food choices from within each food group and make personal dietary choices that contribute to good health. The image is easy to conceptualize and makes a good educational tool as well.

Please note that MyPlate, like other food guides, is not absolute. As will be learned in later chapters, an individual's nutritional needs vary throughout the stages of life. In addition, medical conditions can affect what constitute "ideal" dietary choices for any

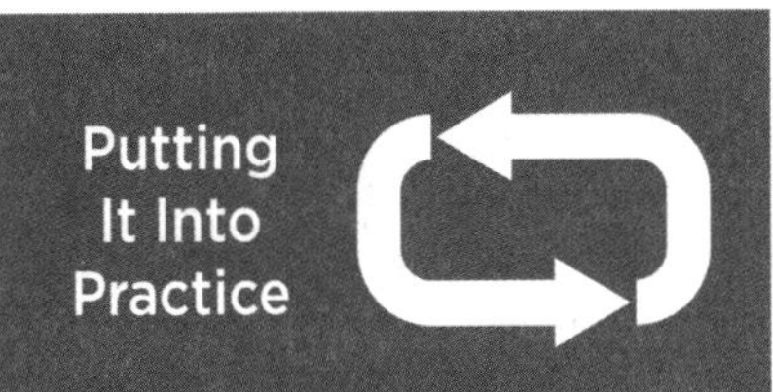

3. How could the following meal be modified to better fit MyPlate guidelines?
   - Roast beef
   - Mashed potatoes
   - Corn
   - Bread
   - Milk

Figure 1.9
Examples of Counting Mixed Dishes

FOOD AND SAMPLE PORTION	AMOUNT FROM FOOD GROUP IN THIS PORTION					
	Grains Group	Vegetable Group	Fruit Group	Dairy	Protein	Estimated Total Calories
Cheese Pizza—Thin Crust (1 slice from medium pizza)	1 oz.-eq.	1/8 cup	0	1/2 cup	0	215
Macaroni and Cheese (1 cup made from package mix)	2 oz.-eq.	0	0	1/2 cup	0	260
Tuna Noodle Casserole (1 cup)	1-1/2 oz.-eq.	0	0	1/2 cup	2 oz.-eq.	260
Chicken Pot Pie (8 oz. pie)	2-1/2 oz.-eq.	1/4 cup	0	0	1-1/2 oz.-eq.	500
Beef Taco (2 tacos)	2-1/2 oz.-eq.	1/4 cup	0	1/4 cup	2 oz.-eq.	370
Egg Roll (1)	1/2 oz.-eq.	1/8 cup	0	0	1/2 oz.-eq.	150
Chicken Fried Rice (1 cup)	1-1/2 oz.-eq.	1/4 cup	0	0	1 oz.-eq.	270
Stuffed Peppers with Rice and Meat (1/2 pepper)	1/2 oz.-eq.	1/2 cup	0	0	1 oz.-eq.	190
Clam Chowder-New England (1 cup)	1/2 oz.-eq.	1/8 cup	0	1/2 cup	2 oz.-eq.	165
Cream of Tomato Soup (1 cup)	1/2 oz.-eq.	1/2 cup	0	1/2 cup	0	160
Large Cheeseburger	2 oz.-eq.	0	0	1/3 cup	3 oz.-eq.	500
Peanut Butter & Jelly Sandwich (1)	2 oz.-eq.	0	0	0	2 oz.-eq.	375
Tuna Salad Sandwich (1)	2 oz.-eq.	1/4 cup	0	0	2 oz.-eq.	290
Chef Salad (3 cups—no dressing)	0	1-1/2 cups	0	0	3 oz.-eq.	230
Pasta Salad with Vegetables (1 cup)	1-1/2 oz.-eq.	1/2 cup	0	0	0	140
Apple Pie (1 slice)	2 oz.-eq.	0	1/4 cup	0	0	280

Source: U.S. Department of Agriculture and U.S. Department of Heath and Human Services

individual. In later chapters, the focus will be to learn more about how diets may need to be modified for certain disease states.

Other Significant Dietary Recommendations

Today's nutrition advice indicates a need to make some adjustments to the usual American diet. Here are more tips for making healthy choices based on the Dietary Guidelines for Americans, the USDA Food Plans, and MyPlate.

Carbohydrate: Limit Sugar

The Dietary Guidelines for Americans recommend using sugars only in moderation. Foods containing large amounts of refined sugars should be eaten in moderation by most healthy people, and sparingly by people with low calorie needs. For very active people with high calorie needs, sugars can be an additional source of calories. The following tips can help reduce sugar in the diet:

- Instead of regular soft drinks or powdered drink mixes, choose diet soft drinks, 100 percent fruit juices, bottled waters such as seltzer, or iced tea made without added sugar or with non-nutritive sweeteners.
- Instead of desserts such as cake, emphasize fruits. Fresh fruit can be baked (baked apples), poached (poached pears), broiled, or made into compote. Choose canned fruits that are packed in fruit juice or water and avoid those packed in syrup.
- Make cakes, cookies, pies, and other baked goods from scratch and reduce the sugar by one-quarter to one-third. It usually does not affect the quality of the product. Use recipes that contain fruits to sweeten and sweet spices such as cinnamon, nutmeg, and cloves.
- Try a cookie that uses less sugar, such as graham crackers, vanilla wafers, ginger snaps, or fig bars.
- Choose 100 percent pure fruit juices. They do not contain added sugars. Products labeled as fruit drinks, fruit beverages, or flavored drinks usually contain only small amounts of fruit juice, with added water and much refined sugar.
- Choose whole grain, unsweetened breakfast cereals with less than four grams of sugar per serving (unless the sugar comes from a dried fruit such as raisins) and top with fresh fruit.
- Jams, jellies, and pancake syrup contain considerable amounts of refined sugar. Select jams and jellies made without (or with less) sugar and pancake syrup labeled "reduced calorie." Other suggested toppings for toast or pancakes are chopped fresh fruit, applesauce, part-skim ricotta cheese, peanut and other nut butters, and fruit.

Mixed Dishes: Look for Fats and Sugar

Some mixed foods contain a lot of fat, oil, or sugar, which adds calories (see Figure 1.10).

SoFAs is a term that refers to the addition of solid fats (like butter, shortening, margarine, and the like) and added sugars. The addition of SoFas on a regular basis in the American diet is significant. Look again at the foods listed in Figure 1.10. Hidden

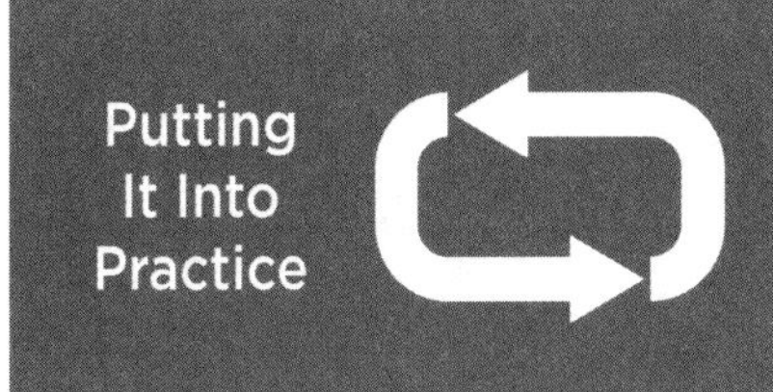

4. Which foods and beverages contain natural sugars, and which contain added sugars?
   - Canned fruit
   - Plain milk
   - Eggs
   - Bread
   - Soda
   - Chocolate milk
   - Fresh fruit
   - Flavored oatmeal packets
   - Sweet potatoes

fats, sugars, and calories are in common foods. These foods (like cheese, for example) are often added to other foods, thus increasing the fat of an entrée. Make some healthier substitutions. Consider these easy substitutions:

- Instead of sweetened breakfast pastries such as Danish, try a bagel, English muffin, roll, or fruited muffin and make them whole grain.
- Use less table (refined) sugars in coffee, tea, cereals, etc., or use sugar substitutes.
- Try fresh or dried fruit for a sweet snack instead of candy.
- Cut back on the fat in a baked product by substituting applesauce for some of the butter or margarine in the recipe.

Figure 1.10
Examples of Solid Fats and Added Sugars in Current American Diets

SOLID FATS	ADDED SUGARS
• Grain-based desserts, including cakes, cookies, pies, doughnuts, and granola bars	• Soda
• Regular cheese	• Grain-based desserts
• Sausage, franks, bacon, and ribs	• Fruit drinks
• Pizza	• Dairy-based desserts
• Dairy-based desserts such as ice cream	• Candy

Source: U.S. Department of Agriculture, Center for Nutrition Policy and Promotion. Dietary Guidelines for Americans, 2015-2020

Figure 1.11
Good Sources of Fiber

FOOD	GRAMS	FOOD	GRAMS
Breakfast Cereals (1 cup)		**Breads and Pastas (1 ounce)**	
Bran-type Cereals	10	Whole Wheat Bread	2
Raisin Bran-type Cereals	8	Bran Muffin	5
Whole Wheat Breakfast Cereals	4	Whole Wheat Pasta	1-6
Whole Oat Breakfast Cereals	2	**Fruits**	
Dried Beans and Peas (1/2 cup)		Apple	3
All Cooked Beans and Peas	7	Banana	3
Vegetables (1/2 cup)		Blackberries (1 cup)	8
Broccoli	3	Cherries (10 each)	2
Brussels Sprouts	3	Figs (10 each)	2
Carrots	3	Grapefruit	2
Peas	4	Kiwi Fruit	3
Potatoes with Skin (1 each)	5	Orange	3
Spinach, Raw	< 1	Pear	4
Sweet Potatoes (1 each)	3	Prunes (1 cup)	16
		Raspberries (1 cup)	8
		Strawberries (1 cup)	3

Source: U.S. Department of Agriculture, Center for Nutrition Policy and Promotion, www.ChooseMyPlate.gov

Increase Your Fiber: Eat Fiber-Rich Foods

General recommendations for fiber intake are from 20 to 35 grams daily. The Daily Value used for Nutrition Facts Labeling is 25 grams. For children, use the "age + 5" rule, which recommends that children consume an amount of fiber equal to their age plus an additional 5 grams of fiber. Unfortunately, the average American takes in less than 20 grams of fiber a day. Figure 1.11 lists good sources of fiber. When increasing fiber intake, do so slowly to avoid problems with cramps, diarrhea, and excessive gas. Also, it's important to chew foods well and drink at least 8 to 10 glasses of water each day, because fiber takes water out of the body. Make at least half of your grains whole grains.

Fat: Limit Solid Fats, Saturated Fats, Trans-Fat, and Cholesterol

The Dietary Guidelines for Americans recommend a diet moderate in total fat and low in saturated fat and cholesterol. Guidelines generally suggest that no more than 30 percent of daily calories should come from fat. Figure 1.12 gives the recommendations for saturated fat intake according to various calorie levels.

Additional recommendations for Americans without cardiovascular disease include:

- No more than 10 percent of total calories should be in the form of saturated fat with an eventual goal of <7 percent.
- Avoid trans-fatty acids (trans-fat) from processed food sources.
- Cholesterol intake should be less than 300 milligrams daily.
- Increase total amount of fish consumption to two times per week, especially those fish high in omega-3 fatty acids.

This advice does not apply to infants and toddlers below the age of two years. After age two, children should gradually adopt a diet that, by about five years of age, contains no more than 30 percent of calories from fat. As they begin to consume fewer calories

Figure 1.12
Recommended Saturated Fat intake

Total Daily Calories	Saturated Fat @ 10%
1600	18 grams or less
2000	20 grams or less
2200	24 grams or less
2400	25 grams or less
2800	31 grams or less

Source: U.S. Department of Health and Human Services and U.S. Department of Agriculture, Center for Nutrition Policy and Promotion, Dietary Guidelines for Americans, 2010

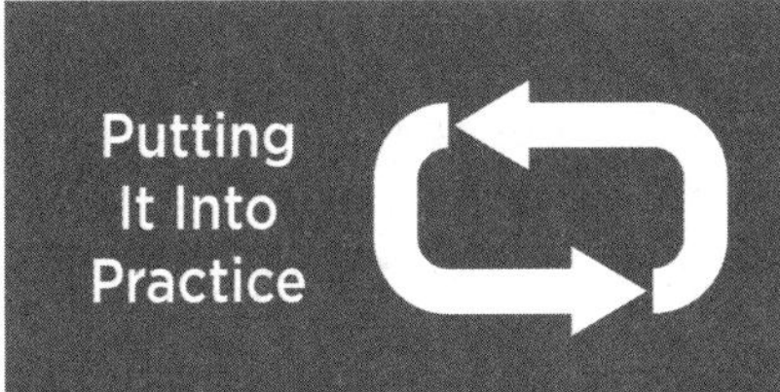

5. Which foods or beverages have more fiber:
   - A bagel or a vegetable omelet?
   - Vegetable juice or a baked potato?
   - White rice or pinto beans?

from fat, children should replace these calories by eating more grain products, fruits, vegetables, low-fat milk products or other calcium-rich foods, beans, lean meat, poultry, fish, or other protein-rich foods.

Meat, poultry, fish, and shellfish contain saturated fat and/or cholesterol. Luckily, some choices are quite low in saturated fat. In general, poultry is low in saturated fat, especially when the skin is removed. When buying fresh ground turkey or chicken, find a product that says "light meat" or "breast" on the label. Poultry products that include the skin and/or dark meat are much higher in fat. Goose and duck are also high in fat. Most fish is lower in saturated fat and cholesterol than meat and poultry. Fatty fish (such as salmon and tuna) are rich in omega-3 fatty acids, which may protect against heart disease and certain forms of cancer. Shellfish varies in cholesterol content.

Figure 1.13 lists lean cuts of meat. High-fat processed meats, such as many luncheon meats and sausages, provide a hefty 60 to 80 percent of their calories from fat, much of which is saturated. Other examples of processed meats are bacon, bologna, salami, hot dogs, and sausage. In some cases, processed meats are made from turkey or chicken and are lower in fat. Look for low-fat processed meats. Organ meats, like liver and kidneys, are relatively low in fat. However, these meats are high in cholesterol.

Figure 1.13
Lean Cuts of Meat

Beef	Veal	Pork	Lamb
• Eye of the Round • Top Round	• Shoulder • Ground Veal • Cutlets • Sirloin	• Tenderloin • Sirloin • Top Loin	• Leg-shank

Source: U.S. Department of Agriculture, Center for Nutrition Policy and Promotion

When cooking meats, poultry, and fish, use cooking methods that use little or no fat, such as roasting, baking, broiling, grilling, boiling, stir frying, or poaching. Do not fry. When making pan gravy, refrigerate the drippings first so the fat will solidify and can be removed. One may also extend meat with pasta, beans, or vegetables for hearty dishes. For less saturated fat and cholesterol and more variety, dried beans or legumes are an excellent meat alternative.

Although many people believe that meats have the highest cholesterol and saturated fat content, dairy products can also be high in saturated fat and cholesterol. As dairy products are often added to foods like casseroles, cakes, or pies, it's easy to eat a significant amount of them without knowing it. Both 1 percent and skim milk provide much less saturated fat and cholesterol and fewer calories than whole milk, as shown in Figure 1.14.

6. What could be a better choice when limiting saturated fats:
    - Bologna sandwich or tuna sandwich?
    - Ribeye steak or sirloin steak?

Figure 1.14

Comparison of Milk, Poultry, Meat, and Cheese

MILK	TOTAL FAT	SATURATED FAT	CHOLESTEROL	CALORIES
Skim Milk	0.4 g	0.3 g	4 mg	86
1% Milk	2.6 g	1.6 g	10 mg	102
2% Milk	4.7 g	2.9 g	18 mg	121
Whole Milk	8.2 g	5.1 g	33 mg	150
CHICKEN				
Roasted Chicken (no skin, light meat, 3 oz.)	3.1 g	.9 g	72 mg	140
MEAT				
Beef (top round, broiled, 3 oz.)	4.8 g	1.7 g	65 mg	158
CHEESE				
Natural Cheddar (1 oz.)	9.4 g	6.0 g	30 mg	110

Source: National Institutes of Health

Often, when people cut back on meat, they replace it with cheese, thinking they are cutting back on their saturated fat and cholesterol. However, most cheeses are prepared from whole milk or cream, which are also high in saturated fat and cholesterol. Cheeses are particularly high in saturated fat (Figure 1.14). Fortunately, manufacturers offer low-fat versions of cheese favorites like cheddar, Swiss, and mozzarella. They use skim milk and vegetable oils to replace some of the cream and other fat. The result is reduced-fat or fat free cheese.

Americans love ice cream. Ice cream is made from whole milk and cream, and therefore contains a considerable amount of saturated fat and cholesterol. Some frozen desserts such as ices, popsicles, and sorbet are generally made without fat. Ice milk contains less fat and saturated fat than regular ice cream, as does frozen low-fat yogurt. With the wide variety of frozen desserts, it's a good idea to read nutrition labels.

Egg yolks are high in cholesterol. The average large egg yolk contains 185 milligrams of cholesterol, about two-thirds of the suggested daily intake. To lower cholesterol and fat content, use egg substitutes with less than 60 calories per one-quarter cup serving, or egg whites, which contain no cholesterol. Two egg whites can be substituted for one whole egg in most recipes.

Most breads and bread products contain only small amounts of fat, with less than two grams per slice or serving—that is, if margarine or mayonnaise is not spread on them. Some breads typically have significant fat added in their preparation. Examples include biscuits, croissants, cornbread, dinner rolls, scones, and muffins. Also note that most granolas are high in fat. Commercial cakes, pies, cookies, donuts, and pastry are often high in fat, saturated fat, and calories. In addition, some are quite high in cholesterol. Tasty alternatives include angel food cake, sponge cake, fig bars, ginger snaps, and baked goods made with little or no fat. Recipe substitution ideas appear in Figure 1.15. Many desserts can also be made with less fat. Simply reduce the fat called for by one-fourth to one-third the original amount. When decreasing the fat in a recipe, it is important to note that the quality of the product may be affected. Be sure to test recipes prior to serving.

Figure 1.15
Lower Fat Baking Substitutions

INSTEAD OF...	...USE THIS
1 cup shortening, butter, or margarine	1/2 cup oil and 1/2 cup applesauce
1 whole egg	2 egg whites
1 cup sour cream	1 cup reduced-fat sour cream
1 cup whole milk	1 cup skim milk
1 Tbsp. cream cheese	1 Tbsp. fat-free or light cream cheese
1 cup cream	1 cup low-fat yogurt
1 oz. baking chocolate	3 Tbsp. cocoa and 1 Tbsp. vegetable oil

Source: U.S. Department of Agriculture, Food and Nutrition Service

Protein

Proteins are especially important because they provide both energy and essential amino acids, which will be discussed in the next chapter. Unlike fats, the amount required per day is based on grams of protein per kilogram of body weight. The Recommended Dietary Allowance (RDA) for protein is 0.8 g protein/kg body weight/day for ages 19 and above. Average protein intake for most Americans is considered adequate. As Americans decrease their calorie intake to fight obesity, there is a shift in the percentage of calories from protein. Percent of proteins may need to increase. Figure 1.16 indicates how the percentage of calories from protein changes for a 150 lb. person based on the total daily calorie intake.

High quality protein sources are animal proteins. In the past few years, many consumers have adopted high-protein diets for weight-loss purposes. This has resulted in some Americans consuming diets high in protein, especially animal sources. According to the Report of the DGAC on the Dietary Guidelines for Americans 2020, "In shorter-term studies, low-calorie, high-protein diets may result in greater weight loss, but these differences are not sustained over time." Eating too much protein has no health benefits. In fact, eating excess protein from animal products may add excessive fat and calories.

Lower quality protein sources are plant-based. Review the complementary protein sources in Chapter 2. Consuming lower-quality proteins is of greater concern when protein needs are high, such as pregnancy, lactation, childhood, and during illness

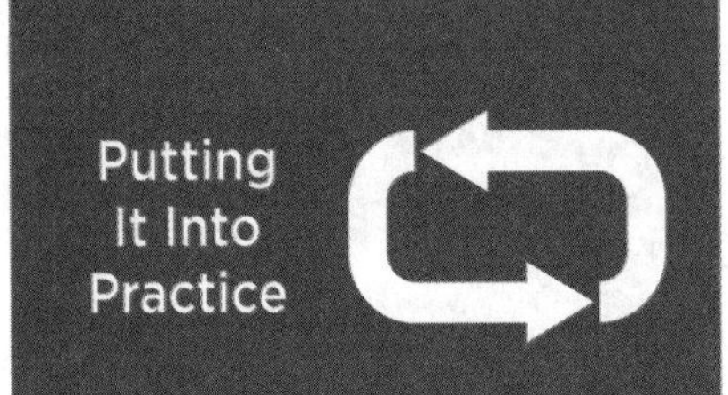

7. What are some ways to reduce saturated fat intake to 7% of total calories while also increasing the meal's nutrient value?
   - 4 oz. ribeye steak
   - Small baked potato with 1 Tbsp. butter and 1 tsp. sour cream
   - 1/2 cup green beans with 1 tsp. butter
   - 1 cup whole milk
   - 1/2 cup ice cream

Figure 1.16
Changes in Protein Needs by Calorie Level

CALORIE LEVEL	% OF CALORIES
1200	18%
1500	14.4%
1800	12%
2000	10.8%
2500	8.5%

Protein needs for 150 lb. person @ 0.8gm/kg = 54 grams. That amount stays the same regardless of the different level of energy intake.

Source: U.S. Department of Agriculture and U.S. Department of Health and Human Services

or injury. The Report of the DGAC on the Dietary Guidelines for Americans 2010, indicated moderate evidence linking a plant-protein diet to lower blood pressure.

The best way to manage protein intake is to follow the Dietary Guidelines and MyPlate. Also, note that many of the recommendations for reducing dietary fat and saturated fat are based on following recommended portion sizes.

Drink Enough Water: Meeting Daily Fluid Requirements

Water is an essential nutrient. In the past, there was no dietary guideline or Dietary Reference Intake for water. Some people have even referred to it as the "forgotten nutrient." Since nearly all bodily systems depend on water and proper hydration, let's look at the recommendation for water and how to calculate daily fluid requirement. How much is needed depends upon health, physical activity, and even where a person lives. Humans lose about 10 cups of water each day through breathing, sweating, and urine and bowel movements. Most physicians recommend drinking 8-10, 8-ounce glasses of water each day. Approximately 20 percent of fluid needs come from food that is consumed, and the other 50 percent from beverage consumption (which will be discussed at length in other chapters).

Sources of water from food plus the 8-10 glasses of water would help to replace what is lost each day. Additional water may be needed for high temperature and humidity. In the effort to fight the obesity epidemic, replacing other fluids such as soda, sports drinks, and juice with water will help reduce calories. On average, Americans consume over 130 calories each day from soda, sports drinks, and juice.

Food or Supplements? Real Food First

A common nutritional question concerns multivitamin preparations or supplements. Should one rely on a balanced diet or pills to ensure good nutrition? While nutrition science is quite advanced, scientists are only beginning to understand the many components of foods that are active in the human body. The emerging concept of functional foods makes this quite evident. Beyond vitamins, minerals, protein, lipids, and carbohydrates, foods provide other compounds. Some appear to offer health benefits. Already, some functional ingredients in foods have been incorporated into nutritional supplements. But this is not a complete answer for sound nutrition. The bottom line is that real food is preferred. With real food, provided through a balanced diet and based on established dietary guidance, one can obtain necessary nutrients, as well as compounds that may not be fully understood. Real food also gives people pleasure, offers fiber (not present in all supplemental products), and water. It provides a sense of satiety or fullness when eaten.

Real Food First is a concept that has gotten much notice in long-term care. With liberalized diets in long-term care, real food should always be the first food offered between meals, prior to beginning any nutritional supplements.

Multivitamins or nutritional supplements can be important for an individual who wishes to ensure adequate nutrition, or who needs to correct a deficiency. Iron supplements, for example, may be important to supplement dietary intake of iron. Iron-deficiency anemia is common in the U.S. and it is not easy for everyone to consume adequate iron through food. Calcium is another nutrient that may be worth supplementing—especially for adult women. The AI level is not easy for every woman to achieve and calcium plays a role in preventing osteoporosis. These are just examples of situations in which supplementation may be useful. However, it's prudent to consider supplements for what they are— supplements—not replacements for healthy eating habits. It is also important to review DRIs for nutrients and pay particular attention to the UL levels for nutrients. Excessive supplementation of some nutrients can cause health problems.

The Dietary Guidelines emphasize real foods over nutrition supplements, saying, "A basic premise of the Dietary Guidelines is that nutrient needs should be met primarily through consuming foods. Foods provide an array of nutrients and other compounds that may have beneficial effects on health. In certain cases, fortified foods and dietary supplements may be useful sources of one or more nutrients that otherwise might be consumed in less than recommended amounts. However, dietary supplements, while recommended in some cases, cannot replace a healthful diet." Figure 1.17 provides guidelines for minimizing nutrient loss during cooking. The human diet is complex. So much nutrition information bombards a person that sorting through it all can be challenging. Looking to the Dietary Guidelines for Americans, the USDA Food Plans, and MyPlate to translate the science to what is consumed is the best way to ensure a healthy diet. Remember, for menu planning and in-depth assessment, the DRIs offer a science-based standard of reference.

8. Why might a nutritional shake, such as an oral nutrition supplement or a smoothie, not align with the Real Food First concept?

Figure 1.17
Tips for Protecting Nutrients

- Minimize storage time. Do not store foods longer than necessary.
- Keep foods wrapped or covered for storage.
- Do not soak foods in water unless absolutely necessary. If you need to soak a food, use as little water as possible. If practical, add the water to the product (e.g. boiling vegetables, if possible, use the water in soups instead of throwing it away).
- Cut and cook vegetables in large pieces to minimize contact between surface area and air.
- To cook vegetables, steam rather than boil. This helps them retain nutrients.
- Cook vegetables as soon as possible after cutting. If preparing for later use, keep in airtight bag or container and keep in the refrigerator.
- Use raw vegetables (rather than boiled) whenever possible.
- Avoid adding baking soda to vegetables during cooking. Some people use this practice to retain color. However, it destroys thiamin and vitamin C.
- Avoid overcooking food, as heat can destroy vitamins (especially vitamin C). Cook just until tender and serve as soon as possible.
- Do not rinse enriched rice before cooking and do not discard the water during cooking.
- Do not brown undercooked rice before adding water. This destroys thiamin.
- After cooking rice, pasta, or other grain-based foods, do not rinse; just drain.
- Store food away from light or in dark containers. This is important for milk, since riboflavin and B vitamin in milk is destroyed by light.
- In foodservice operations, cook food as close to service times as possible. Cook in small batches as appropriate. For example, steamed vegetables may be prepared in small batches throughout an extended meal service time.

Source: U.S. Department of Agriculture

Chapter References

RESOURCES	
American Cancer Society*	http://www.cancer.org
Centers for Disease Control and Prevention*	https://www.cdc.gov/
Centers for Disease Control and Prevention. Survey Results and Products from the National Health and Nutrition Examination Survey. National Center for Health Statistics. Updated February 13, 2018.*	https://www.cdc.gov/nchs/nhanes/nhanes_products.htm
International Food Information Council Foundation*	https://foodinsight.org
Office of Disease Prevention and Health Promotion. Healthy People 2020.*	https://www.healthypeople.gov
U.S. Department of Agriculture*	https://www.usda.gov/
U.S. Department of Agriculture. Food and Human Nutrition. National Agricultural Library.*	https://www.nal.usda.gov/food-and-human-nutrition
U.S. Department of Agriculture. MyPlate.*	https://www.choosemyplate.gov
U.S. Department of Agriculture. Scientific Report of the 2015 Dietary Guidelines Advisory Committee. Published February, 2015. Accessed September 16, 2020.	https://health.gov/sites/default/files/2019-09/Scientific-Report-of-the-2015-Dietary-Guidelines-Advisory-Committee.pdf
U.S. Department of Agriculture. What We Eat in America. Agricultural Research Service. Updated August 15, 2019.*	https://www.ars.usda.gov/northeast-area/beltsville-md-bhnrc/beltsville-human-nutrition-research-center/food-surveys-research-group/docs/wweia-usual-intake-data-tables/
U.S. Department of Health and Human Services*	https://www.hhs.gov/
U.S. Department of Health and Human Services. DASH Eating Plan. National Heart, Lung, and Blood Institute.*	https://www.nhlbi.nih.gov/health-topics/dash-eating-plan
U.S. Department of Health and Human Services and U.S. Department of Agriculture. 2015–2020 Dietary Guidelines for Americans, 8th Edition. Office of Disease Prevention and Health Promotion. Published December 2015.*	https://health.gov/dietaryguidelines/2015/resources/2015-2020_Dietary_Guidelines.pdf.
U.S. Department of Health and Human Services and U.S. Department of Agriculture. Dietary Guidelines for Americans, 2010. 7th Edition. Office of Disease Prevention and Health Promotion. Published December 2010*	https://health.gov/dietaryguidelines/dga2010/DietaryGuidelines2010.pdf
U.S. Department of Health & Human Services. Nutrient Recommendations: Dietary Reference Intakes (DRI). National Institutes of Health Office of Dietary Supplements.*	https://ods.od.nih.gov/Health_Information/Dietary_Reference_Intakes.aspx
U.S. Department of Health and Human Services. USDA Food Patterns. National Institute on Aging. Updated April 29, 2019.*	https://www.nia.nih.gov/health/usda-food-patterns

**Accessed September 18, 2019*

The Building Blocks of Nutrition

Overview and Objectives

In order to plan and implement menus, a Certified Dietary Manager®, Certified Food Protection Professional® (CDM®, CFPP®) needs to master nutrition concepts. An understanding of basic nutrients is also essential for planning modified diets. CDM, CFPPs apply information from the six nutrient categories. After completing this chapter, you should be able to:

- Identify six groups of nutrients
- Define calorie
- List the energy content of nutrients
- Differentiate between simple and complex carbohydrates
- Explain nutrient density of foods
- Calculate energy content of a simple food

People eat foods for many different reasons. Many people have feelings and beliefs regarding the foods they choose. Most people care about their body...how they feel and look. Each person has a relationship with nutrition. Nutrition is all about how food nourishes the body. When properly combined, nutrients from the foods that are eaten help to provide optimum health.

Nutrition is also about food energy, which affects how a person looks and feels. Energy is needed every day to work and play. That energy comes either directly or indirectly from the sun in the form of nutrients in food. Plants convert the sun's rays into stored energy and when plants become food, the body releases that stored energy from the plants. Animals that eat plant foods get their energy in the same way, so both plant and animal foods provide energy.

GLOSSARY

Nutrients
Food components that supply the body with energy, promote growth and maintenance of tissues, and regulate body processes

Essential Nutrients
Nutrients that cannot be made in the body or cannot be made in the quantity needed by the body. Humans must get them via food

Nutrients, or food components, supply the body with energy, promote the growth and maintenance of tissues, and regulate body processes. There are about 50 known nutrients that are categorized into six groups:

- Carbohydrates
- Fats (lipids)
- Proteins
- Vitamins
- Minerals
- Water

The functions of each group of nutrients are shown in Figure 2.1.

Most foods are a mixture of carbohydrates, proteins, and fats and contain smaller quantities of other nutrients, such as vitamins, minerals, and water. It's been said many times: "You are what you eat." Indeed, the nutrients within the foods we eat, once eaten, are in the body. Water accounts for about 50-70 percent of body weight. Fats (lipids) account for about 4-27 percent of body weight, and protein accounts for about 14-23 percent of body weight. Carbohydrates comprise only 0.5 percent. (Even though carbohydrates are important nutrients, most do not remain as carbohydrates in the body.) The remainder of body weight includes minerals, like calcium (in bones, teeth) and vitamins.

Most, but not all, nutrients are considered **essential nutrients.** Essential nutrients either cannot be made in the body or cannot be made in the quantities needed by the body; therefore, they must be obtained through food. Thus, "essential" in this term

Figure 2.1
Functions of Each Group of Nutrients

NUTRIENT GROUP	FUNCTION
• Carbs, Fats, Protein	• Provide energy
• Fats, Protein	• Promote growth and maintenance of tissue and bone
• Minerals, Water, Vitamins	• Maintain and regulate body processes
• Minerals	• Provide structural function

means it is essential (necessary) that these nutrients be consumed; they are essential components of the diet. Carbohydrates, vitamins, minerals, water, and some parts of lipids and proteins are considered essential. Remember, the nutrients are not usually eaten by themselves, nutrients are components of foods.

SECTION A MACRONUTRIENTS

The Energy Nutrients

The macronutrients ("macro" means "big") are the nutrients that are found in the greatest amounts in the diet and in the body. In addition, macronutrients are those that provide the fuel that the body needs to function. These are called **energy-yielding nutrients**—carbohydrates, lipids (fats), and protein. All of the energy a human uses in a day are one of these energy-yielding nutrients that are metabolized by the body, yielding energy in the form of Adenosine Triphosphate (ATP). ATP is the form of energy the body uses as fuel. The other three nutrient groups—vitamins, minerals, and water—do not provide any calories, but do promote other important functions, which will be discussed later in this chapter.

A **calorie** is a unit of measurement of heat or energy. Although the term "calorie" is commonly used, a calorie is actually a shortened form of the term "kilocalorie," which means 1,000 calories. Of the six categories of nutrients, only carbohydrates, lipids, and protein provide energy, as follows:

- Carbohydrates: 4 calories per gram
- Lipids (Fat and Oils): 9 calories per gram
- Protein: 4 calories per gram

Remember from chapter one, a gram is a unit of weight; there are 28 grams in one ounce. To determine calories from grams, this is how it is done: Let's say we needed to calculate the calories in 1 pat of butter (about 5 grams by weight). How would we do that?

- 1 pat of butter = 5 grams of fat
- 5 grams of fat x 9 calories per gram = 45 calories

There are 3500 calories in a pound. So when an extra 3500 calories are consumed, one could gain one pound of body weight. Another calorie-contributor is alcohol. While it is definitely not a macronutrient, alcohol contributes seven calories per gram of alcohol consumed.

As can be seen in Figure 2.1, energy-yielding nutrients can also serve as building blocks for body tissue and bone. This is particularly true of proteins and lipids (fats). Because these nutrients give the body energy and are used for building body tissue and bone, a large amount of these nutrients are needed. Now, let's take a closer look at the macronutrients—carbohydrates, lipids, and protein.

GLOSSARY

Energy-Yielding Nutrients
Nutrients that provide energy or calories to the body, such as carbohydrates, fats, and protein

Calorie
A measurement of heat or energy

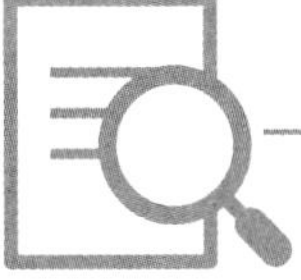

View the Supplemental Material for the Focus on Formulas video: Calorie Exchange.

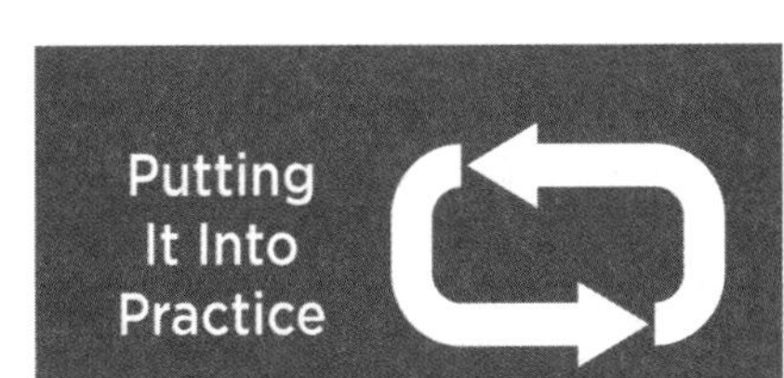

1. Describe which of the six nutrient categories are found in a snack consisting of an apple. Are all six nutrient categories present? If not, what could be included in this snack to account for the remaining nutrient categories?

Carbohydrates

Carbo means carbon and *hydrate* means water. **Carbohydrates** (CHO) contain carbon and the two chemical elements that make up water: hydrogen and oxygen. The main function of carbohydrates is to provide energy or fuel to the body. In fact, the central nervous system, including the brain and nerve cells, relies almost exclusively on a form of carbohydrate called glucose for energy.

Carbohydrates (CHO) fall into two categories: **simple carbohydrates** (commonly called sugars) and **complex carbohydrates** (commonly called starch and fiber). All digestible forms of CHO are converted to glucose in the body. The number of molecules of glucose linked together determines the type of carbohydrate. If a food is a simple carbohydrate, it "melts" or dissolves in the mouth. Simple CHO also have fewer glucose molecules linked together and the chemical bonds are easily broken. Think of foods that are high in sugar (i.e. frostings, marshmallows, hard candy). Complex carbohydrates include nutritious foods such as whole grain breads and cereals, fruits and vegetables, dried beans and peas. They are complex because there are many carbohydrate molecules linked together. To better understand carbohydrates, let's take a closer look at simple and complex carbohydrates.

GLOSSARY

Carbohydrates
Nutrients made up of carbon, hydrogen, and oxygen that primarily provide energy to fuel the body

Simple Carbohydrates
Carbohydrates with a simple chemical structure, commonly called sugars

Complex Carbohydrates
Carbohydrates with a complex chemical structure that is more difficult to break down, such as starch and fiber

Monosaccharide
Simple carbohydrate containing one sugar molecule

Glucose
A simple sugar used for energy—also called blood sugar or blood glucose

Disaccharide
Simple carbohydrate containing two sugar molecules

Simple Carbohydrates: Sugars

Simple carbohydrates are so named because their chemical structure is fairly simple. In fact, the simple carbohydrates are building blocks for the complex carbohydrates. There are six forms of simple carbohydrates, or sugars, that are nutritionally important (see Figure 2.2).

Mono means one and *saccharide* means sugar. A **monosaccharide**, like a **glucose** molecule is absorbed without further breakdown when eaten. In the body, glucose is called "blood sugar" or "blood glucose" because it circulates in the blood at a relatively constant level. Glucose (also known as dextrose) is the most common form of sugar in the body. It is the preferred energy source for brain functions, the central nervous system, and for performing physical activity.

Di means two and *saccharide* means sugar. A **disaccharide** is two monosaccharides linked by a chemical bond. When disaccharides are eaten, the body must break them down (digest) them first. Enzymes split the two sugar molecules apart so they can be more easily absorbed into the bloodstream. Because of the need for every cell to use glucose and because our bodies can't make them, carbohydrate is an essential nutrient. There is no substitute for carbohydrate in the body.

Sugar in Food

The sugars listed in Figure 2.2 have differing levels of sweetness. Fructose is more than twice as sweet as glucose. Fructose, also known as fruit sugar, is found in ripe fruits and honey; it is also found in other foods. There are two primary types of simple carbohydrates in food. There are naturally-occurring sugars in fruits (fructose) and

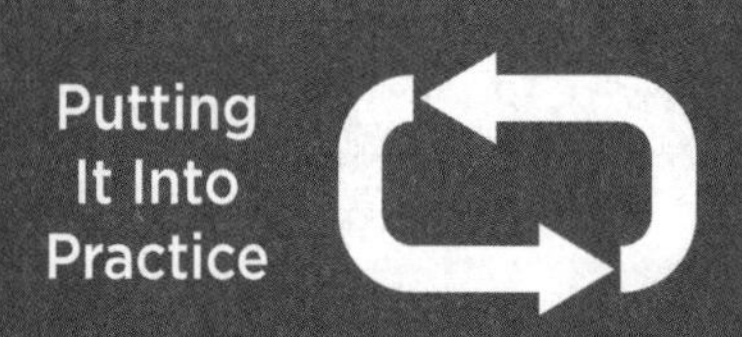

2. If there are about 7 grams of protein in one ounce of meat, how many calories are in a 4 ounce portion of meat?

Figure 2.2
Six Sugar Molecules Important in Nutrition

Molecule	Characteristics	Known As
Glucose	Mono (one) saccharide	Blood sugar in the body; commonly found in nature and used for energy
Fructose	Mono (one) saccharide	Fruit sugar or the sugar in honey
Galactose	Mono (one) saccharide	Combines with glucose to make lactose or milk sugar
Sucrose	Di (two) saccharide comprised of glucose and fructose	Table sugar
Lactose	Di (two) saccharide comprised of glucose and galactose	Milk sugar
Maltose	Di (two) saccharide comprised of two molecules of glucose	Malt sugar

dairy products (lactose), and there are added sugars, such as sucrose. Sweeteners come in different forms, from powdered and crystalline to syrup (see Figure 2.3).

Some compounds used to sweeten foods are not sugars at all. Instead, they are "artificial sweeteners." Sucralose and aspartame, for example, are artificial sweeteners, not sugars. However, they can substitute for sugars in food by providing a sweet taste.

In addition to sweetening foods, sugars help to prevent spoilage in jams and jellies and perform several functions in baking. These include browning the crust and retaining moisture in baked goods. Sugar also acts as a food for yeast in breads. When yeast "eats" sugar, carbon dioxide (a gas) is produced. Carbon dioxide makes bread rise and gives it an airy texture.

As well as occurring naturally in some foods, sugar is often added to foods to sweeten them. Some of the added sugars include table sugar, high fructose corn syrup, and corn syrup. Although a natural sugar, honey is primarily made of fructose and glucose, the same two components as table sugar. Honey and table sugar both contribute only energy (calories), but no other significant amounts of nutrients. However, because honey is more concentrated, it has more calories than an equal amount of table sugar. Fruits are an excellent source of natural sugar (fructose). Canned fruits are packed in four different ways: in water, fruit juice, light syrup, and/or heavy syrup. Both light syrup and heavy syrup have sugar added (usually sucrose or high fructose corn syrup), with heavy syrup containing more added sugar, and thus, more calories. Dried fruits,

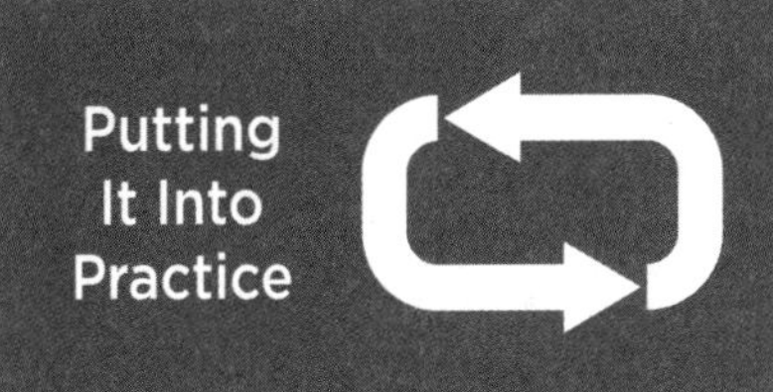

3. Explain which would affect diabetes management more, consuming honey in coffee or regular sugar. Why?

Figure 2.3

Common Forms of Added Sugars

Table Sugar (granulated sugar, sucrose)	Obtained in crystalline form from cane and beets; is about 99.9% pure; is sold in granulated or powdered form.
Corn Syrup	Made from cornstarch; mostly glucose. Only 75% as sweet as sucrose; less expensive than sucrose. Used extensively in baked goods; also used in canned goods.
High Fructose Corn Syrup	Corn syrup treated with an enzyme that converts glucose to fructose, which results in a sweeter product. Used in soft drinks, baked goods, jelly, syrups, fruits, and desserts.
Brown Sugar	Sugar crystals contained in a molasses syrup with natural flavor and color; 91 to 96% sucrose.
Molasses	Thick syrup left over after making sugar from sugar cane. Brown in color with a high sugar concentration.
Turbinado Sugar	Sometimes viewed incorrectly as raw sugar. Produced by separating raw sugar crystals and washing them with steam to remove impurities.

Nutrition Facts

Serving Size 1 Container (150g)

Calories 120	**Calories from Fat** 0
Amount/Serving	**%DV***
Total Fat 0g	0%
Saturated Fat 0g	0%
Trans Fat 0g	
Cholesterol 5mg	2%
Sodium 50mg	2%
Total Carbohydrate 19g	6%
Dietary Fiber 0g	0%
Sugars 18g	
Added Sugars 0g	
Protein 12g	24%
Vitamin A 0% • **Vitamin C** 0% • **Vitamin D** 15%	
Calcium 15% • **Iron** 0%	

INGREDIENTS: CULTURED GRADE A NON FAT MILK, WATER, STRAWBERRY, SUGAR, FRUCTOSE, CONTAINS LESS THAN 1% OF MODIFED CORN STARCH, NATURAL FLAVOR, CARRAGEENAN, CARMINE AND BLACK CARROT JUICE CONCENTRATE (FOR COLOR), SODIUM CITRATE, POTASSIUM SORBATE (TO MAINTAIN FRESHNESS), MALIC ACID, VITAMIN D_3.

CONTAINS ACTIVE YOGURT CULTURES.

having had much of their water removed, are much more concentrated sources of sugar than fresh fruits, and again, more calories for the same volume of fresh fruits. As seen in Figure 2.4, lactose, or milk sugar, is present in large amounts in milk, ice cream, ice milk, sherbet (which also contains sucrose and/or other forms of sugars), cottage cheese, cheese spreads and other soft cheeses, eggnog, and cream. Hard cheeses contain only traces of lactose.

In addition to the "artificial sweeteners" mentioned above, sugarless gums and many sugar-free products use sweeteners such as sorbitol, xylitol, and mannitol. These substances are called sugar alcohols. Sorbitol is 60 percent as sweet as sucrose, with about the same number of calories per gram. Sorbitol is used in such products as sugarless hard and soft candies, chewing gums, jams and jellies. Xylitol is about as sweet as table sugar and is absorbed very slowly. Finally, mannitol is poorly digested, so it does not contribute a full four calories per gram. Mannitol occurs naturally in pineapple, olives, sweet potatoes, and carrots, and is added to sugarless gums. Both mannitol and sorbitol, when taken in large amounts, may cause diarrhea. Products "whose reasonably foreseeable consumption may result in a daily ingestion of 20 grams of mannitol [or 50 grams of sorbitol] shall bear the labeling statement, 'Excess consumption may have a laxative effect'" (Code of Federal Regulations Title 21, April 2016, Section 180.25, [e]).

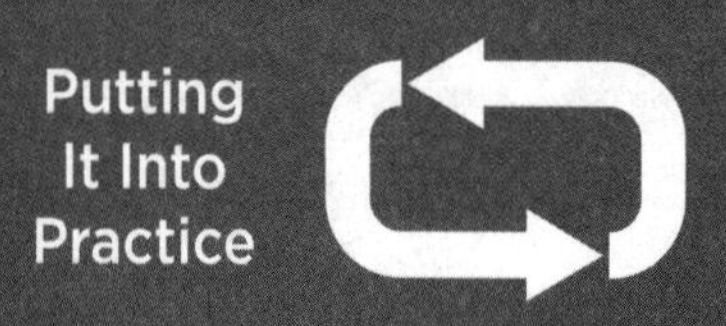

4. Using the food label above, how would we know if the 18 grams of sugar in this food is from added or natural sugars?

Figure 2.4
Sugar Content of Foods

FOOD/PORTION	TEASPOONS OF SUGAR
Dairy	
Skim Milk*, 1 cup	3
Swiss Cheese*, 1 ounce	Less than 1
Vanilla Ice Cream**, 1/2 cup	4
Meat, Poultry and Fish	
Meat, Poultry, or Fish, 3 ounces	0
Eggs	
Egg, 1	0
Grains	
White Bread*, 1 slice	Less than 1
English Muffin*, 1	Less than 1
White Rice*, Cooked, 1/2 cup	Less than 1
Circular-shaped Oat Cereal*, 1 cup	Less than 1
Honey-flavored, Circular-shaped Oat Cereal**, 1 cup	3
Square-shaped Oatmeal Cereal**, 1 cup	2
Fruits	
Apple*, 1 medium	4.5
Banana*, 1 medium	7
Orange*, 1 medium	3
Raisins*, 1/2 ounce	2.5
Vegetables	
Broccoli*, 1/2 cup raw, chopped	Less than 1 gram
Mixed Vegetables*, 1/3 cup, chopped	Less than 1 gram
Beverages	
Cola Soft Drink**, 12 fluid ounces	10
Cakes, Cookies, Candies, and Pudding	
Brownie**, 1 average	6
Chocolate Graham Crackers**, 8 squares	2
Chocolate Chip Cookies**, 3	3
Lemon Drops**, 4 pieces	2.5
Candy-coated Chocolate Pieces**, 70	7
Vanilla Pudding**, 1/2 cup	6
Sweeteners	
White Sugar*, 1 tablespoon	4
Honey*, 1 tablespoon	4
High Fructose Corn Syrup**, 1 tablespoon	4

*Source: U.S. Department of Agriculture   * Naturally-occurring sugars ** Added sugars*

Sugar on the Food Label

Sugar content is listed on the nutrition label of food. Both the naturally-occurring sugars in food, such as the fruit sugar or milk sugar, as well as added sugars, such as table sugar, are reported on the food label. These are lumped together so it is difficult to determine the amount of added sugars. Read the food label carefully and look for any and all of the sugars listed in Figure 2.3. Limit foods that are high in added sugars. Be sure to read the food label and look at the ingredient list to see what types of sugars have been added.

Complex Carbohydrates: Starches

Whereas simple sugars are chemically made up of one or two units of monosaccharides, starch is much more complex. Chemically, starch and fiber—both forms of complex carbohydrates—consist of many glucose molecules strung together. This is why they are referred to as *complex*. Another term for complex carbohydrates is polysaccharides. *Poly* means many, *saccharide* means sugar [glucose] so a polysaccharide is made up of many glucose units. A single starch molecule (or chain) may contain 300 to 1,000 or more glucose molecules. The giant molecules are packed side by side in a plant root or seed, providing energy for the plant. All forms of starch are plant materials.

Cereal grains, which are the fruits or seeds of cultivated grasses, are rich sources of starch. Examples include wheat, corn, rice, rye, barley, and oats. Wheat and other grains consist of three parts: the starchy endosperm, the vitamin-rich germ, and the bran—the protective outer coat that contains fiber. Figure 2.5 is a diagram of a grain of rice. Cereal grains are used to make breads, breakfast cereals, and pastas. Starches are also found in potatoes, vegetables, and dried beans and peas. Figure 2.6 identifies common sources of starch in the diet.

Starch is a key component of a healthful diet. Some starch is broken down immediately after a meal and is used as sugar (glucose) to fuel body functions. If blood sugar goes too high, the body can take the excess and store it as **glycogen**, a readily available source of glucose. Glycogen is stored in muscles and in the liver. Glycogen is not really a food component; it is a special form of carbohydrate the body makes.

GLOSSARY

Glycogen
A particular form of carbohydrate storage found in animal tissue and used by the body for quick energy

Figure 2.5
Whole Grain Kernel

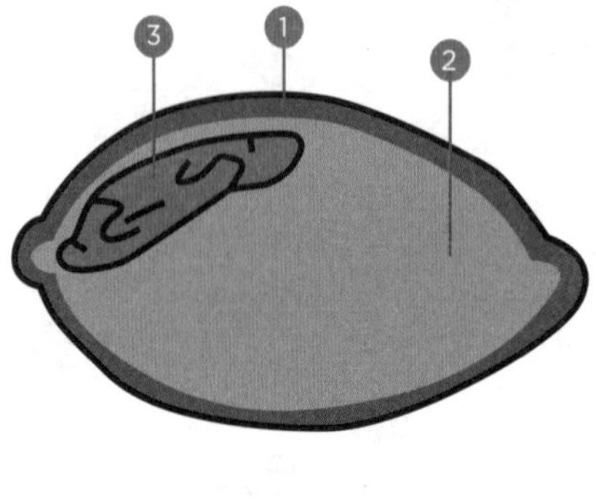

3 1 2

1 **Bran:** Outer shell protects seed (fiber, B vitamins, trace minerals)

2 **Endosperm:** Provides energy (carbohydrates, protein)

3 **Germ:** Nourishment for the seed (antioxidants, vitamin E, B vitamins)

Source: U.S. Department of Agriculture

Figure 2.6
Sources of Starch

Sources of Starch	Sources of Soluble Fiber	Sources of Insoluble Fiber
• Breads • Cereals • Flour • Grains • Legumes • Pasta • Starchy Vegetables	• Dried Beans and Peas • Some Grains (oats, barley) • Some Fruits and Vegetables (apples, grapes, citrus, and carrots)	• Whole Grains with Bran • Products Made with Whole Grains (whole wheat bread, brown rice) • Many Vegetables (corn, celery, green beans)

Complex Carbohydrates: Dietary Fiber

The term **dietary fiber** describes a variety of carbohydrate compounds from plants that are not digestible. Like starch, most fibers are chains of glucose units bonded together, but what's different is that the chains can't be broken down or digested. In other words, most fiber passes through the stomach and intestines unchanged and is excreted in the feces. Unlike sugars or starches, fiber does not give rise to blood sugar in the body. Fiber is found only in plant foods where it supports the plant's stems, leaves, and seeds.

There are two major types of fiber—soluble and insoluble. **Soluble fiber** simply means fiber that dissolves in hot water, forming a gel. **Insoluble fiber** is the tough, fibrous part of plants that is not digestible and does not dissolve in water.

Soluble fibers include gums, mucilages, pectin, and some hemicelluloses. Soluble fiber is found in foods like apples, oats, and dried beans (see Figure 2.6). In the body, soluble fiber slows down the movement of food through the lower part of the digestive tract. Fiber also slows down the release of glucose from other foods into the body, which may be beneficial to someone with diabetes who needs to control blood sugar. Soluble fibers also help control blood cholesterol levels.

Insoluble fibers include cellulose, lignin, and some hemicelluloses. Insoluble fiber is found in foods like bran (wheat bran, corn bran, whole grain breads) and vegetables. Insoluble fibers form the structures of plants, such as skins and the bran of the wheat kernel. Insoluble fiber can be seen in the skin of whole kernel corn and the strings of celery. Insoluble fibers speed up the movement of food through the lower digestive tract and can help prevent constipation. Like soluble fibers, they also help to slow down the release of glucose from other foods into the body. People need both types of dietary fiber for proper nutrition and digestion.

The amount of fiber in a plant varies from one kind of plant to another and may vary within a species or variety, depending on growing conditions and maturity of the plant at the time of harvest. Like starch, fiber is found abundantly in plants, especially in the outer layers of cereal grains and the fibrous parts of legumes (e.g. dried beans and peas), fruits, vegetables, nuts, and seeds. Fiber is not found in animal products such as meat, poultry, fish, dairy products, and eggs. Most plant foods contain both soluble and insoluble fibers.

Whenever the fiber-rich bran and the vitamin-rich germ are left on the endosperm of a grain, the grain is called whole grain. Examples of whole grains include whole

GLOSSARY

Dietary Fiber
A polysaccharide made up of many molecules of sugar; plant materials that are not digested by the body

Soluble Fiber
Fiber that forms a gel when combined with water (i.e., fruits, oats, and dried beans)

Insoluble Fiber
Outer covering (bran) of plants or fibrous inner parts that are not soluble in water (i.e., bran, celery, and corn)

wheat, whole corn, whole rye, bulgur (i.e. whole wheat grains that have been steamed and dried), oatmeal, whole cornmeal, whole hulled barley, popcorn, and brown rice. There are many others, but these are the most common. The milling of whole wheat to produce white flour removes the bran and germ and leaves behind mostly starch.

During the milling process, bran and germ are removed to produce **refined grains**. Much of the fiber and vitamins (especially the B vitamins) are lost in this process. By law, white flour and other refined grain products must be **enriched**, meaning that certain nutrients (thiamin, riboflavin, niacin, and iron) are added in amounts approximately equivalent to those originally present in the whole grain but were lost through milling. Enrichment does not replace the fiber removed by milling, it only replaces some of the other nutrients that were lost. Whole wheat flour retains most of the original nutrients and has more fiber, vitamin B6, magnesium, and zinc than enriched white flour.

As a general rule, *unrefined* (unprocessed) foods contain more fiber than *refined* foods because fiber is usually removed in processing. For example, raw apples contain much fiber in the skin (a whole, raw apple contains about 5 grams of fiber), but if the skin is removed to make applesauce or canned sliced apples, its fiber content drops to about 2-3 grams. When apples are processed further to make apple juice, all of the fiber is lost. Whole foods contain a greater variety of fibers, as well as many other nutrients.

Since insoluble fiber holds water and speeds the movement of waste through the intestines, stools produced by a high fiber diet tend to be bulkier and softer and pass more quickly and more easily through the intestines. A diet high in insoluble fiber helps reduce the risk of hemorrhoids; it is also important for those who have diverticulosis, a disease of the large intestine in which the intestinal walls become weakened and bulge out into pockets. Insoluble fibers may also reduce the risk of colon cancer.

Eating adequate soluble and insoluble fiber has many benefits, including increasing a sense of fullness (satiety), when part of an overall health plan that includes eating less dietary fat and cholesterol.

GLOSSARY

Refined Grain
A grain in which, during the milling process, the bran and germ are removed leaving behind the starchy endosperm

Enriched
Adding B vitamins and iron back into refined flour and grain products

Lipids
Nutrient category that includes both fats, such as butter, shortening, and oils (i.e. olive or canola oil)

Fats

Lipid is the scientific name for a diverse family of compounds that are characterized by their insolubility in water. Lipids include fats, oils, and cholesterol. Except for cholesterol, these compounds are important for providing energy and for helping the body absorb fat-soluble vitamins (discussed later in this chapter). Fats and oils are the most plentiful lipids in nature. It is customary to call a lipid a *fat* if it is a solid at room temperature and an *oil* if it is a liquid at the same temperature. Fats from animal sources, such as butter, are usually solid, whereas oils are liquid and generally of plant origin (such as corn or canola oil). There are a few exceptions to this rule: Coconut oil and palm/palm kernel oil have a plant origin, but are solid at room temperature. It is common to hear the general category of fats referred to as "animal fats" and "vegetable oils." For the purposes of this book, the word "fat" will refer to both fats and oils.

In recent years, there has been much discussion about fats and cholesterol including what kind of fat is eaten and the relationship between dietary fats and cholesterol and cardiovascular (heart and artery) disease. A high level of blood cholesterol has been identified as one of the major risk factors for having a heart attack or a stroke. This is important because diet, particularly fat intake, influences blood cholesterol levels.

Functions of Fats

Fat serves a variety of functions.

- Some fat is needed in the diet to provide the essential fatty acids. Fat in food also contains the fat-soluble vitamins (A, D, E, and K).
- Fat provides a concentrated source of energy (9 calories per gram). It is also a great way for the body to store extra calories. About 15-20 percent of the weight of healthy normal-weight men is fat; for women, it's about 18-25 percent.
- Fat cushions parts of our body for protection: At least half of fat deposits are located just beneath the skin, where they help to cushion body organs (acting like shock absorbers).
- Fat acts as insulation: fat provides insulation to help maintain a constant body temperature.
- Lipids are also an important component of cells, including the cell membrane (the outer layer of the cell).
- Because fats slow digestion and the emptying of the stomach, they help delay the onset of hunger.
- In addition to creating a feeling of fullness, fats increase the palatability of foods by enhancing their aroma, taste, flavor, juiciness, and tenderness.

Triglycerides

The bulk of the body's fat tissue is in the form of **triglycerides**. Likewise, most of the fats found in foods are in the form of triglycerides. Figure 2.7 shows what a triglyceride molecule looks like. It is composed of three fatty acids attached to glycerol. Each fatty acid is made up of carbon atoms joined like links on a chain. The carbon chains vary in length, with most fatty acids containing 4 to 20 carbon atoms. Each carbon has hydrogen attached, much like charms on a charm bracelet.

GLOSSARY

Triglycerides
Common form of fats in foods; comprised of three fatty acids and glycerol

Figure 2.7
Triglyceride Molecule

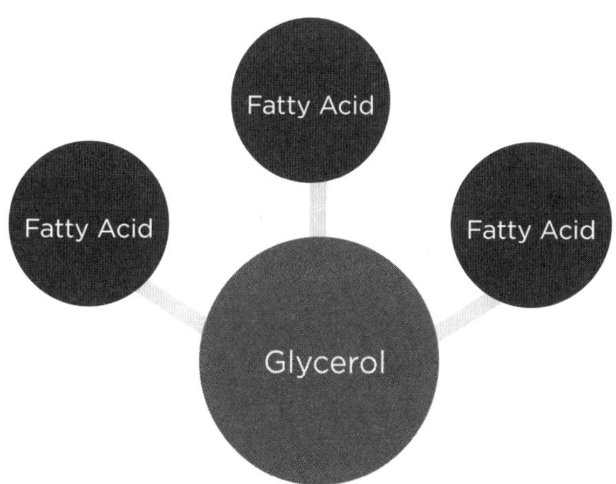

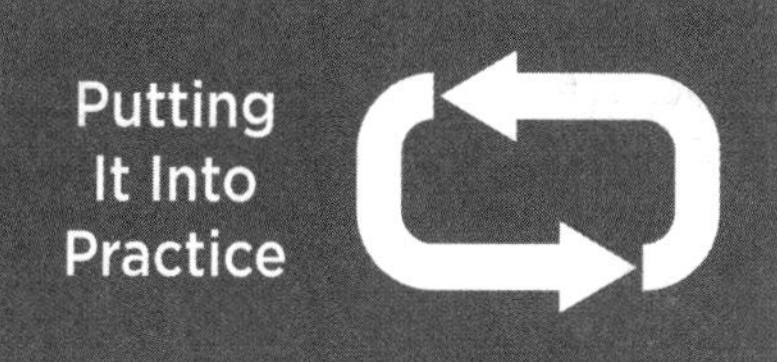

5. How would using a "fat-free" salad dressing affect how we use the nutrients from dark, leafy greens?

GLOSSARY

Saturated Fat
Fatty acid that is filled with hydrogen, making it solid or semisolid at room temperature

Unsaturated Fat
Fatty acid that contains one or more double bonds

Monounsaturated Fatty Acid
Fatty acid that contains one double bond and is found in foods like olive oil, almonds, and most hydrogenated margarines

Polyunsaturated Fatty Acid
A fatty acid that contains more than one double bond and is found in foods like corn oil, soybean oil, and soft margarines

Trans-Fatty Acid or Trans Fat
A fatty acid where hydrogen atoms have been added and chemically rearranged to make them more solid—found in hydrogenated oils, margarines, shortening, and many snack foods

Hydrogenated
A process of adding hydrogen to oils in order to make them more solid

Essential Fatty Acid
Fatty acids that cannot be made by the body, so much come from the diet

Types of Fatty Acids

Fatty acids may be one of three different types:

- Saturated
- Monounsaturated
- Polyunsaturated

The terms *saturated* and *unsaturated* relate to the chemistry and chemical structure of fats. "Saturated" means each carbon atom in the chain holds as many hydrogen atoms as it can (two). It is called a **saturated fatty acid** or saturated fat because it is filled or *saturated* with hydrogens. When a double bond forms between two neighboring carbons, two hydrogens are missing, so the carbons are not fully saturated. This type of fatty acid is called an **unsaturated fatty acid**. A fatty acid that contains one double bond in the chain is a **monounsaturated fatty acid** or unsaturated fat (mono means one). A fatty acid containing more than one double bond is a **polyunsaturated fatty acid** (PUFA). *Poly* means many, so this term means that the fatty acid is unsaturated in many places. Another fatty acid, **trans-fatty acid** (sometimes referred to as *trans fat*), has hydrogen atoms that have been added and chemically rearranged. Trans-fatty acids are made during the process in which vegetable oils are partially **hydrogenated** (adding hydrogen and saturation) to make them more solid at room temperature. Hydrogenated oils are used in margarines and shortening.

Hydrogenated oils in margarines and shortening extend the shelf life of the fat. The health risk of transfat has been widely publicized in the past decade. Consuming trans fat can increase your LDL "bad" cholesterol, and at the same time, decrease your HDL "good" cholesterol. This combination of increasing LDL and decreasing HDL cholesterol increases the risk of heart disease. In 2008, a law went into effect that requires trans fats to be listed on the Nutrition Facts Panel for all foods. In addition, some cities and states have banned all trans fat use in food products. Trans-fatty acids are found in vegetable shortenings and some margarines. Trans fats are also found in foods that contain shortening or margarines, such as crackers, cookies, canned frosting, and foods fried in partially hydrogenated fats.

Two of the fatty acids in food are considered to be **essential fatty acids** (EFA). Because the body can't make EFA, it is essential to get them from the diet. The names of the two essential fatty acids are linoleic acid and alpha-linolenic acid. Linoleic acid is polyunsaturated and is found in corn, cottonseed, soybean, and safflower oil. It is also found in nuts, seeds, and whole grain products. Alpha-linolenic acid is also polyunsaturated and appears in some vegetable oils such as canola, walnut, soybean oils, and in fatty fish.

Triglycerides in Foods

Fat in the diet is both visible and invisible. When thinking about fats, most think about only the visible fats—butter, margarine, and cooking oils. But much of the fat in the diet comes from less visible sources—the fatty streaks in meat (also known as marbling), the fat under the skin of poultry, the fat in milk and cheese, the fat in many baked goods, fried foods, nuts, and the fat contained in many processed foods such as candy, chips, crackers, canned soups, and convenience foods. Unprocessed cereal grains, fruits and vegetables (except avocados and olives), flour, pasta, breads, and most cereals have little or no fat.

All fats in foods are made up of mixtures of fatty acids. If a food contains mostly saturated fatty acids, it is considered a main source of saturated fat. If it contains mostly polyunsaturated fatty acids, it is a main source of polyunsaturated fat. Monounsaturated fats contain mostly monounsaturated fatty acids. Regardless of the type of fat used— saturated, monounsaturated, or polyunsaturated—all contain nine calories per gram.

Animal fats are generally more saturated than liquid vegetable oils. Saturated fat raises blood cholesterol more than anything else in the diet. Animal products are a major source of saturated fat in the typical American diet. The fat in whole dairy products (like butter, cheese, whole milk, ice cream, and cream) contains high amounts of saturated fat. Saturated fat is also concentrated in the fat that surrounds meat and in the white streaks of fat in the muscle of meat (marbling). Well-trimmed cuts from certain sections of the animal, such as the round and loin, are lower in saturated fat than well-marbled, untrimmed meat. Poultry without the skin and most fish are lower in saturated fat.

A few vegetable fats—coconut oil, cocoa butter, and palm oil—are high in saturated fat. These may be used for commercial deep-fat frying and in foods such as cookies and crackers, whipped toppings, coffee creamers, cake mixes, and even frozen dinners. Chocolate products, such as chocolate candy bars and baking chips, contain cocoa butter and sometimes also palm kernel oil or palm oil.

Recommendations for Daily Fat Intake

As discussed in chapter one, there are specific dietary recommendations for how much of these fats should be consumed. Total fat intake should be no more than 30 percent of total daily calories. Of that 30 percent, less than 7 percent should come from saturated fat. The American Heart Association recommends less than one gram per day of trans fat and less than 300 milligrams per day of dietary cholesterol. See Figure 2.8 for ways to choose healthy fats.

Cholesterol

Cholesterol is a type of sterol the body needs to function. Cholesterol is made in the liver of the human body, so it is technically not an essential nutrient. The body uses cholesterol to build cell membranes and brain and nerve tissues. It also helps the body produce steroid hormones needed for body regulation, bile acids needed for digestion, and for vitamin D synthesis.

Cholesterol is found only in foods of animal origin: egg yolks, meat, poultry, fish, milk, and milk products. Egg yolks and organ meats (liver, kidney, brain) are major sources of cholesterol. Cholesterol is found in both the lean and fat sections of red meat and the meat and skin of poultry. In milk products, cholesterol is mostly in the fat, so lower fat products contain less cholesterol. Egg whites and foods that come from plants have no cholesterol. Figure 2.9 shows the cholesterol content of selected foods.

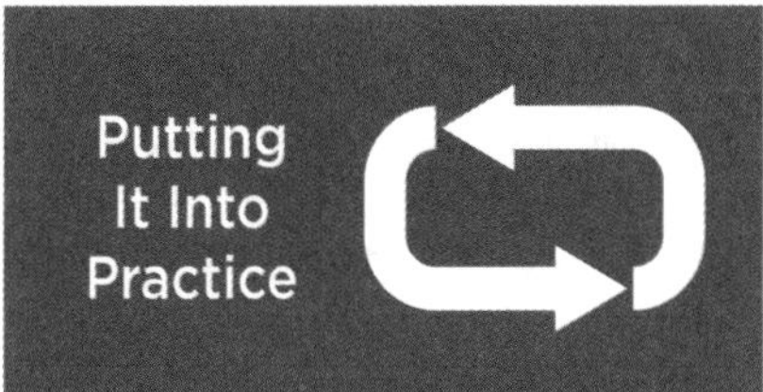

6. A person following a vegan diet asks you what she can do to obtain omega-3 fats. What would you tell her?

Figure 2.8
Dietary Fats

TYPE OF FAT	INCREASE Your Intake of These Foods
Polyunsaturated Fats	Most low-fat or soft margarines, soybean oil, corn oil, sunflower oil, safflower oil, walnuts, sunflower seeds
Monounsaturated Fats	Peanuts and peanut oil, olive oil, canola oil, almonds, avocado, some seeds
Omega-3 Fatty Acids	Cold water finfish, flaxseed products, flaxseed oil, walnuts

TYPE OF FAT	DECREASE Your Intake of These Foods
Saturated Fats	Animal products, high-fat cheese and other dairy products, lard, butter, coconut and palm oil
Trans Fats	Foods fried in trans fat oils, foods made with partially hydrogenated oils, shortening, some margarines
Dietary Cholesterol	Eggs, animal products, shellfish

Figure 2.9
Cholesterol in Foods

FOOD	PORTION	CHOLESTEROL IN mg
Liver, braised	3 ounces	333
Egg	1 whole	185
Beef, Short Ribs, braised,	3 ounces	80
Beef, ground, lean, broiled	Medium, 3 ounces	74
Beef, Top Round, broiled	3 ounces	73
Chicken, roasted, no skin, light meat	3-1/2 ounces	75
Haddock, baked	3 ounces	63
Mackerel, baked	3 ounces	64
Swordfish, baked	3 ounces	43
Shrimp, moist heat	3 ounces	167
Milk, whole	8 ounces	33
Milk, 2% fat	8 ounces	18
Milk, 1% fat	8 ounces	10
Milk, skim	8 ounces	4
Cheddar Cheese	1 ounce	30
American Processed Cheese	1 ounce	27
Cottage Cheese, low-fat	1/2 cup	5

Source: National Institutes of Health

Protein

Carbohydrate and fat can both be independent food sources, such as sugar or butter, or they can be combined together to form other foods like cookies. Protein is rarely found by itself; it is usually found in combination with fat. The word *protein* comes from a Greek word that means "of prime importance." Protein has been considered to be "of prime importance" for centuries because of the essential functions in our bodies. In the United States, most people eat too much protein, which generally means a diet higher in fat.

To most Americans, the term "protein" means meat, poultry, or fish. These foods are all excellent sources of complete protein. In addition, there are other less well-known sources like dried beans and peas, whole grains, and vegetables. Protein-rich meats, poultry, and fish are the "main course" in the diets of Americans. In other parts of the world, plant-based protein sources are the foundation of the diet.

Like carbohydrates and fats, proteins contain carbon, hydrogen, and oxygen. But unlike these other nutrients, proteins contain the chemical element *nitrogen*. **Amino acids** are the nitrogen-containing building blocks of proteins. Proteins are strands of amino acids (Figure 2.10). This allows for an endless number of combinations and sequences in the amino acid chains and, therefore, a great variety of proteins in plants and animals.

Each protein has a unique sequence of amino acids, which are the *building blocks* of proteins. These amino acids build proteins and have a unique way of bending and coiling that is necessary for the protein to function normally. Different tissues in the body, such as hair and skin, each have their own characteristic proteins. Some amino acids, called **essential amino acids**, must be provided by the foods eaten, because the body can't make them. Other amino acids are considered **nonessential amino acids** because they can be made by the human body. If essential amino acids are not consumed regularly, the body isn't able to synthesize proteins.

GLOSSARY

Amino Acids
Building blocks of protein

Essential Amino Acids
Amino acids that cannot be made in the body; must come from foods

Nonessential Amino Acids
Amino acids that can be made in the body

Figure 2.10
Complete and Incomplete Proteins

COMPLETE PROTEINS

Meat, Dairy Products, Eggs
Animal sources contain all essential amino acids.

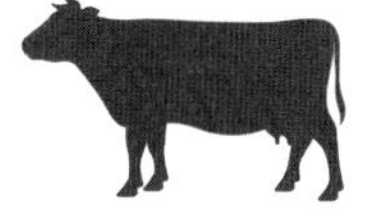
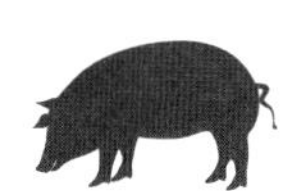
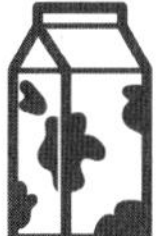
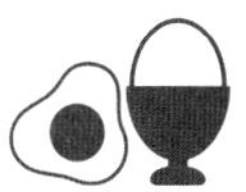

INCOMPLETE PROTEINS

When combined foods from two or more of these categories make a complete protein and provide all of the essential amino acids. If eaten alone, they do not provide all of the essential amino acids.

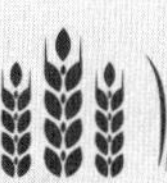
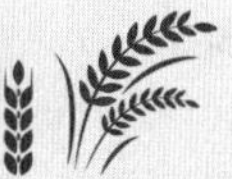

Grains
Whole grain bread, barley, corn, corn-meal, oats, rice, pasta

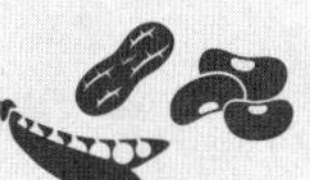

Legumes
Dried beans and peas, peanuts, soy products

Seeds/Nuts
Nut butters, nuts, sunflower seeds, sesame seeds

Functions of Protein

Building Blocks. Amino acids are required by the body for building new cells. For instance, proteins are found in the skin, bone, cartilage, and muscles. The greatest amount of proteins are needed when the body is building new cells rapidly, like during pregnancy, infancy, or lactation. Building new cells is also important after burns, surgery, healing, and for growing new hair or nails (like after chemotherapy).

Amino acids are combined to build **enzymes**, some of the most important proteins formed in cells. Enzymes act as a catalyst that helps make the chemical reactions in the body. **Hormones** are also built from proteins and act as messengers that regulate metabolism.

Proteins build **antibodies** that fight infection. Antibodies travel in the blood, where it is their job to attack any foreign bodies that do not belong there. These foreign bodies could include viruses, bacteria, or toxins. Antibodies actually combine with these foreign bodies, producing an immune response that helps ward off harmful infections.

GLOSSARY

Enzymes
Catalysts that speed up chemical reactions in the body

Hormones
Chemical messengers that regulate metabolism—such as thyroid hormones

Antibodies
Blood proteins required for an immune response to foreign bodies

Maintaining

Besides building cells, proteins also maintain tissues by replacing worn-out cells. The body is constantly sloughing all kinds of cells (e.g. red blood cells, cells lining our intestinal tract, or skin cells), and these cells need to be replaced continually, thus maintaining balance.

Protein also assists in maintaining water and electrolyte balance. There must be a constant amount of fluid both inside and outside of the cells. Protein is important in the maintenance of fluid levels. Edema is a condition that occurs if this fluid balance fails.

Protein is also important in maintaining an acid-base (pH) balance within the body. Protein in the blood keeps the blood neutral, meaning that the blood is neither too acidic nor too basic. Normal processes of the body produce acids and bases that, if left unchecked, can cause major problems such as coma and death. Blood proteins buffer these acids and bases to keep the blood pH neutral.

Providing Energy

While protein does provide energy (four calories per gram), this is not one of its major functions. However, if the diet does not supply enough calories from carbohydrates or fats, proteins can be used for energy, though this would be at the expense of tissue building and maintenance functions. Some amino acids can be converted to glucose, the sole fuel of the brain.

Unlike fat, the body has few protein reserves, so we need to consume it daily. However, if more protein is eaten, and thus more calories than is needed by the body, the extra protein is used for energy, or converted to body fat and stored in fat cells. The recommended daily amount of protein is 0.8 grams per kilogram of body weight. That converts to about 40-60 grams of protein per day for a person weighing between 110 and 165 pounds. The average daily protein intake is about 1½ - 2 times more than we need.

During digestion, proteins are broken down into amino acids that are then absorbed into the blood. Amino acids travel through the blood into the body's cells. There is an amino acid pool in the body that provides the cells with a supply of amino acids for making protein. The amino acid pool refers to the overall amount of amino acids distributed in the blood, the organs (such as the liver), and the body's cells. Amino acids from foods, as well as amino acids from body proteins that have been dismantled, stock these pools. In this manner, the body recycles its own proteins. If there is a shortage of a nonessential amino acid during production of a protein, the cell will make it and add it to the protein strand. If there is a shortage of an essential amino acid, the protein can't be completed.

Protein deficiency in the United States is usually due to illness, injury, or economic factors. Protein deficiency may cause wasting of muscles, weight loss, delayed wound healing, or lowered immunity due to fewer antibodies being made and edema. **Edema** is the abnormal pooling of fluid in the tissues, causing swelling of the part of the body where the pooling occurs. Edema is often seen with malnutrition because protein helps to maintain fluid balance. In protein deficiency, fluids collect outside the cells. With appropriate nutritional intervention, extra protein can be given where there is a loss of body protein due to burns, surgery, stress, infections, skin breakdown, and similar situations. Protein deficiency commonly occurs in developing countries where children do not have enough to eat. It is rarely seen without a deficiency of calories and other nutrients as well. **Protein-Calorie Malnutrition** is the name for a group of diseases characterized by both protein and energy deficiency. Protein-calorie malnutrition is also called Protein-Energy Malnutrition (PEM). Protein-deficiency disease is called kwashiorkor, and energy-deficiency disease is called marasmus. Kwashiorkor is characterized by retarded growth and development, a protruding abdomen due to edema, peeling skin, a loss of normal hair color, irritability, and sadness. Marasmus is characterized by gross underweight, no fat stores and wasting away of muscles, and apathy. There is no edema, as seen in kwashiorkor. Whereas marasmus is usually associated with severe food shortage, prolonged semi-starvation, or early weaning, kwashiorkor is associated with poor protein intake.

GLOSSARY

Edema
Abnormal pooling of fluid in the tissues causing swelling

Protein-Calorie Malnutrition
A name for a group of diseases characterized by protein and energy deficiency

Complete or High-Quality Protein
Protein that provides all of the essential amino acids

Incomplete Protein
Plant protein that lacks one or more essential amino acids

Sources and Quality of Protein

Protein is in all foods of animal origin, and in most foods of plant origin. Animal sources of protein in the American diet include meat, poultry, seafood, eggs, milk, and cheese. Plant sources include legumes, cereal grains, and products made with them, such as bread and ready-to-eat cereals, vegetables, nuts, and seeds. The legumes (beans, peas, and lentils) contain larger amounts and better quality proteins than other plant sources. Fruits and fat contain little-to-no protein. Animal sources of protein often also contain fat, especially saturated fat, while plant sources contain very little fat.

The quality of a particular protein depends on its content of essential amino acids. Food proteins providing all of the essential amino acids in the proportions needed by the body are called **complete or high-quality proteins**. Meat, poultry, fish, milk and milk products, and eggs are all sources of complete proteins. Animal proteins are more readily absorbed than plant proteins.

Complete proteins have a high *biological value* (BV). BV measures how effectively the body can use a particular protein source. Plant proteins are usually low, or lacking one or more of the essential amino acids, and are called **incomplete proteins**. The amino

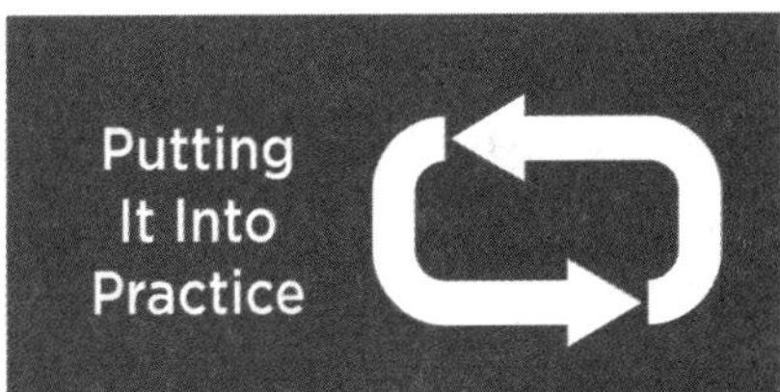

7. A friend of yours mentions he read in a bodybuilding magazine that he should be eating 1 gram of protein per pound of body weight to be healthy. Is he right?

GLOSSARY

Complementary Proteins
The combination of two protein sources so that all of the essential amino acids are present

acid that is in short supply is called the *limiting amino acid*. Although plant proteins are incomplete proteins, they are the major source of protein for many people around the world. **Complementary proteins** combine either some animal protein (such as milk or eggs) with vegetable protein, or combine two plant sources, such as grains and legumes, so that the essential amino acids deficient in one are present in the other. See Figure 2.10 for examples of complete and incomplete proteins.

SECTION B VITAMINS

Vitamins are essential in small quantities for growth and good health. Vitamins are similar to each other because they are made of the same elements—carbon, hydrogen, oxygen, and sometimes nitrogen or cobalt. They are different in that their elements are arranged differently and each vitamin performs one or more specific functions in the body. In the early 1900s, scientists thought they had found the compounds needed to prevent two diseases caused by vitamin deficiencies: scurvy and pellagra. These compounds originally were believed to belong to a class of chemical compounds called *amines*. Their name comes from the Latin *vita*, or life, plus *amine*—vitamine. Later, the "e" was dropped when it was found that not all of the substances were amines. At first, no one knew what they were chemically and they were identified by letters. Later, because nutrition science is continuously emerging, what was thought to be one vitamin turned out to be many, and numbers were added instead. The vitamin B complex is the best example of this. The B complex vitamins are numbered from vitamin B1 to vitamin B12. When some were found unnecessary for human needs, they were removed from the list (e.g. B4 and B5). This accounts for some of the gaps in the numbers. Additionally, vitamin B8, adenylic acid, was later found not to be a vitamin, so it was removed from the numbered list. Others, originally designated as different from each other, were found to be one and the same. For example, vitamins H, M, S, W, and X were all shown to be biotin, now vitamin B7. Let's start with some basic facts about vitamins.

- Very small amounts of vitamins are needed by the human body and very small amounts are present in foods. Some vitamins are measured in international units (IUs), a measure of biological activity; others are measured by weight in micrograms (μg) or milligrams (mg). Some vitamins, such as vitamin D, can be measured in both IUs and micrograms. To illustrate how small these amounts are, remember that one ounce is 28 grams. A milligram is 1/1000 of a gram and a microgram is 1/1000 of a milligram.
- Although vitamins are needed in small quantities, the roles they play in the body are enormously important.
- Vitamins must be obtained through foods because they are either not made in the body or not made in sufficient quantities (i.e. they are essential).
- There is no perfect food that contains all the vitamins in just the right amounts. The best way to assure an adequate intake of vitamins is to eat a varied and balanced diet.
- Vitamins do not have any calories, so they do not directly provide energy to the body. However, they are involved in how the body uses energy and performs many of its necessary functions.
- Some substances considered to be vitamins in foods are not actually vitamins, but rather are precursors. In the body, the precursor chemically changes to the active form of the vitamin, under proper conditions.

Figure 2.11
Vitamins—Quick Glance

CATEGORY	VITAMIN NAME	
Fat-Soluble	Vitamin A Vitamin D	Vitamin E Vitamin K
Water-Soluble	Vitamin C B2 Riboflavin B3 Niacin	B5 Pantothenic Acid B7 Biotin B9 Folate Vitamin B12

Vitamins are classified according to solubility; they are either fat-soluble or water-soluble. Figure 2.11 lists the fat-soluble and water-soluble vitamins. The fat-soluble vitamins generally are found in foods containing fat and can be stored in the body, in fat tissue. The water-soluble vitamins are not stored appreciably in the body.

Now let's take a closer look at 13 vitamins.

Vitamin A

Vitamin A is involved in many different functions. It plays a role in the formation and maintenance of healthy skin and hair, as well as in proper bone growth and tooth development in children. Vitamin A is also needed for the immune system to work properly (for fighting infections) and for maintenance of the protective linings of the lungs, intestines, urinary tract, and other organs. Vitamin A is essential for normal reproduction and, when eaten generously in the form of fruits and vegetables, may protect against certain forms of cancer. Vitamin A is well known for its part in helping us to see properly. Vitamin A is necessary for the health of the eye's *cornea*, the clear membrane that covers the eye. Without enough vitamin A, the cornea becomes cloudy and dry. Vitamin A is also necessary for night vision, the ability of the eyes to adjust after seeing a flash of bright light at night. With night blindness, it takes longer than normal to adjust to dim lights. This can be an early sign of vitamin A deficiency. If the deficiency continues, it can eventually lead to overall blindness.

The form of vitamin A found in fruits and vegetables is actually a precursor of vitamin A called *beta-carotene*. In the body, beta-carotene is converted to vitamin A. Beta-carotene often gives food an orange color. Vitamin A is abundant in deep orange fruits and vegetables, such as apricots, carrots, and sweet potatoes. It is also found in dark green vegetables, such as spinach, kale, and Romaine lettuce (see Figure 2.12).

Other sources of vitamin A include animal products such as liver (a very rich source), egg yolk, butter, whole milk, and fortified cereals. Low-fat and skim milk are often fortified with vitamin A, because the vitamin is removed from the milk when the fat is removed. **Fortified** foods have one or more nutrients added. Most ready-to-eat and

GLOSSARY

Fortified
Foods that have one or more nutrients added

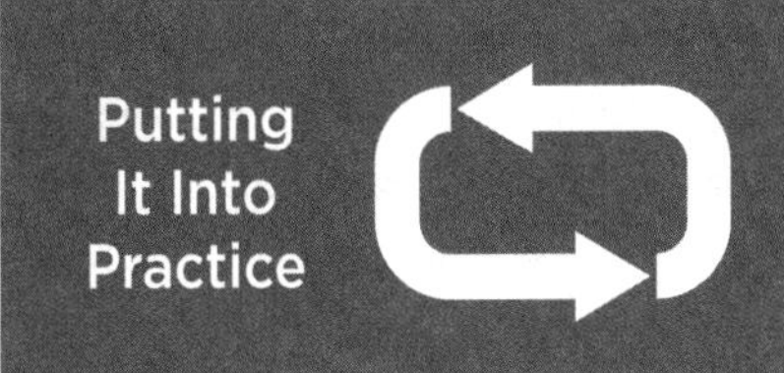

8. What would be the benefit of obtaining vitamin A from whole foods rather than from a supplement?

Figure 2.12
Vitamin A in Foods

FOOD	PORTION	RETINOL EQUIVALENTS
Liver, Beef	3 ounces	9,011
Sweet Potato, baked	1 small	2,488
Carrots, raw	1	2,025
Spinach, cooked	1/2 cup	875
Squash, Butternut	1/2 cup	857
Cantaloupe	1/4 melon	516
Fortified Milk, 2%	1 cup	140
Apricots, dried	4 large halves	127
Broccoli, cooked	1/2 cup	110
Egg Yolk	1	97
Cheese, Cheddar	1 ounce	86
Peach	1 medium	47
Orange	1 medium	27

Source: U.S. Department of Agriculture

instant-prepared cereals are also fortified with vitamin A. Retinol, the active form of vitamin A found in animal foods, is used in fortification.

Nutrient needs for vitamin A are expressed in *retinol equivalents* (REs). Retinol equivalents measure the amount of retinol the body will actually absorb and utilize from eating foods with various forms of vitamin A (e.g. retinol or beta-carotene).

Because the body stores vitamin A, it is not absolutely necessary to eat a good source every day. Vitamin A deficiency is not often seen in the United States. Unfortunately, it is of concern in third-world countries. Vitamin A deficiency may cause poor growth, infection, blindness, and death. Although there may not be agreement on exactly how much vitamin A can be considered a toxic dose, excessive use of vitamin A may cause dry, scaly skin, bone pain, soreness, stunted growth, liver damage, nausea, and diarrhea. Tolerable Upper Intake Levels (UL) have been established and vary with gender and age. Megadoses of supplemental vitamin A (more than 10 times the estimated nutrient need) are particularly dangerous for pregnant women and for children.

Vitamin D

Vitamin D differs from the other fat-soluble vitamins in that it can be made in the body and it acts more like a hormone than like a vitamin. Acting like a hormone or chemical messenger, vitamin D maintains blood calcium and phosphorus levels so that there is enough calcium and phosphorus present for building bones and teeth. Vitamin D also helps the body absorb calcium and phosphorus from the digestive tract. Only small amounts of vitamin D are found in most foods. For this reason, milk is usually fortified with vitamin D. Other significant food sources of vitamin D include liver, egg yolks, and fish liver oils. When ultraviolet rays shine on the skin, a cholesterol-like compound is converted into a vitamin D precursor and absorbed into the blood. The precursor is then transformed into vitamin D. A light-skinned person needs only 10 to 15 minutes of sun each day to make enough vitamin D; a dark-skinned person may need several hours. Vitamin D deficiency causes *rickets* in children and infants. With rickets, bones are soft and pliable because they lack enough calcium and phosphorus to become strong. When this happens, several problems develop: bowlegs, knock knees, chest deformities, and curving of the spine. Deficiency may also occur in adults and is a condition known as *osteomalacia*. Adults at risk include those who have little exposure to the sun and low intakes of vitamin D, calcium, and phosphorus. Osteomalacia is seen most commonly in the Middle East and Asia. It is characterized by soft bones that break and/or bend easily, causing deformities of the spine.

New research over the past decade suggests that vitamin D may provide protection from osteoporosis, hypertension (high blood pressure), cancer, dementia, and several autoimmune diseases. Although further research is needed, vitamins D and E might help to protect against dementia and Parkinson's Disease. The Adequate Intake (AI) levels of vitamin D were established by the U.S. Institute of Medicine of the National Academy of Sciences: the Recommended Dietary Allowance (RDA) for vitamin D was established by the U.S. Institute of Medicine of the National Academy of Sciences. The RDA has been set at 600 IU (International Units) per day for all individuals (males, females, pregnant/lactating women, and children) from the age of 1 year up to the age of 70 years. For those over the age of 70, the RDA is 800 IU daily.

Vitamin D, when taken in excess from supplements, is the vitamin most likely to cause noticeable symptoms of toxicity. Symptoms include nausea, vomiting, diarrhea, fatigue, and thirst. Toxicity can lead to calcium deposits in the heart and kidneys, which can cause severe health problems. Megadoses of vitamin D in infants and young children can cause growth failure.

Vitamin E

Vitamin E has an important function in the body as an *antioxidant*. **Antioxidants** combine with the oxygen molecule so that it is not available to oxidize, or destroy, important substances. Vitamin E prevents the destruction of cells. Today, scientists suggest that antioxidants can slow down the normal aging process and provide important protections against cancer. Vitamins A (beta-carotene), E, and C are considered antioxidant vitamins. Vitamin E is also important for the health of the cell (especially the red blood cells), the proper functioning of the immune system, and the metabolism of vitamin A.

GLOSSARY

Antioxidants
Anti means against and oxidant means oxygen—An antioxidant prevents oxygen from destroying important substances

Vitamin E is widely distributed in plant foods. Rich sources include vegetable oils, margarine and shortening made from vegetable oils, and wheat germ. In oils, vitamin E acts like an antioxidant and thereby prevents the oil from going rancid or bad. Other good sources include whole grain cereals, green leafy vegetables, nuts, and seeds. Animal foods are poor sources, except for liver and egg yolk. Vitamin E deficiency is rare, as is toxicity.

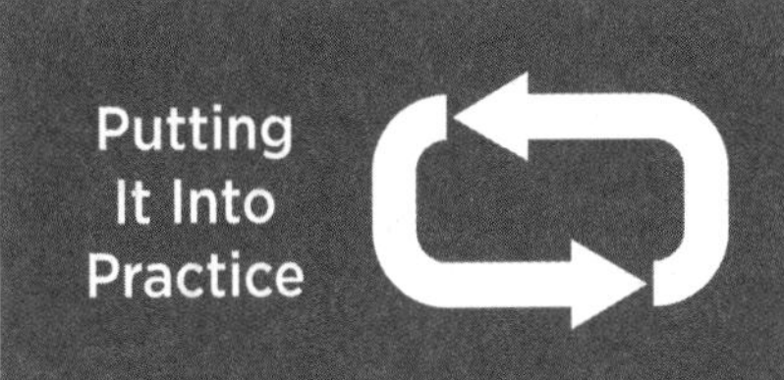

9. Your elderly neighbor has been told by his doctor he is at risk for vitamin D deficiency What, besides supplements, are some ways to get vitamin D?

Vitamin K

Vitamin K has an important role in the production of the proteins that are involved in blood clotting. When the skin is broken, blood clotting is vital to prevent excessive blood loss. Vitamin K is also involved in calcium metabolism. Vitamin K appears in certain foods and is also made in the body. There are billions of bacteria that normally live in the intestines and some of these produce vitamin K. It is thought that the amount of vitamin K produced by the bacteria is significant and may meet about half of the body's need; food sources of vitamin K are needed to provide the rest. Excellent sources of vitamin K include green leafy vegetables such as kale, spinach, and cabbage. Other sources include liver, milk, and eggs. A deficiency of vitamin K is rare in adults. An infant is normally given this vitamin after birth to prevent bleeding, because the intestines do not yet have the bacteria to produce vitamin K.

Water-Soluble Vitamins

The water-soluble vitamins include vitamin C and the B-complex vitamins. The B vitamins work in every cell of the body where they function as *coenzymes*. A coenzyme works with an enzyme to make it active. An enzyme boosts chemical reactions in the body to support all kinds of body functions. The body stores only limited amounts of water soluble vitamins; excesses are excreted in the urine. However, many water-soluble vitamins taken in excess through massive supplementation can cause toxic side effects.

Vitamin C

Vitamin C (also called ascorbic acid) is important in forming collagen, a protein that gives strength and support to bones, teeth, muscle, cartilage, blood vessels, and skin tissue. It has been said that vitamin C acts like cement or glue, holding together our cells and tissues. Vitamin C also helps absorb iron into the body and strengthens resistance to infection. Like vitamins A (beta-carotene) and E, vitamin C is an important antioxidant, preventing the oxidation of vitamin A and polyunsaturated fatty acids in the intestine. Because of its antioxidant properties, vitamin C has been widely used in foods as an additive to help preserve freshness. It may appear on the food label as sodium ascorbate, calcium ascorbate, or simply ascorbic acid.

Foods rich in vitamin C include fruits (e.g. oranges, grapefruits, limes, lemons, as well as cantaloupe, strawberries, and tomatoes). Other good food sources include white potatoes, sweet potatoes, broccoli and other green and yellow vegetables, as well as cantaloupe and strawberries (See Figure 2.13). There is little or no vitamin C in meats or dairy foods. Some juices are fortified with vitamin C, as are most ready-to-eat cereals. Certain situations raise the body's need for vitamin C. These include pregnancy and nursing, growth, fevers, infections, burns, fractures, surgery, cancer, heavy alcohol intake, and cigarette smoking. Megadoses of supplemental vitamin C often cause nausea, abdominal cramps, and diarrhea; it can also interfere with clotting medications (such as warfarin and dicoumarol); and it can cause incorrect urine test results for diabetes. A deficiency of vitamin C can cause a disease called scurvy. Symptoms of

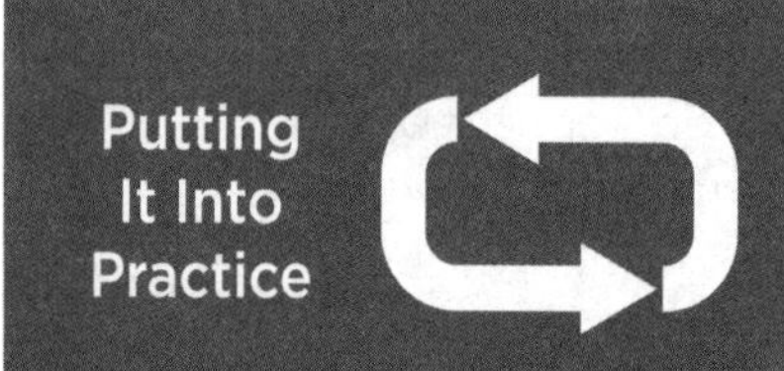

10. You overhear a new cook commenting to one of the more experienced trayline cooks about how his broccoli always looks so much more vibrantly green than what she cooks at home. He proudly mentions his secret, which is to sprinkle a little baking soda in the cooking water. Why might this be a problem?

Figure 2.13
Vitamin C in Foods

FOOD	PORTION	VITAMIN C (in mg)
Fruits		
Orange	1 medium	80
Kiwi	1 medium	75
Cranberry Juice Cocktail	3/4 cup	67
Orange Juice, from concentrate	1/2 cup	48
Papaya	1/2 cup cubes	43
Strawberries	1/2 cup	42
Grapefruit	1/2 each	41
Grapefruit Juice, canned	1/2 cup	36
Cantaloupe	1/2 cup cubes	34
Tangerine	1 medium	26
Mango	1/2 cup slices	23
Honeydew Melon	1/2 cup cubes	21
Banana	1 medium	10
Apple	1 medium	8
Nectarine	1 medium	7
Vegetables		
Broccoli, chopped, cooked	1/2 cup	49
Brussels Sprouts, cooked	1/2 cup	48
Cauliflower, cooked	1/2 cup	34
Sweet Potato, baked	1 small	28
Kale, cooked, chopped	1/2 cup	27
White Potato, baked	1 medium	26
Tomato, fresh	1 medium	22
Tomato Juice	1/2 cup	22
Cereals		
Corn Flakes (Fortified)	1 cup	15

Source: U.S. Department of Agriculture

scurvy include bleeding gums, weakness, growth failure, delayed wound healing, easy bruising, and iron-deficiency anemia. Many of these symptoms are due to the faulty formation of collagen.

Thiamin (B1), Riboflavin (B2), and Niacin (B3)

Thiamin (B1), riboflavin (B2), and niacin (B3) all play key roles as *coenzymes* in energy metabolism. Coenzymes are chemical compounds that help *enzymes* work. Enzymes are specialized proteins that speed up specific chemical reactions in the body. Vitamins B1, B2, and B3 help to release energy from glucose, fatty acids, and amino acids. B1 also plays a vital role in the normal functioning of the nervous system and appetite; B2 is important for healthy skin and normal functioning of the eyes; and B3 is needed for the maintenance of healthy skin and the normal functioning of the nervous system and digestive tract.

B1 is widely distributed in foods. Pork is an excellent source of this nutrient; other sources include liver, dry beans and peas, peanuts, peanut butter, seeds and whole grains, and enriched breads and cereals.

Milk is a major source of B2, as are yogurt and cheese. Other sources include organ meats like liver (very high), whole grain and enriched breads and cereals, and some meats.

The main sources of B3 are meat, including organ meats, poultry, and fish. Whole grains and enriched breads and cereals also supply vitamin B3. All foods containing complete proteins, including milk and eggs, are good sources of *tryptophan*, which is the precursor of vitamin B3.

Though vitamin B deficiencies are rare, they can occur with chronically reduced dietary intake. For example, B1 deficiency is linked to a disease called *beriberi*, which is characterized by poor appetite, depression, confusion, weakness, muscle wasting, heart problems, and deterioration of the nervous system. Most deficiencies of B vitamins include more than just one vitamin, so it is not surprising to find a B2 deficiency along with B1. Signs of a B2 deficiency include cracks at the corner of the mouth, skin rash, poor healing, burning and itching eyes. B3 deficiency first appears as fatigue, poor appetite, indigestion, and a skin rash. A chronic B3 deficiency can lead to a disease known as *pellagra*. Symptoms include diarrhea, *dermatitis* (skin inflammation), dementia, and ultimately death.

Toxicity is not a problem with these vitamins, except for megadoses of B3. Typical symptoms include flushing, rashes, tingling, itching, hives, nausea, diarrhea, and abdominal discomfort. More serious side effects of large doses include liver malfunction, high blood sugar levels, and abnormal heart rhythm. Whole grains and enriched breads and cereals supply the majority of the starch in many diets today. It is important to understand that grains are an excellent source of vitamins, but processing results in both vitamin and mineral losses. Processing removes the germ and the bran from the grain, taking with it many vitamins and minerals that are not replaced through enrichment or fortification (See Figure 2.14).

Pyridoxine (B6)

Vitamin B6 plays an important role as part of a coenzyme involved in carbohydrate, fat, and protein metabolism. It is particularly important in protein metabolism. Vitamin B6 is also used to make red blood cells, which transport oxygen around the body. And it helps convert the amino acid tryptophan to niacin (B3).

Figure 2.14
Processing Effects on Grain

Vitamins & Minerals Lost During Processing		
Thiamin (B1)	Pantothenic Acid (B5)	Copper
Riboflavin (B2)	Vitamin E	Calcium
Niacin (B3)	Fiber	Zinc
Pyridoxine (B6)	Iron	Manganese
Folate (B9)	Magnesium	Potassium

Vitamins & Minerals Replaced with Enrichment	
Thiamin (B1)	Niacin (B3)
Riboflavin (B2)	Iron

Good sources of vitamin B6 include organ meats, meat, poultry, and fish. Vitamin B6 also appears in plant foods, though it is not as well absorbed from these sources. Plant sources include whole grains, potatoes, some fruits (such as bananas and cantaloupe), and some green leafy vegetables (such as broccoli and spinach). Fortified ready-to-eat cereals are also good sources of B6. A chronic deficiency of B6 can lead to muscle twitching, rashes, greasy skin, and *microcytic* (small cell) anemia. Excessive intake (i.e. more than two grams daily for two months or more) of supplemental B6 can lead to irreversible nerve damage and symptoms such as numbness in hands and feet and difficulty walking.

Folate (B9)

Folate is part of a coenzyme used to make new cells, including red blood cells, white blood cells, and digestive tract cells. Folate occurs naturally in a variety of foods, including liver, dark-green leafy vegetables such as collards, turnip greens and Romaine lettuce, broccoli and asparagus, citrus fruits and juices, whole grain products, wheat germ, and dried beans and peas, such as pinto, navy, and lima beans, and chickpeas and black-eyed peas. Folic acid is the synthetic form of folate, which is used in fortified foods and supplements. By law, many grain products are fortified with folic acid.

A deficiency of folate can lead to *megaloblastic anemia*, a condition in which the red blood cells are oversized and function poorly. Other deficiency symptoms may include digestive tract problems (e.g. diarrhea) and depression. During pregnancy, the need for folate increases because of its vital role in producing new cells. Folate is needed both before and during pregnancy to help reduce the risk of certain serious and common birth defects called neural tube defects, which affect the brain and spinal cord. The tricky part is that neural tube defects can occur in an embryo before a woman realizes she's pregnant.

Cobalamin (B12)

Vitamin B12, also called cobalamin and cyanocobalamin, is present in all body cells. Along with folate, vitamin B12 is involved in making new cells in the body and in the growth of healthy red blood cells. It also helps in the normal functioning of the nervous system by maintaining the protective cover around nerve fibers. Vitamin B12 is found only in animal products such as meat, poultry, fish, shellfish, eggs, milk, and milk products. Plant foods do not contain any B12. *Vegans*, vegetarians who do not consume any animal products, must include fortified foods, such as soy milk, or take supplements of B12, in order to meet this nutrient need.

In order to be absorbed, vitamin B12 requires a compound called *intrinsic factor* (IF), which is produced in the stomach. B12 deficiencies can be because of poor intake or poor absorption. A condition known as pernicious (macrocytic, megaloblastic) anemia can develop if there is a problem with the IF.

B12 deficiency can cause poor cell division, which leads to abnormally large cells (megaloblastic) and the condition of pernicious anemia. Pernicious anemia is also characterized by deterioration in the functioning of the nervous system that, if untreated, could cause significant and sometimes irreversible damage. Vitamin B12 toxicity rarely if ever occurs.

Pantothenic Acid (B5) and Biotin (B7)

Both pantothenic acid and biotin are involved in energy metabolism. Pantothenic acid is part of a coenzyme used in energy metabolism; biotin is part of a coenzyme used in energy metabolism, amino acid metabolism, fat synthesis, and glycogen synthesis. Both pantothenic acid and biotin are widespread in foods and deficiency is rare. There is no known toxicity of either pantothenic acid or biotin.

Vitamins and Food Preparation

Food preparation and storage techniques affect the vitamin content of food. Using too much water, too high a temperature, or too long a cooking time for vegetables significantly reduces the content of vitamins B and C. Too much acidity or base can also affect the nutrient content of fruits and vegetables. For example, some chefs use baking soda (a base) to enhance the green color of vegetables. This process significantly reduces the vitamin content of vegetables. To help decrease the loss of vitamins in vegetables, use *batch* cooking (cooking small amounts of vegetables) immediately prior to service. For dairy products, vitamin loss can be diminished during storage by keeping products at a constant, cold temperature and out of the light. Thawing and refreezing causes nutrient loss as well as loss of quality. Figure 2.15 summarizes the functions and food sources of vitamins.

SECTION C MACRO MINERALS

If one were to weigh all the minerals in the body, they would only amount to four or five pounds. The human body needs only small amounts of minerals in the diet, but they perform enormously important jobs—such as building bones and teeth, regulating heartbeat, and transporting oxygen from the lungs to tissues.

Some minerals are needed in relatively large amounts (macro or major minerals) in the diet—over 100 milligrams daily. (A paper clip weighs about 1 gram. A milligram is 1/1000 of a gram.) **Macro minerals** include calcium, chloride, magnesium, phosphorus, potassium, sodium, and sulfur. Other minerals, called **trace minerals** or trace elements, are needed in smaller amounts—less than 100 milligrams daily. Iron, fluoride, and zinc are examples of trace minerals. Figure 2.16 lists macro and trace minerals.

Minerals have some distinctive properties not shared by other nutrients. For example, whereas over 90 percent of the carbohydrate, fat, and protein in the diet is absorbed into the body, the percentage of minerals absorbed varies tremendously. Here are some

GLOSSARY

Macro or Major Minerals
Calcium, chloride, magnesium, phosphorous, potassium, sodium, and sulfur

Trace Minerals
Minerals needed in less than 100 mg a day

Figure 2.15
Vitamins—Functions and Food Sources

VITAMIN	FUNCTIONS	FOOD SOURCE
Vitamin A	Forming skin, hair, teeth, protective linings; immune function	Orange/yellow vegetables and fruits, dark green vegetables, dairy products
Vitamin D	Aids absorption of calcium and phosphorous; bone health; used in hormones	Fortified milk, liver, egg yolks, fish liver oil
Vitamin E	Antioxidant; protects red and white blood cells	Vegetable oils, margarine, shortening, seeds, nuts, wheat germ, whole grain and fortified breads and cereals, soybeans
Vitamin K	Blood clotting; makes protein used in making bones	Dark green leafy vegetables, cabbage
Vitamin C	Antioxidant; formation of collagen; wound healing; iron absorption; functioning of immune system	Citrus fruits, bell peppers, kiwifruit, broccoli, strawberries, tomatoes, potatoes, juices and cereals fortified with vitamin C
Thiamin (B1)	Coenzyme in energy metabolism; functioning of nervous system; normal growth	Pork, sunflower seeds, wheat germ, peanuts, dry beans, whole grain and enriched/fortified breads and cereals
Riboflavin (B2)	Coenzyme in energy metabolism; healthy skin; normal vision	Milk and milk products, whole grain and enriched/fortified breads and cereals, some meats, eggs
Niacin (B3)	Coenzyme in energy metabolism; healthy skin; normal functioning of nervous system	Meat, poultry, fish, whole grain and enriched/fortified breads and cereals, eggs
Pyridoxine (B6)	Coenzyme in carbohydrate, fat and protein metabolism; synthesis of blood cells	Meat, poultry, fish, fortified cereals, some leafy green vegetables, potatoes, bananas, watermelon
Folate (B9)	Formation of new cells	Green leafy vegetables, legumes, orange juice, enriched/fortified breads and cereals
Cobalamin (B12)	Activation of folate; normal functioning of the nervous system	Meat, poultry, seafood, eggs, dairy products, fortified breads and cereals
Pantothenic Acid (B5)	Energy metabolism	Widespread
Biotin (B7)	Energy metabolism; carbohydrate, fat and protein metabolism	Widespread

examples: only 5-10 percent of dietary iron is normally absorbed; about 30 percent of calcium is absorbed; yet almost all of dietary sodium is absorbed. Unlike some vitamins, minerals are not easily destroyed in storage or preparation. Like vitamins from dietary supplements, minerals from dietary supplements can be toxic when consumed in excessive amounts.

Figure 2.16
Minerals At-A-Glance

MACRO MINERALS			
Body contains approximately five teaspoons or 25 grams			
Calcium	Magnesium	Potassium	Sulfur
Chloride	Phosphorus	Sodium	
TRACE MINERALS			
Body contains less than 1/2 teaspoon or 3 grams			
Iron	Copper	Iodine	Zinc
Manganese	Fluoride	Selenium	

Calcium

Calcium, along with phosphorus, is used for building bones and teeth and are the most abundant minerals in the body. They give rigidity to the structures. Bone is being constantly rebuilt, with new bone being formed and old bone being taken apart, every day.

Calcium also circulates in the blood and appears in other body tissues, where it helps blood clot, muscles (including the heart muscle) contract, and nerves transmit impulses. Calcium also helps maintain normal blood pressure and immune defenses.

The major sources of calcium are milk and other dairy products. Not all dairy products are as rich in calcium as milk (see Figure 2.17). As a matter of fact, butter, cream, and cream cheese contain very little calcium. Other good sources of calcium include canned salmon and sardines (containing bones), oysters, calcium-fortified foods such as orange juice, and greens such as broccoli, collards, kale, and mustard and turnip greens. Other greens such as spinach, beet greens, Swiss chard, sorrel, and parsley are rich in calcium but also contain a binder (called oxalic acid) that prevents much of the calcium from being absorbed. Dried beans and peas and certain shellfish contain moderate amounts of calcium, but are usually not eaten in sufficient quantities to make a significant contribution. Meats and grains are poor sources.

Ordinarily, only about 30 percent of the calcium that is eaten is absorbed. However, the body is able to increase calcium absorption (up to 60 percent) during times when it is needed, such as during growth and pregnancy, and also when there is inadequate calcium in the diet. When there isn't enough calcium in the diet, calcium can be removed from the bones. However, one problem with relying on this process is that, over time, this will weaken the bone structure and increase the risk of developing a disease called osteoporosis, or bone loss. Many calcium supplements provide mixtures of calcium with other compounds, such as calcium carbonate. Research has also shown increased absorption when taken with vitamin D. Calcium supplements should not be taken without guidance from a physician or Registered Dietitian Nutritionist (RDN).

Phosphorus

Phosphorus is involved in the release of energy from fats, proteins, and carbohydrates during metabolism and in the formation of genetic material and many enzymes. Phosphorus also helps in the absorption and transport of fats, and assists in keeping blood chemistry neutral. Phosphorus has the ability to buffer or neutralize both acids and bases.

Phosphorus is widely distributed in foods and is not likely to be lacking in the diet. Milk and dairy products are excellent sources. Additional sources of phosphorus include meat, poultry, fish, eggs, legumes, and whole grain foods. Fruits and vegetables are generally low in this mineral.

Sodium

Sodium is a critical mineral that helps the body maintain water balance and acid-base balance. It also plays an important role in helping contract muscles and transmit nerve impulses. Meat, poultry, fish, eggs, and milk are high in natural sodium when compared to fruits and vegetables, but are still quite low compared to processed foods.

Deficiency of sodium is not a problem in the United States. The estimated minimum requirement is 500 mg per day, however an intake of ≤1500 mg per day is adequate. This may also be compared to the Tolerable Upper Limit of 2300 mg for those ≤14 years of age. The sodium intake of Americans is easily six times this amount—varying from 3000 mg to 8000 mg daily, much of it coming from processed foods. Overconsumption of sodium increases the risk of developing chronic diseases such as high blood pressure and cardiovascular disease.

Potassium

Potassium (one of three **electrolytes**, along with sodium and chloride) is found mainly inside the body's cells. All three electrolytes conduct electricity within the body. Potassium is also needed to release energy from carbohydrates, fats, and proteins. In the blood, potassium assists in muscle contraction, helps maintain a normal heartbeat, and helps send nerve impulses. Along with sodium and chloride, potassium helps maintain water balance and acid-base balance.

Potassium is distributed widely in foods, both plant and animal. Unprocessed, whole foods such as fruits and vegetables, as well as milk, grains, meat, poultry, fish, and legumes, are the best sources of potassium.

A potassium deficiency is very uncommon in healthy people, but may result from dehydration or from using a certain class of blood pressure medications called **diuretics**. Diuretics cause increased urine output. In addition, some diuretics cause an increased excretion of potassium. Symptoms of a deficiency include weakness, nausea, and abnormal heart rhythms that can be very dangerous, even fatal.

GLOSSARY

Electrolytes
Substances that produce an electrically conducting solution when dissolved in a polar solvent

Diuretic
A chemical that causes the body to increase urine output

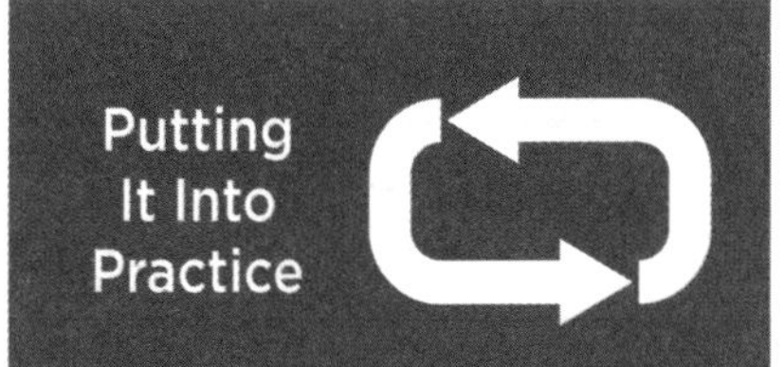

11. A client tells you she is lactose intolerant; because she can't have dairy foods, she asks if she should take a calcium supplement. What are some food sources of calcium besides dairy?

Figure 2.17
Calcium in Selected Foods

FOOD	PORTION	CALCIUM CONTENT (mg)
Milk		
Skim	8 ounces	302
2%	8 ounces	297
Whole	8 ounces	291
Cheese		
Cottage Cheese, creamed	1 cup	147
Swiss	1 ounce	272
Parmesan	1 ounce	390
Cheddar	1 ounce	204
Mozzarella	1 ounce	183
American	1 ounce	174
Yogurt		
Low-Fat	1 cup	415
Low-Fat with Fruit	1 cup	345
Frozen	1 cup	200
Fish		
Sardines with Bones	3 ounces	372
Oysters	1 cup	226
Shrimp	3 ounces	98
Vegetables		
Turnip Greens, frozen and cooked	1 cup	249
Kale, frozen and cooked	1 cup	179
Mustard Greens	1 cup	104
Broccoli, frozen and cooked	1 cup	94
Miscellaneous		
Ice Cream	1 cup	176
Cheese Pizza	1/4 of 14" pie	332
Macaroni and Cheese	1/2 cup	181
Orange Juice, calcium-fortified	8 ounces	300
Tofu	3-1/2 ounces	128
Dried Navy Beans, cooked	1 cup	95

Source: U.S. Department of Agriculture

Excessive potassium is equally dangerous and megadoses of it can cause numbness, abnormal heart rhythms and cardiac failure, in which the heart stops beating. It is not recommended to take potassium supplements without the advice of a physician.

Chloride

Chloride is another important electrolyte in the body. It helps maintain water balance and acid-base balance. Chloride is also part of hydrochloric acid, found in high concentration in the juices of the stomach. Hydrochloric acid aids in protein digestion. The most important source of chloride in the diet is sodium chloride (NaCl), or table salt. If dietary sodium intake is adequate, there will be ample chloride as well.

Magnesium

Magnesium is found in all body tissues, with about 50-60 percent being in the bones and the remainder in the muscles and other soft tissues. It is an essential part of many enzyme systems responsible for energy conversions in the body. Magnesium is used in building bones and teeth and works with calcium, potassium, and sodium to contract muscles and transmit nerve impulses. Magnesium also has a role in making fatty acids and protein.

Magnesium is a part of the green pigment called chlorophyll that is found in plants. Good sources include dark green leafy vegetables, nuts (especially almonds and cashews), seeds, whole grain cereals, and legumes such as soybeans. Deficiency and subsequent symptoms are rare.

Sulfur

Sulfur is found in three of the amino acids (cysteine, homocysteine, and methionine).

The protein in hair, skin, and nails is particularly rich in sulfur. Sulfur is also a part of two vitamins, thiamin and biotin. High protein foods supply adequate amounts of sulfur. A deficiency is not known to occur.

SECTION D TRACE MINERALS

Most of the trace minerals do not occur in the body in their free form, but are bound to organic compounds on which they depend for transport, storage, and function. The true understanding of many trace minerals is just starting to emerge.

Fluoride

Fluoride is the term used for the form of fluorine as it appears in drinking water and in the body. The terms fluoride and fluorine are used interchangeably. Fluoride contributes to solid tooth formation and results in a decrease of dental caries (cavities), especially in children. Although fluoride is not an essential element, there is also evidence that fluoride helps retain calcium in the bones of older people.

The major source of fluoride is drinking water. Some supplies of drinking water are naturally fluoridated; many have fluoride added, usually at a concentration of one part fluoride to one million parts water. In nearly all areas where **fluoridation** of water has been introduced, the incidence of dental caries in children has been reduced by at least 50 percent. In areas where there is too much natural fluoride in the water, teeth become discolored (mottled), but there are no undesirable health effects.

GLOSSARY

Fluoridation
The addition of fluoride to municipal water systems

Iodine

Iodine is required in extremely small amounts for the normal functioning of the thyroid gland. The thyroid gland is located in the neck and is responsible for producing important hormones that maintain a normal level of metabolism in the body. These hormones are essential for normal growth and development.

With a deficiency of dietary iodine, thyroid enlargement (called goiter) occurs. Iodine deficiency goiter used to be common in areas of the U.S. where the soil contains little iodine. Iodized salt was introduced in 1924 to combat iodine deficiencies.

Iron

Iron is an important part of compounds necessary for transporting oxygen to the cells and making use of the oxygen when it arrives. It is widely distributed in the body, where much of it is in the blood as the heme portion of hemoglobin. Hemoglobin is the oxygen carrier found in red blood cells. Iron is also part of the protein myoglobin in muscles, which makes oxygen available for muscle contraction. Iron works with many enzymes in energy metabolism.

Liver is an excellent source of iron. Other sources are meats, egg yolks, seafood, green leafy vegetables, legumes, dried fruits, and whole grain and enriched breads and cereals. The ability of the body to absorb and utilize iron from different foods varies from 3 percent for some vegetables to up to 30 percent for red meat. The iron in animal foods such as meat, poultry, and fish is absorbed and utilized more readily than iron in plant foods. The presence of these animal products in a meal increases the availability of iron from plant sources (non-heme iron), as well. The presence of vitamin C in a meal also increases iron absorption. Some foods actually decrease iron consumption: coffee, tea, calcium supplements, wheat bran, and other forms of fiber. The body adjusts its own iron absorption according to need.

Iron deficiency, which may be a result of inadequate dietary intake or from blood loss, can lead to **iron deficiency anemia**, a condition in which the size and number of red blood cells are reduced. Symptoms of iron deficiency anemia include fatigue, pallor, irritability, and lethargy. Iron deficiency anemia is a real concern in the U.S., more so for women than men. Iron requirements are higher for women of childbearing age than for men, because women have to replace menstrual blood losses.

GLOSSARY

Iron Deficiency Anemia
A condition resulting from insufficient dietary iron intake or blood loss

Selenium

It was not known that selenium was an essential mineral until 1979. Selenium is part of an enzyme that acts like an antioxidant and prevents oxidative damage to tissues, much like vitamins A, C, and E. Major food sources include Brazil nuts, seafood, meat, and liver. Because selenium is sometimes found in the soil, whole grains may be a good source of selenium as well, depending on where they are grown. Deficiency and toxicity in the U.S. are rare.

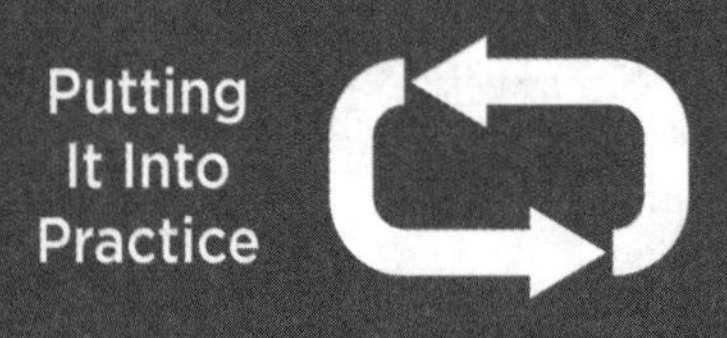

12. For clients who have an iron deficiency, what are two dietary practices that would improve iron absorption?

Zinc

Zinc is involved in enzymes that promote at least 50 metabolically important reactions in the body. Zinc assists in wound healing, bone formation, development of sexual organs, and general growth and maintenance of all tissues. Zinc is also important for taste perception and appetite.

Protein-containing foods are all good sources of zinc, particularly meat, shellfish, eggs, and milk. Whole grains and some legumes are good sources as well, but zinc is much more readily available in animal foods. In general, iron and zinc are both found in the same foods.

Children, pregnant and premenopausal women, and the elderly are most at risk for being deficient in zinc. Children who are deficient in zinc typically have poor growth and little appetite. Other symptoms of zinc deficiency include diarrhea, impaired immune response, slowed metabolism, loss of taste and smell, confusion, and poor wound healing. Though zinc toxicity is rare, excess supplemental intake can interfere with copper metabolism and can cause other serious problems.

Other Trace Minerals

Chromium participates in carbohydrate, protein, and fat metabolism. Chromium works with insulin to get glucose into the body's cells. Good sources of chromium are liver, meat, the dark meat of poultry, whole grains, and brewer's yeast. A chromium deficiency results in a condition much like diabetes, in which the glucose level in the blood is abnormally high.

Cobalt is a part of vitamin B12 and is, therefore, needed to form red blood cells. We take in the cobalt we need by eating vitamin B12-rich foods. (Remember that vitamin B12 is found only in animal foods.)

Copper is necessary along with iron for the formation of hemoglobin. As a part of many enzymes, it also helps make the protein collagen, assists in wound healing, and keeps nerves healthy. Good sources of copper include organ meats, meats, shellfish, whole grain cereals, nuts, and legumes. Copper deficiency is generally rare, except in cases of malnutrition or malabsorption diseases; excessive supplemental copper intake can be toxic.

Manganese is needed for blood formation and bone structure, and as part of many enzymes involved in energy metabolism. Manganese is found in many foods, especially whole grains, legumes, nuts and seeds, and green leafy vegetables. A deficiency is unknown.

Molybdenum is a cofactor in a number of enzyme systems and is possibly involved in the metabolism of fats. Deficiency does not seem to be a problem.

As time goes on, more trace minerals will probably be recognized as essential to human health. There are currently several trace minerals that are essential to animals and are likely to be essential to humans, as well. They include arsenic, nickel, silicon, and boron. Figures 2.18 and 2.19 summarize this section on minerals.

Figure 2.18
Macro Minerals—Function and Food Sources

MINERAL	FUNCTION	FOOD SOURCES
Calcium	• Mineralization of bones and teeth • Blood clotting muscle contractions • Transmission of nerve impulses	• Milk and milk products • Calcium-set to calcium-fortified foods • Collards, kale, mustard greens, turnip greens • Legumes • Whole wheat bread
Phosphorus	• Mineralization of bones and teeth • Energy metabolism • Formation of DNA and many enzymes • Buffer	• Milk and milk products • Meat and poultry • Eggs • Legumes
Magnesium	• Energy metabolism • Formation of bones and maintenance of teeth • Muscle contraction and nerve transmission • Immune system	• Green leafy vegetables • Potatoes • Nuts and legumes • Whole grain cereals
Sodium	• Water balance • Acid-base balance • Buffer, muscle contraction • Transmission of nerve impulses	• Salt • Processed foods • MSG
Potassium	• Water balance • Acid-base balance • Buffer, muscle contraction • Transmission of nerve impulses	• Many fruits and vegetables (oranges, grapefruit, potatoes) • Milk and yogurt • Legumes • Meats
Chloride	• Water balance • Acid-base balance • Part of hydrochloric acid in stomach	• Salt
Sulfur	• Part of some amino acids • Part of thiamin	• Protein foods

Figure 2.19
Trace Minerals—Function and Food Sources

MINERAL	FUNCTION	FOOD SOURCES
Copper	• Iron metabolism • Formation of hemoglobin • Collagen formation • Energy release	• Seafood • Whole-grain breads and cereal • Legumes, nuts, and seeds
Fluoride	• Strengthening of developing teeth	• Water (naturally or artificially fluoridated) • Tea • Seafood
Iodine	• Normal functioning of thyroid gland • Normal metabolic rate • Normal growth and development	• Iodized salt • Salt-water fish
Iron	• Part of hemoglobin and myoglobin • Part of some enzymes • Energy metabolism • Needed to make amino acids	• Red meats • Shellfish • Legumes • Whole-grain and enriched breads and cereals • Green leafy vegetables
Selenium	• Activation of antioxidant	• Seafood • Meat and liver • Eggs • Whole grains • Vegetables (if soil is rich in selenium)
Zinc	• Co-factor of many enzymes • Wound healing • DNA and protein synthesis • Bone formation • Development of sexual organs • General growth and maintenance • Taste perception and appetite	• Protein foods • Legumes • Dairy products • Whole-grain products • Fortified cereals

SECTION E WATER

Nothing survives without water and virtually nothing takes place in the body without water playing a vital role. While variations may be great, the average adult's body weight is generally 50 to 60 percent water—enough, if it were bottled, to fill 40 to 50 quarts. For example, in a 150-pound man, water accounts for about 90 pounds; fat about 30 pounds; with proteins, carbohydrates, vitamins, and minerals making up the balance. Men generally have a higher percentage of water than women. Some parts of the body have more water than others. Human blood is about 92 percent water; muscle and the brain are about 75 percent; and bone is about 22 percent.

The body uses water for virtually all its functions: digestion, absorption, circulation, excretion, transporting nutrients, building tissue, and maintaining temperature. Almost all of the body's cells depend on water to perform their functions; water carries nutrients to the cells and carries away waste materials to the kidneys; water is needed in each step of the process of converting food into energy and tissue; digestive secretions are mostly water, acting as a solvent for nutrients; water in the digestive secretions softens, dilutes, and liquefies the food to facilitate digestion; water also helps move food along the gastrointestinal tract.

Additionally, water serves as an important part of lubricants, helping to cushion the joints and internal organs, keeping body tissues, such as the eyes, lungs, and air passages moist, and surrounding and protecting the fetus during pregnancy.

The body gets rid of the water it doesn't need through the kidneys (as urine) and skin (as perspiration) and, to a lesser degree, from the lungs and gastrointestinal tract. The largest amount of excess water, between 2-8 cups, is excreted as urine by the kidneys. The amount of urine reflects, to some extent, the amount of fluid intake of the individual, although no matter how little water one consumes, the kidneys will always excrete a certain amount each day to eliminate waste products generated by the body's metabolic actions. See Figure 2.20 for food sources of water. See Figure 2.21 for factors that upset water balance. Calculating fluid needs will be discussed as part of Nutrition Screening, found in Chapter 7.

Figure 2.20
Food Sources of Water

FOOD SOURCES	%
Coffee and tea (brewed)	100
Clear broth; boiled vegetables such as celery, cabbage, cauliflower, and broccoli; cucumber slices; iceberg lettuce; pumpkin; beer	95-99
Cider, cola drinks, lemonade, canned juice, skim milk, most broth-based soups, green peppers	90-94
Whole milk, wines, spaghetti canned in tomato sauce, boiled potatoes, canned grapefruit, fresh orange juice, strawberries, low-fat yogurt, eggplant, mango, cooked spinach, peas, stewed apples	80-89
Milkshake, yogurt, mashed potato, baked beans, sweet potato, cooked oatmeal, rice, poached fish, peaches, banana, boiled egg, cottage cheese	70-79
Pizza, fried and scrambled egg, tuna in oil, stewed prunes, roast beef and poultry, cheese spread, cream	50-69
Pork, lunch meat, cheddar cheese, processed cheese, hazelnuts	30-49
Most other nuts, salad dressings, honey syrup	10-29
Peanut butter, candy and sugar, oils, potato chips	< 10

Figure 2.21
Factors that Upset Water Balance

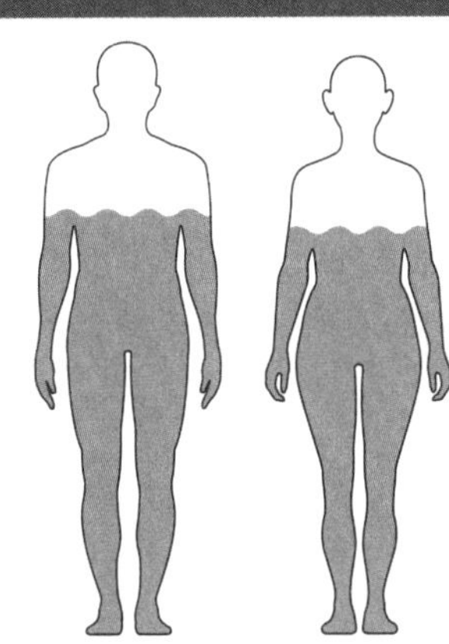

- Surgery
- Physical activity
- Illness with prolonged vomiting, diarrhea, or fever
- Amount of alcohol consumed
- Diuretic consumption
- Pregnancy or breastfeeding
- Hot weather or hot environments
- Increased intake of fiber, salt, protein, or sugar

SECTION F NUTRIENT DENSITY

Foods vary in how rich they are in nutrients. Foods that are nutrient-rich relative to their calorie (energy) content are said to be high in **nutrient density**. For example, one cup of broccoli has 25 calories and proportionally high levels of vitamins and minerals. Thus, it has a high nutrient density. In contrast, one cup of cola has 100 calories and no vitamins, thus low nutrient density. Think of these calories as a "price" paid for the lack of vitamins, minerals, and other essential nutrients. If a high calorie price was "paid" for a food that has little or no nutrients when eaten, that food is not nutrient-dense. Sometimes people use the term **empty calories** to describe a food that has low nutrient density. See the sample in Figure 2.22. In the "price" analogy, if you pay a low price (caloric intake) and receive many nutrients, the food you are consuming is nutrient-dense. Sound dietary habits rely on nutrient-dense foods for many of the daily food choices.

GLOSSARY

Nutrient Density
Foods that have many nutrients relative to their calorie or energy content

Empty Calories
Foods that are not nutrient-dense and may contain many calories

Figure 2.22
Example of Empty Calories

Homemade Cupcake with Icing

Information per Serving:
Serving Size = 1 Cupcake

Calories	170
Total Fat	5 grams
Sodium	110 milligrams
Carbohydrates	30 grams
Protein	2 grams
Vitamin A	*
Vitamin C	*
Calcium	*
Iron	*

There is a high calorie price for very little of the essential nutrients, Vitamins A and C, and minerals calcium and iron, with this cupcake.

Yogurt Parfait with Fruit and Granola

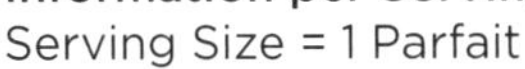

Information per Serving:
Serving Size = 1 Parfait

Calories	162
Total Fat	2 grams
Sodium	78 milligrams
Carbohydrates	31 grams
Protein	6 grams
Vitamin A	46 IU
Vitamin C	1.5 milligrams
Calcium	210 milligrams
Iron	75 milligrams

The yogurt parfait is a better dessert option, as it is lower in fat and sodium. It contains more protein, vitamins, and minerals while providing fewer calories.

Chapter References

RESOURCES	
Association of Nutrition & Foodservice Professionals	www.ANFPonline.org
U.S. Department of Agriculture. Food and Nutrition Information Center. National Agricultural Library*	https://www.nal.usda.gov/fnic
U.S. Department of Agriculture. Scientific Report of the 2015 Dietary Guidelines Advisory Committee. Published February, 2015*	https://health.gov/dietaryguidelines/2015-scientific-report/pdfs/scientific-report-of-the-2015-dietary-guidelines-advisory-committee.pdf
U.S. Department of Agriculture. What We Eat in America. Agricultural Research Service. Updated August 15, 2019.*	https://www.ars.usda.gov/northeast-area/beltsville-md-bhnrc/beltsville-human-nutrition-research-center/food-surveys-research-group/docs/wweia-usual-intake-data-tables/
U.S. Department of Health & Human Services. History of Dietary Guidelines for Americans. Dietary Guidelines for Americans*	https://health.gov/dietaryguidelines/history.htm

**Accessed September 18, 2019*

Digestion, Absorption, and Utilization of Nutrients

Overview and Objectives

An understanding of how digestion occurs helps a Certified Dietary Manager®, Certified Food Protection Professional® (CDM®, CFPP®) plan and modify menus for individuals who have unique nutrition needs. After completing this chapter, you should be able to:

- Follow the path of digestion
- Relate digestion to nutrition
- Describe the organs involved in digestion
- Differentiate between digestion of protein, fat, and types of carbohydrate
- Discuss absorption and its relationship to other body systems
- Explain the concepts of absorption and availability of nutrients

The body is made up of many complex systems that work together to make a whole person. The word *system* describes groups of organs working together to perform functions. Systems are made up of organs. Organs are made up of body tissues. In turn, tissues are made up of cells. Cells are the basic unit of life and the building blocks of the human body. Each cell has a membrane that surrounds and protects it. Most cells also have a nucleus, which directs the work going on in the cell. The body contains many types of cells: nerve, bone, muscle, and fat. Each type of cell has a unique structure related to what it does in the body.

Tissues are groups of similar cells that work together to perform a certain function. For example, epithelial tissue lines many body surfaces and one of its functions is to protect the body. Organs are made of several kinds of tissue. Examples of body organs include the liver, stomach, intestines, gallbladder, kidney, brain, and heart. Even skin is considered an organ. Organs work together as part of body systems. Systems include:

- The digestive system, which digests food
- The circulatory system, which circulates blood and lymph (a body fluid)
- The musculoskeletal system, essential for body movement
- The nervous and endocrine (hormone) systems, which control body functions
- The respiratory system, responsible for breathing
- The immune system, which protects against illness and infection
- The reproductive system, responsible for new life
- The urinary system, which excretes waste (urine)

How the Digestive System Works

Ever wondered how food that is eaten becomes the nutrients needed for the body to function? What controls what happens to the food? The human body controls what is eaten. The brain and hormones alert and cue hunger and eating. The brain and hormones also guide the digestive system after food has been eaten.

Digestion occurs through the digestive system. The digestive system is made up of organs and a long, looped tube from the mouth to the anus (about 30 feet long when stretched out; however, this may vary widely—see Figure 3.1). The digestive system feeds the rest of the body, which is why it is so important that foods are chosen wisely. When food is eaten, it goes through three different processes: digestion, absorption, and metabolism. **Digestion** is the process of breaking food into smaller components, in some cases, converting those components into nutrients and eliminating solid wastes. That long, looped tube is known as the **gastrointestinal tract (GI tract)**. It starts in the mouth, which is connected to the throat or pharynx, esophagus, stomach, small intestine, large intestine, rectum, and anus, where solid waste leaves the body. These organs are hollow so that digested food can pass through them. The mouth, stomach, and small intestine are lined with **mucosa** that produces digestive enzymes that help digest food. There is also a layer of smooth muscle in the GI tract that helps food move along and further break down food.

The liver, pancreas, and gallbladder are also involved in the digestive process. The liver produces bile that emulsifies fat, and the pancreas also produces digestive juices. These digestive juices are sent from the liver and the pancreas to the intestine through small tubes called ducts. The gallbladder is the holding tank and stores the liver's digestive juices until they are needed in the intestine. Figure 3.2 lists the organs and their role in the digestion of food.

GLOSSARY

Digestion
The process of breaking food into nutrients for the body to use

Gastrointestinal Tract (GI Tract)
The tubular organs used for digestion from the mouth to the anus, plus the liver, pancreas, and gallbladder

Mucosa
The lining of the mouth, stomach, and small intestine that contain tiny glands that produce digestive enzymes

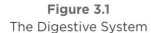

Figure 3.1
The Digestive System

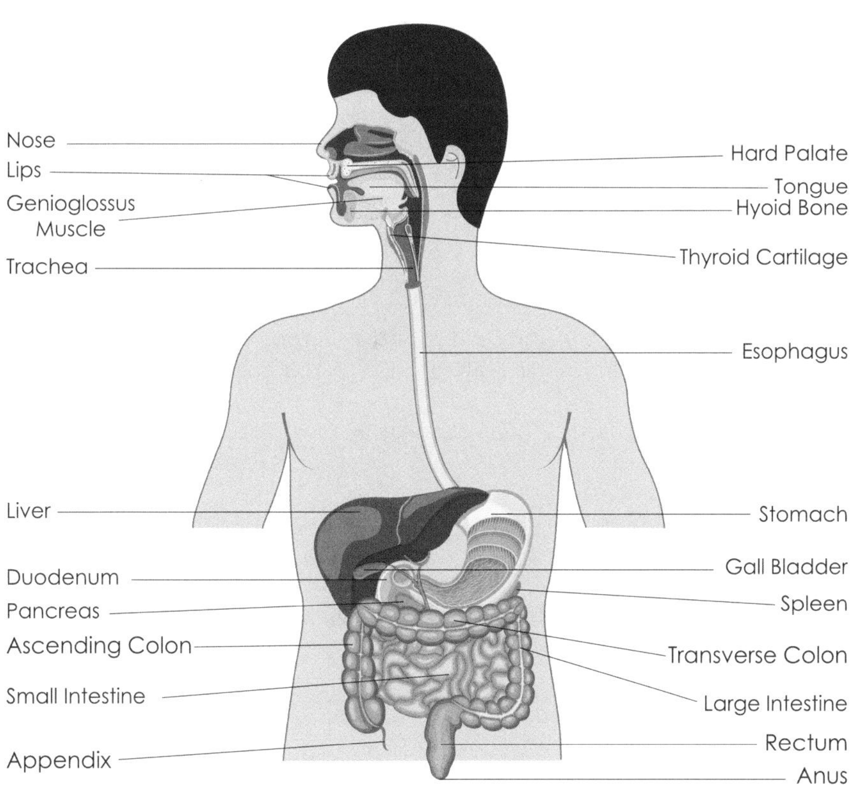

As discussed in previous chapters, the body uses nutrients. Most foods contain multiple nutrients that need to be broken down into useable parts. This is what digestion does. For example, body cells cannot use a peanut butter and jelly sandwich as a whole. Instead, it needs to be broken down into protein (amino acids), lipids (triglycerides), carbohydrates (complex and simple sugars), along with the vitamins and minerals present. Thus, to convert food into nutrients, the body needs to break it down into smaller components. Essentially, the body takes food apart so that it can use the pieces to rebuild exactly what it needs for life.

During the process of digestion, food is broken down two ways: mechanically and chemically. **Mechanical breakdown** is the physical breaking of food into smaller pieces. In the digestive system, this is the job of the mouth, the esophagus, and the stomach. When chewing food, the teeth, tongue, and jaw break bites of food into smaller pieces. After chewing, the food is swallowed and enters the esophagus on its way to the stomach, for more mechanical digestion. As food moves through the esophagus towards the stomach, strong muscular action that moves the food through also breaks it down a little bit more. When food is in the stomach, it stays there for a time and the stomach (a muscle) churns the food into even smaller pieces.

Chemical breakdown of food occurs with the help of digestive enzymes. Enzymes are substances that speed up chemical reactions and help in the breakdown of complex nutrients. Enzymes break complex proteins into simpler amino acids. They break disaccharides, as well as complex carbohydrates like starch, into monosaccharides. Enzymes also break large fat molecules down to fatty acids and glycerol. Figure 3.3 lists some of the digestive enzymes.

GLOSSARY

Mechanical Breakdown
The physical breakdown of food into smaller pieces using teeth, tongue, jaws, and the smooth muscles in the esophagus and stomach

Chemical Breakdown
The breakdown of food from digestive enzymes (gastric juices)

Figure 3.2
Organs in the Digestive System

ORGAN	WHAT HAPPENS HERE
Mouth	Chewing and mixing of food with salivary fluids.
Esophagus	Delivers swallowed food to the stomach.
Stomach	Food is churned and mixed with hydrochloric acid and pepsin for further breakdown. The food mixture that leaves the stomach is called chyme. Alcohol and certain drugs are absorbed from the stomach.
Duodenum (first part of the small intestines)	Mixes food with secretions from the liver and pancreas to neutralize stomach acid and further digest food. Much absorption of food occurs here.
Jejunum (second part of the small intestines)	Continues chemical digestion. Much absorption of food occurs here.
Ileum (third part of the small intestines)	Reabsorbs bile salts used to digest fats earlier in the small intestines.
Colon	Absorbs water and vitamins. Collects indigestible residue (waste) to form feces.
Rectum	Controls release of waste (feces).
Liver	Produces bile, a chemical that emulsifies fat, i.e. it breaks fat down into smaller globules so that digestive enzymes can go to work.
Gallbladder	Stores bile and secretes it into the duodenum during digestion.
Pancreas	Produces many digestive enzymes.

Figure 3.3
Examples of Digestive Enzymes

ENZYME	WHERE IT IS	WHAT IT DOES
Salivary Amylase	Mouth (made by salivary glands)	Breaks down starch and complex sugars.
Pepsin	Stomach	Breaks down protein.
Lipase	Secreted by the pancreas into the small intestine	Breaks down fat.
Protease	Secreted by the pancreas into the small intestine	Breaks down protein.

The digestive system starts with the mouth or oral cavity. There are 32 permanent teeth in the mouth that grind and break down the food. Chewing is important because it breaks the food up into smaller pieces so that enzymes can get in and do their job. Saliva, a fluid secreted into the mouth from the salivary glands, not only contains salivary amylase to begin breakdown of starches, it also lubricates the food so that it may readily pass down the throat and esophagus. The tongue, which extends across the floor of the mouth, moves food around the mouth during chewing and rolls it into a ball to be swallowed. The mucous-like substance in saliva coats food and helps to form a mass of chewed food called a bolus. Food in the form of a bolus can safely be swallowed. Even though the food is inside the digestive track, nutrients and food components are not inside the body until they are absorbed by the gastrointestinal tract. The body is able to purge unabsorbed food components by vomiting or diarrhea.

How does swallowing work? There are two steps. In the first step, the tongue pushes the bolus back towards the pharynx, or the back of the oral cavity (see Figure 3.4). Then, an involuntary (occurs automatically, a reflex) muscular contraction pushes the bolus into the esophagus. During this second step, the epiglottis, a muscular flap by the trachea (or breathing tube), automatically closes the respiratory passages so that the food will not be breathed into the respiratory tract. From time to time, this process doesn't work (commonly referred to the "food going down the wrong pipe"). Think of a time when a little bit of food or drink has accidentally entered the respiratory system. This is called aspiration. In a healthy person, the result is coughing to clear it out. In some patients, aspiration may lead to respiratory problems such as pneumonia; therefore, it is important to avoid aspiration in all patients.

Food enters the esophagus, a muscular tube about 10 inches long that connects the throat to the stomach. Food is propelled down the esophagus by rhythmic contractions of circular muscles in the wall of the esophagus. These contractions are called peristalsis. Peristalsis also helps break up food into smaller and smaller particles. Think of it as squeezing a marble (the bolus) through a rubber tube. Food passes down the esophagus through the lower esophageal sphincter (LES), a muscle that relaxes and contracts to move food from the esophagus into the stomach. The LES works like a gatekeeper into the stomach. Normally, it allows only a one-way movement. When a person experiences heartburn, the LES has mistakenly allowed stomach acid contents to shoot back up into the esophagus. This backflow of stomach contents is also called reflux or "heartburn." Heartburn actually has nothing to do with the heart. It acquired its name because the discomfort sufferers feel is close to the position of the heart.

The stomach has three digestive tasks. The first is that it is a muscular sac that holds about one liter of food. Within the folds of the mucous membranes are digestive glands that make the enzyme pepsin, as well as hydrochloric acid. Hydrochloric acid makes stomach contents very acidic (pH about 2.0, more acidic than vinegar), which activates the pepsin for protein digestion. Hydrochloric acid also destroys harmful bacteria and increases the ability of calcium and iron to be absorbed. People sometimes wonder why the stomach does not digest itself. The stomach has several forms of protection from

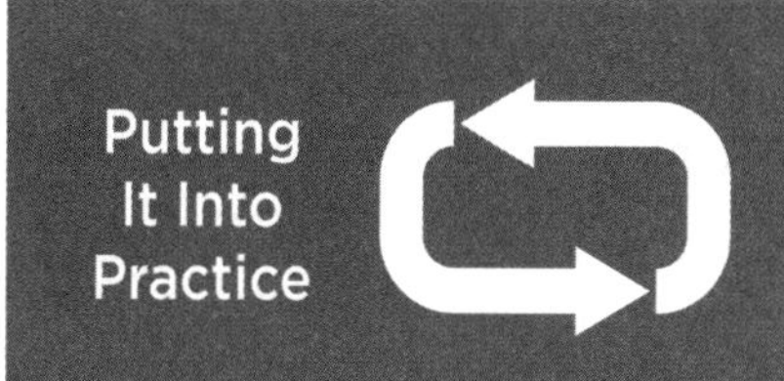

1. You notice one of your clients seems to always develop a cough after each meal, but it subsides between meals. Today he seems to really be under the weather, and he feels a little warm. What might be the problem?

Figure 3.4
Anatomy Involved in Swallowing

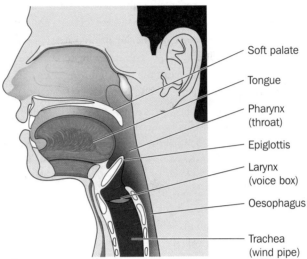

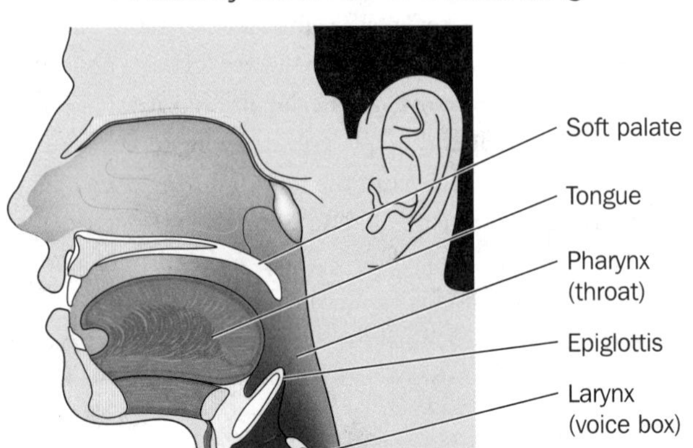

these strong chemicals. It has a mucous lining that can neutralize hydrochloric acid and it keeps the enzyme pepsin ready in a safer state called pepsinogen. Only after food arrives does it release acid and make pepsin active.

The second digestive task of the stomach is to churn food so that it can be passed into the first part of the small intestine. When the food is ready, it reaches a liquid consistency known as chyme. The stomach functions like a holding tank and takes approximately two to six hours to empty. A high amount of fat in a meal slows stomach emptying. Remember that little absorption of nutrients takes place in the stomach. However, this is the site where alcohol and aspirin are absorbed.

The third digestive task of the stomach is to empty the chyme slowly into the small intestine. Several factors determine how quickly the stomach empties, including the kind of food and the degree of muscle action. Carbohydrates are the easiest to digest, and therefore spend the least amount of time in the stomach. Carbohydrate digestion begins in the mouth, so it is already partly digested when it arrives in the stomach. Protein digestion begins in the stomach so protein stays in the stomach longer. Fat takes the longest to digest and stays in the stomach the longest.

A specialized muscle called the pyloric sphincter allows chyme to travel from the stomach into the small intestine. The small intestine is about 20 feet long and has three parts: the duodenum, the jejunum, and the ileum. It is called the small intestine because the diameter is smaller than that of the large intestine. The pancreas plays a key role in digestion. Pancreatic juices containing enzymes are added into the small intestine by the pancreas. These juices include enzymes and other chemicals produced by the pancreas. Sodium bicarbonate neutralizes the acidic chyme that is arriving from the stomach. Also present are an array of digestive enzymes that continue the breakdown of carbohydrate, protein, and fat. The duodenum, about one-foot long, receives the digested food from the stomach. A small organ above the intestines, the pancreas, releases enzymes into the duodenum to help digest carbohydrate, protein, and fat.

Before enzymes can work on fat, however, the fat must be broken down into smaller parts. This is the job of bile, a compound produced by the liver and stored in the gallbladder. The gallbladder releases bile into the small intestine. Bile works like detergent to emulsify fat into little droplets. What does this mean? Imagine hands that are greasy from rubbing oil on a turkey, or changing oil in the car. The fat cannot be rinsed off of the hands with water. Soap or detergent must be used to split fat globules into smaller parts to be washed away. Bile works quite similarly. Its action produces smaller pieces of fat, so that enzymes can get at them and digest the fat. See Figure 3.5 to review digestion.

Simple carbohydrates pass through the stomach into the small intestine where they are broken down into glucose, galactose, and fructose. Starch digestion begins in the mouth with an enzyme in saliva, then passes quickly through the stomach into the small intestine where digestion is completed. Protein foods such as meat and eggs are large molecules so the stomach must break these molecules into smaller molecules. When they are small enough, they are passed into the small intestine and broken down further into amino acids. Fat digestion also begins in the stomach.

Vitamins are also absorbed through the small intestine. Fat-soluble vitamins are dissolved with the fat and stored in the liver and fatty tissues of the body. Water-soluble vitamins are not easily stored and are, for the most part, passed into the urine.

In the wall of the duodenum—and throughout the entire small intestine—are tiny fingerlike projections called villi. The muscular walls of the small intestine mix the chyme with the digestive juices and bring the nutrients into contact with the villi for absorption. Most nutrients pass through the villi of the duodenum and jejunum into either the intestinal cell, into the bloodstream or lymph system, where they are transported to the liver and to the cells of the body. The duodenum connects with the second section or the small intestine, the jejunum, which connects to the ileum.

Figure 3.5
Digestion and Absorption Summary

FOOD	DIGESTION LOCATIONS	OUTCOME
Sucrose/ Lactose	Small Intestine	Glucose, Fructose, Galactose
Starch	Mouth and Small Intestine	Glucose
Fiber	No Digestion Action	Binds some molecules; most are excreted in feces
Protein	Stomach and Small Intestine	Peptides → Amino Acids
Fats	Milk fat begins in mouth; small amount in stomach; most is in the small intestine	Fatty Acids and Glycerol

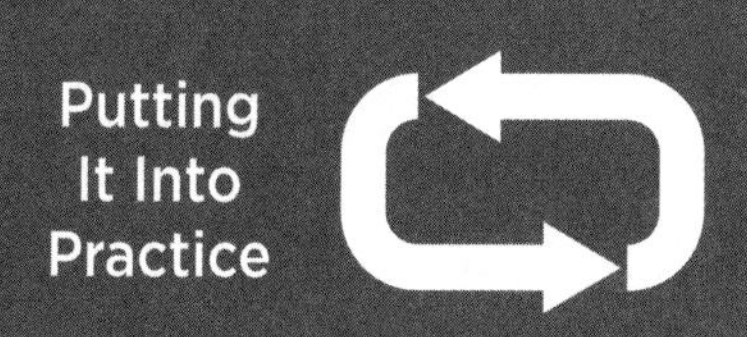

2. List at least two ways a gallbladder removal surgery affects nutrient digestion and absorption.

The large intestine or colon is four to five feet long and extends from the end of the ileum to the rectum. Water and some minerals are absorbed here. In addition, healthful bacteria in the colon actually manufacture vitamin K, as well as some biotin. The body absorbs and uses these nutrients. One of the functions of the large intestine is to receive and store the waste products of digestion; in other words, it handles the material that has not entered the blood or lymph vessels. The waste accumulated here includes indigestible fiber from foods. Bacteria that are naturally present in the colon ferment some of the fiber, producing gases. Indigestible fiber can also attract and hold water. This makes stools softer and helps prevent constipation. The large intestine stores waste material until it is released as solid feces, through the anus, the lower opening of the gastrointestinal tract.

Before the body can use any of the nutrients present in food, the nutrients must pass through the walls of the gastrointestinal tract through a process called **absorption**. Nutrients pass through the cells of the intestinal tract into the circulatory system. There are two parts of the circulatory system that are involved in this process: the blood and lymph. The blood and lymph are two body fluids that deliver needed products to the cells for use. Sugars and amino acids travel into the blood, while fatty acids enter the body through the lymphatic system. Remember that fat and water do not mix. The blood is largely water-based. This is why fat cannot enter the bloodstream. Lymphatic fluid, on the other hand, can hold and carry fat. If nutrients are not absorbed into the blood or lymph at some point along the gastrointestinal tract, they are excreted as feces.

GLOSSARY

Absorption
The process by which nutrients pass through the cells of the intestinal tract into the circulatory system to be utilized by the body

Metabolism
The chemical process in a cell by which nutrients are used to support life

Bioavailability
How well a nutrient is absorbed and utilized by the body

As the blood circulates nutrients through the body, cells begin to use the nutrients in a process called metabolism. **Metabolism** refers to all the chemical processes in a cell by which nutrients are used to support life. Metabolism involves building substances (called anabolism) or breaking down substances (called catabolism). Nutrients such as glucose are converted to energy (ATP) in a catabolic reaction that releases energy to maintain body temperature or to perform work within the cell. Anabolism is the opposite of catabolism. It is the process of building substances, such as proteins, from their amino acid components.

Availability of Nutrients

An important aspect of nutrition is the bioavailability of nutrients. The term **bioavailability** describes how well a nutrient is absorbed and used by the body. When the process of digestion and absorption is complete, the amount of a nutrient a body actually has may differ from the amount consumed. For example, the body typically absorbs only about 10 percent of dietary iron. If the iron is from a meat source (a form called *heme iron*), absorption may rise to about 25 percent. Interestingly, studies demonstrate that individuals who have iron deficiency absorb iron more efficiently during their period of deficiency.

In addition, presence of other nutrients in the intestinal tract can have positive or negative effects on absorption. Vitamin C, for instance, seems to promote iron

3. What are some helpful tips you could give to a client who is having constipation in order to help her become more "regular"?

absorption. A person taking an iron supplement along with a glass of orange juice may enjoy better absorption and a higher bioavailability of the nutrient. Conversely, high amounts of magnesium in the gastrointestinal tract may interfere with absorption of iron and calcium. A natural compound in dark green leafy vegetables, called oxalate, can also decrease iron absorption. Spinach, for example, is considered to be a good source of iron from plant sources. However, the availability of the iron is compromised by the naturally-occurring oxalate present in the spinach. To absorb fat-soluble vitamins, the body generally needs some fat in the intestinal tract, too. In a food-based diet this is easy to accomplish, because fat-soluble vitamins are found in conjunction with dietary fat.

Even after absorption, various factors affect how well the body can use nutrients. For example, alcohol counteracts the effects of vitamin B6 in metabolism. In addition, many drugs and other medicines can affect the metabolism of nutrients. Some increase bioavailability; some decrease it. Some people have trouble absorbing nutrients. One common example is lactose intolerance. About three-fourths of the population loses their ability to digest and absorb lactose as they age. They lose the ability to break milk sugar (lactose) into glucose and galactose. This causes them to remain in the small intestine rather than be absorbed since only monosaccharides can be absorbed. A person who is lactose intolerant doesn't make enough lactase or does not make any enzyme. This may cause the person to experience pain, diarrhea, or bloating due to excessive gas. The gas is due to intestinal bacteria that use lactose for fuel and produces gas in the process.

Gastrointestinal illness can also affect bioavailability of nutrients. If the intestines are inflamed and intestinal villi are damaged, as in Crohn's disease, adequate nutrient absorption may not take place. In another example, a poorly functioning pancreas may fail to make enough of the critical enzymes needed for digestion of carbohydrate, protein and fat, leading to poor bioavailability of these nutrients in the body. In cases of illness, an average diet that is adequate in protein, fat, carbohydrate, vitamins, and minerals may nevertheless not be adequate to maintain good nutritional status. This is due to reduced absorption and reduced availability of nutrients. For healthy people, the Recommended Dietary Allowance (RDA) levels of nutrients address ordinary factors that influence nutrient bioavailability. It's important for a CDM, CFPP to know, however, that established nutrient standards may not always "fit the bill" if there are underlying medical conditions. Thus, individual screening and assessment are important to help a CDM, CFPP address the individual needs of each client. Likewise, communication with medical staff and a Registered Dietitian Nutritionist (RDN) can help assure that meals leaving the kitchen are nutritionally adequate for the population being served.

Remember, the role of the CDM, CFPP is to interview and assist in nutrition screening. The RDN will complete the nutrition assessment. We will discuss this more in depth in Chapters 7 and 8.

4. You notice a client loves to have iced tea with meals. She is found to have iron-deficiency anemia. What do you tell her?

Chapter Reference

RESOURCE	
U.S. Department of Health and Human Services. Your Digestive System & How it Works. National Institute of Diabetes and Digestive and Kidney Diseases. *Accessed September 18, 2019.*	https://www.niddk.nih.gov/health-information/digestive-diseases/digestive-system-how-it-works

Manage Food Allergies and Complementary/ Alternative Medicine

Overview and Objectives

Food allergies and alternative therapies often come up during the provision of nutritional care. A Certified Dietary Manager®, Certified Food Protection Professional® (CDM®, CFPP®) needs to understand food allergies and alternative therapies in order to promote optimal nutrition for clients. After completing this chapter, you should be able to:

- Describe common food allergies and discuss the dietary implications
- Define alternative therapies
- Identify risks and benefits of alternative therapies
- Classify use of alternative therapies in long-term and acute care
- List questions to ask when evaluating dietary supplements and other complementary and alternative treatments
- Differentiate between food allergy and food intolerance
- Identify the role of basic nutrition concepts in assessment and implementation of complementary and alternative therapies
- Explain the role of the CDM, CFPP for assisting clients in alternative therapies

SECTION A FOOD ALLERGIES AND INTOLERANCES

How many people do you know who have a food allergy or intolerance? Are there certain foods you avoid because of allergy or intolerance? It seems like food allergies and intolerances are on the rise in the United States. As a CDM, CFPP, you will need to know the common food that causes allergies and intolerance; and what changes need to be made to care for affected individuals.

According to Food Allergy Research & Education (FARE), food allergies are a medical condition that affect approximately 15 million people in the United States. This number is hard to measure since many people are never diagnosed by a physician. About 4% of the adult population have a clinical diagnosis (by a physician). In addition, about 5% of children (1 in 13 children) have a clinical diagnosis of a food allergy.

What is a Food Allergy?

The immune system in the human body is responsible for the identification and destruction of harmful germs (such as bacteria or viruses). What happens with a **food allergy** is the body's immune system mistakenly targets a harmless food protein—an allergen—as a threat and attacks it. This immune response is considered to be "IgE mediated." IgE—immunoglobulin E—is one of the antibodies produced by the body. The immune system releases abnormally large amounts of IgE to fight the "foreign" protein found in the food. Normally, all food proteins are digested to amino acids before they are absorbed; in some individuals, some of the proteins are not digested completely and are absorbed into the blood stream and they are treated by the body as "foreign" protein. The immune system also releases histamine and other chemicals, which trigger the symptoms of an allergic reaction. Common response time for this immune response can span from immediately to several hours after exposure. Reactions to the food allergy may range from mild (hives, itchiness) to severe (resulting in death).

GLOSSARY

Food Allergy
The adverse allergic reaction resulting in mild to severe symptoms. The immune system mistakenly targets a harmless food protein—an allergen—as a threat and attacks it, causing a reaction

Food Intolerance
The intake of food that cannot be tolerated or digested properly (seen in the case of lactose or gluten intolerance). Food intolerance does not generally produce an immune response

What is a Food Intolerance?

A **food intolerance** differs from a food allergy in one important way. Food intolerances are not true food allergies, because there is no IgE immune and histamine response. Without these responses, an intolerance is not a "true" allergy and usually symptoms are limited to gastrointestinal discomfort in the digestive tract and they can range from acute to chronic. Some symptoms include: bloating, migraines, headaches, cough, runny nose, stomach ache, diarrhea, and general "feeling under the weather." About 1 in 3 people claim a food intolerance or about one-third of the population. Since most intolerances go undiagnosed, it is difficult to determine prevalence. If a person has a reaction to a certain food, many times they just avoid the food that makes them "feel bad."

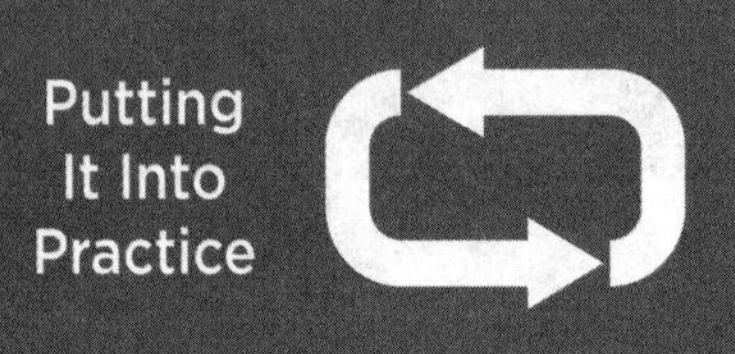

1. Your dad mentions he has suddenly discovered he is allergic to peanuts. He explains he became constipated after the last time he ate them. Is your dad most likely experiencing a food allergy or an intolerance?

Symptoms of Food Allergies

An allergic reaction may present in a variety of ways. It can affect the skin (rash or hives), the gastrointestinal tract (nausea or vomiting), the respiratory tract (difficulty breathing) and, in the most serious cases, the cardiovascular system (affecting the heart). Reactions can range from mild to severe.

Symptoms typically appear almost immediately (within minutes) to several hours after eating the offending food *(Source: Food Allergy Research & Education)*.

- Hives (reddish, swollen, itchy areas on the skin)
- Eczema (a persistent dry, itchy rash)
- Redness of the skin or around the eyes
- Itchy mouth or ear canal
- Nausea or vomiting
- Diarrhea
- Stomach pain
- Nasal congestion or a runny nose
- Sneezing
- Slight, dry cough
- Odd taste in mouth
- Uterine contractions

Anaphylaxis Reaction

Severe symptoms may include one or more of the following *(Source: Food Allergy Research & Education)*:

- Obstructive swelling of the lips, tongue, and/or throat
- Trouble swallowing
- Shortness of breath or wheezing
- Turning blue
- Drop in blood pressure (feeling faint, confused, weak, passing out)
- Loss of consciousness
- Chest pain
- A weak or "thread" pulse
- Sense of "impending doom"

Severe symptoms, alone or in combination with milder symptoms, may be signs of **anaphylaxis** and require immediate treatment. Anaphylaxis is a severe, potentially life-threatening allergic reaction. It can occur within seconds or minutes of exposure to an allergen. The IgE response during anaphylaxis can cause the body to go into shock, causing a sudden drop in blood pressure and narrowing of the airway. Signs and symptoms of anaphylaxis include: rapid and weak pulse, skin rash, and nausea and vomiting. Anaphylaxis requires immediate administration of epinephrine and a visit to the emergency room. If anaphylaxis is not treated immediately, it may lead to unconsciousness or death. In the United States, food allergy symptoms send someone to the emergency room every three minutes.

GLOSSARY

Anaphylaxis
A life-threatening allergic reaction that usually shuts down the respiratory system, sometimes resulting in death

Common Food Allergens

What are the foods that cause the most reactions? That is an interesting question. Worldwide, there are different food allergens and each country has a unique list of top allergens. In the United States, eight foods account for about 90% of food allergies/allergic reactions. Remember that the other 10% of food allergic responses can be just as severe as the common food allergens, and all foods are capable of causing an allergic reaction. The "Big 8" allergens for the United States include:

1. Eggs
2. Fish
3. Shellfish
4. Milk
5. Peanuts
6. Tree Nuts
7. Soy
8. Wheat

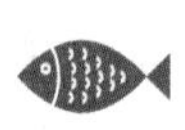
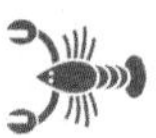
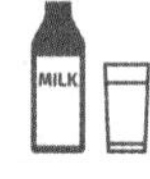
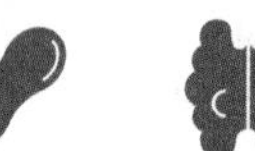

GLOSSARY

Food Allergy Labeling and Consumer Protection Act (FALCPA)
A Federal law that requires manufacturers to disclose the presence of milk, eggs, fish, crustacean shellfish (shrimp, crab, and lobster), tree nuts, wheat, peanuts, and soy/soybeans

The U.S. government passed a law in 2004 that requires food companies to disclose allergen information for the "Big 8" on food labels. In 2006, the **Food Allergy Labeling and Consumer Protection Act (FALCPA)** came into effect. Manufacturers must disclose the presence of milk, eggs, fish, crustacean shellfish (shrimp, crab, and lobster), tree nuts, wheat, peanuts, and soy/soybeans. The label must be in "plain English." Disclosure may take place one of two ways:

1. By placing the word "Contains" followed by the food source of the food allergen immediately after or adjacent to the list of ingredients, *OR*
2. By placing common or usual names of the allergen in the list of ingredients followed by parentheses by the name of the food source from which the allergen is derived.

Example, using the first option for disclosure:

Ingredients: Whey protein, lecithin, vanilla flavoring, natural flavors, and salt
Contains: Milk, soy, and pecans

Example, using the second option for disclosure:

Whey protein (milk), lecithin (soy), vanilla flavoring, natural flavors (pecans), and salt

FALCPA requires that the type of nut must also be listed on the food label. In the case of fish and crustacean shellfish, the manufacturer must specify the type of fish by species. Crustacean shellfish that must be listed include shrimp, lobster, and crab. However, mollusk shellfish such as clams, mussels, etc. are not considered a major allergen and do not have to be declared. It is recommended to read the food label information twice— one time reading the "contains" information and then a second time to read all of the ingredients on the food label to identify the "unusual" names for common food allergens, just to be sure. For further reading on the FDA Food Guidance for the FALCPA go to www.fda.gov and search for FALCPA.

The "Big 8" allergens account for 90% of the food allergens in the United States. It is time to take a more in-depth look at each of these foods.

Allergen: Eggs 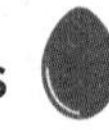

Prevalence of egg allergy in the United States population ranges from 0.5 - 2.5% (Food Allergy Research & Education). The most common type of reaction is atopic dermatitis (rash), but it can range from mild (skin rash) to anaphylaxis. Egg allergy is the most common allergy in young children. Egg allergies are most common in infants and children, and about 70% of children will outgrow the allergy by age 16.

What part of the egg causes the allergic reaction? The white or the yolk? All egg must be strictly avoided. Although allergy to egg whites is most common, the white and the yolk both contain proteins that can cause allergies. However, since the egg can never fully and finally be separated, white from yolk, all egg must be avoided and strict avoidance is necessary. Those with an egg allergy should also avoid eating eggs from other species of birds including duck, goose, turkey, and quail.

When reading food labels, the following ingredients should be avoided: albumin, egg (dried, solid, powdered, white, and yolk), eggnog, lysozyme, mayonnaise, meringue, meringue powder, ovalbumin, and surimi (imitation crab meat made from fish). Also avoid serving baked goods (most contain eggs), egg substitutes, lecithin, marzipan, marshmallow, nougat, and macaroni/pasta (many are made with egg/yolk). If a modification needs to be made, consider this substitution for eggs in a recipe:

- 1 egg = 1-1/2 Tbsp. water + 1-1/2 Tbsp. oil + 1 tsp. baking powder *OR*
- 1 egg = 1 tsp. of yeast dissolved in 1/4 cup warm water
  **Maximum replacement* in a recipe is 3 eggs, depending on the recipe (Food Allergy Research & Education)

Allergen: Fish

There are over 20,000 species of finned fish. Fish allergies affect about 0.4% of the population, with more women being affected than men. Among those having a fish allergy, 40% had their first reaction as an adult. Allergic reactions range from gastrointestinal upset to anaphylaxis. Once the allergy is present, the allergy is usually lifelong. The protein in the flesh of the fish causes most reactions to occur, but fish gelatin (made from bones and skin) may also pose a problem. Salmon, tuna, and halibut are the most common fish allergies. More than half of those allergic to one type of fish are also allergic to another type of fish. Generally, strict avoidance of fish is recommended. Shellfish and finned fish are not related at all, so being allergic to finned fish may not mean that a person should avoid shellfish and vice versa.

Foods to avoid with a fish allergy include: salmon, tuna, and halibut (most common) and avoid all fish and dishes containing fish. Other common fish allergies include: anchovies, bass, catfish, cod, flounder, grouper, haddock, hake, herring, mahi-mahi, perch, pike, pollock, scrod, swordfish, sole, snapper, tilapia, and trout (*This is not an exhaustive list, just the most common in the United States). Other foods that need to be avoided include: Worcestershire sauce, Caesar salad, surimi (imitation fish/crab), fish stock, Asian/African/ Indonesian/Thai/Vietnamese cuisine, bouillabaisse, meatloaf (unless the ingredients are known), barbecue sauce, and capoata (Sicilian eggplant relish).

Cross-contact can happen very easily, since many foods are shipped and stored together. Cross-contact is any instance in which an allergenic food comes in contact with another food either directly or indirectly. Here are some direct cross-contact examples: scraping egg salad off of a sandwich and using chicken instead, removing crab from a salad and still serving it, or touching a cooler door with mayonnaise on

GLOSSARY

Cross-Contact
Any instance in which an allergenic food comes in contact with an allergy-free food, either directly or indirectly

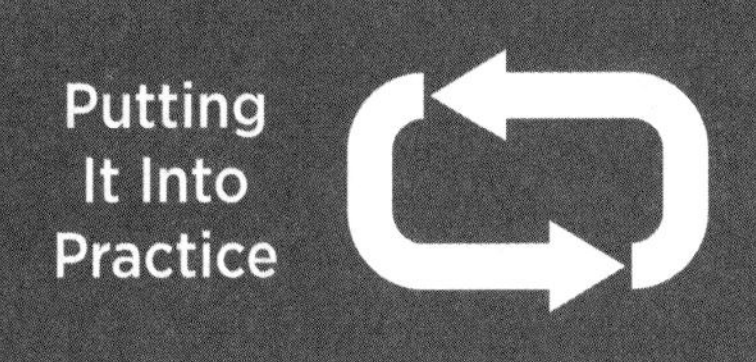

2. While walking through the kitchen, you witness an employee cutting tuna sandwiches and turkey sandwiches with the same knife, on the same surface. What should she be doing differently to prevent food allergen cross-contact?

it and not washing hands prior to handling another order. There also may be indirect cross-contact: using the same tongs to serve sandwiches (that may have allergenic foods present), not washing hands after handling the crab, or using the same knife for butter and mayonnaise. These are some examples of cross-contact. Especially with fish, cross-contact can be an issue since many types of fish are shipped and stored together. They may have direct cross-contact, like fish laying for sale at a fresh seafood market or restaurant. In addition, fish protein may become airborne when boiled, causing issues with certain individuals. (*Source: Food Allergy Research & Education*)

Allergen: Shellfish 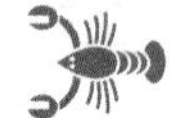

Shellfish allergies are one of the top allergens for adults. Sixty percent of those allergic to shellfish have the first reaction as an adult, and prevalence is approximately 2.3% of the United States population. Shellfish allergic reactions can range from mild (GI issues) to severe (anaphylaxis). (*Source: Food Allergy Research & Education*)

There are two types of shellfish: crustacean and mollusks. Crustacean include shellfish like shrimp, crab, and lobster, and the allergic reaction tends to be more severe. Mollusks include shellfish like clams, mussels, oysters, and scallops. Most people who are allergic to shellfish are usually allergic to more than one type, therefore most are advised to avoid all varieties. Allergy to shellfish is usually a lifelong condition.

The most common shellfish allergies are shrimp, crab, and lobster. Again, if there is an allergy to shellfish, it is advised to avoid all shellfish and shellfish products. Other common crustacean allergies include: barnacle, crab, crawfish (crawdad, crayfish, ecrevisse), krill, lobster (langouste, langoustine, Moreton bay bugs, scampi, tomalley), prawns, and shrimp (crevette, scampi). In addition, it is advised to avoid Asian cuisine since fish sauce is commonly used as a base in cooking.

The Food Allergen Labeling and Consumer Protection Act (FALCPA) requires labeling of the "Big 8" allergens on food packaging, but remember that mollusks are not considered a "major allergen" as part of this act and may not be fully disclosed on a food product. That makes it essential to read the food ingredient information to find mollusk shellfish ingredients.

Common mollusks to look for include: abalone, clams (cherrystone, geoduck, littleneck, pismo, quahog), cockle, cuttlefish, limpet (Lipas, opihil), mussels, octopus, oysters, periwinkle, sea cucumber, sea urchin, scallops, snails (escargot), squid (calamari), and whelk (turban shell). These mollusks should be avoided if allergic to shellfish. There are a few more foods that commonly contain shellfish: bouillabaisse, cuttlefish ink, glucosamine, fish stock, seafood flavoring, crab or clam extract, and surimi. Cross-contact can easily happen for shellfish because, like other fish, it many times is shipped, stored, and prepared with the same equipment. It also becomes airborne when cooked. In addition, mislabeling or omission of a mollusk may occur. (*Source: Food Allergy Research & Education*)

Allergen: Milk 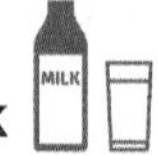

Milk allergy is the most common allergy for infants and young children. About 2.5% of children younger than 3 years are allergic to cow's milk. (Food Allergy Research & Education) Nearly all infants who develop a milk allergy do so before the age of one. However, some studies show that breast feeding may be protective against milk allergy. Infants who are formula fed are more likely to develop an allergy. However, most children (about 80%) will outgrow the allergy by the age of 16. Reactions range from mild (hives, vomiting) to severe (bloody stools, anaphylaxis). With a "true milk allergy" the person is allergic to the proteins found in the milk. That milk protein is what causes the immune (IgE mediated) response. So how is that different from a milk or lactose "intolerance"?

With milk or lactose intolerance, it is a completely different mechanism. As was learned in the previous chapters, the carbohydrate found in milk is called lactose. There is an enzyme, called lactase, which breaks apart the lactose into glucose and galactose in the intestinal lining in order to be absorbed. For those who are milk or lactose intolerant, their body does not have the enzyme lactase. The response is usually cramping, flatulence, and diarrhea—only gastrointestinal response. Lactose intolerance, while unpleasant, is not life-threatening. Some individuals with lactose intolerance may be able to tolerate yogurt, cheese, and some of the fermented dairy products.

Those with a milk allergy must avoid all milk and dairy products. First and foremost, avoid milk in all forms: condensed, derivative, dry, evaporated, low-fat, malted, milk fat, nonfat, powder, protein, skimmed, and whole. Also avoid goat's milk and milk from other animals. Other foods to avoid include: butter, butter fat, butter oil, butter acid, butter esters, buttermilk, casein, casein hydrolysate, caseinates (all forms), cheese, cottage cheese, cream, curd, custard, diacetyl, ghee, half and half, lactalbumin, lactalbumin phosphate, lactoferrin, lactose, lactulose, milk protein hydrolysate, pudding, Recaldent®, and rennet casein. Here are some other foods to avoid with milk allergy: sour cream, sour cream solids, sour milk solids, tagatose, whey (in all forms), whey protein hydrolysate, yogurt, ice cream, artificial butter flavor, baked goods, caramel and caramel candies, chocolate, lactic acid starter culture and other bacterial cultures, luncheon meats, hot dogs, sausages, margarine, nisin, non-dairy products, and nougat. Some brands of canned tuna contain casein and must be avoided. In addition, many non-dairy and meat products contain casein.

Cross-contact is also possible with a milk allergy. Deli meat slicers that cut meats may also cut cheese and may not be properly cleaned to prevent cross-contact. Be aware of other equipment that may be shared with milk products. In some restaurants they use a pat of butter to flavor a steak or may dip shellfish in milk to reduce the "fishy odor." Some medications can also contain milk.

Those with lactose intolerance need to be treated on a case-by-case basis. It is very important to determine the extent of the intolerance. Some people are able to consume small amounts of milk, especially if consumed with other non-dairy foods. Others can tolerate milk that has been heated, like in baked products. The nutrition screening and interview process will help determine what foods can be tolerated.

There is one additional topic to be discussed when talking about milk allergies, which is the topic of Kosher Dairy and Kosher Pareve to determine the presence of dairy or milk in the Jewish tradition. Kosher means "fit to eat" and Orthodox Jewish tradition does not allow for the consumption of meat and dairy in the same meal. Therefore, some people with a milk allergy have started to use the Kosher designation as a hint

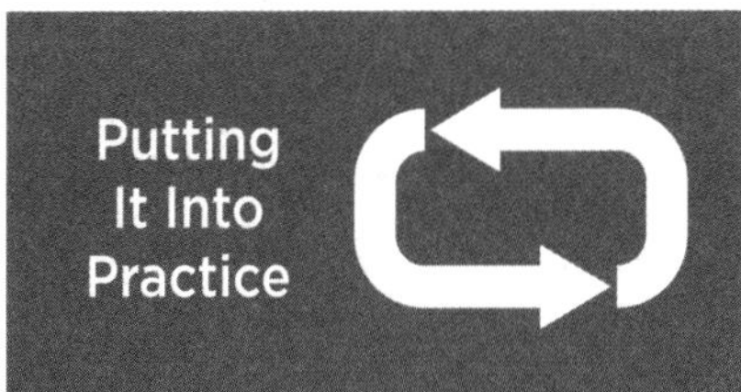

3. What modifications or replacements would you make to the following menu items to omit the top 8 allergens?
   - Peanut butter & jelly sandwich on whole wheat bread
   - Asian shrimp stir-fry with slivered almonds
   - Chocolate cake
   - Tuna salad with mayonnaise and boiled eggs

for the presence of milk/dairy in a product. Kosher Dairy, signified by a "D" or the word "dairy" following the circled K or U on a product label, indicates the presence of milk protein or risk that the product has been contaminated with milk protein. Kosher Pareve (meaning neither dairy nor meat)- a product labeled "pareve" is considered milk neutral—neither dairy or meat— under kosher dairy law. However, a food product may be considered pareve even if it contains very small amounts of milk protein. Do not assume pareve products will always be safe! (*Source: Food Allergy Research & Education*)

Allergen: Peanuts 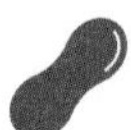

A peanut is "technically" not a nut, it is a legume. Peanut allergies affect about 0.5% of the population in the United States, with about 400,000 of those allergies belonging to children. From 1997-2008 the incidence of peanut allergies in the United States has tripled. Only about 20% of those diagnosed with a peanut allergy will outgrow the allergy. The allergic reaction for a peanut allergy is usually severe and potentially fatal, leading quickly to anaphylaxis. Studies are showing that there is an increased risk of peanut allergy if there are others in the family with the allergy. There is no additional risk for being allergic to other legumes like beans, peas, lentils, and soybeans. In many cases, trace amounts can cause a reaction (including peanut oil or residue).

s there a connection between peanuts and tree nuts? It is estimated that 25-40% of those who have a peanut or tree nut allergy are allergic to *both* peanuts and tree nuts. One of the biggest obstacles is that manufacturers often share equipment for manufacturing of product and when/how products are served.

What foods should be avoided for individuals with a peanut allergy? The list includes: artificial nuts, beer nuts, cold pressed peanut oil, expeller pressed peanut oil, extruded peanut oil, goobers, ground nuts, mandelonas (peanuts soaked in almond flavoring), mixed nuts, monkey nuts, nutmeat, nut pieces, peanut butter, peanut flour, and peanut protein hydrolysate. Arachis oil is another name for peanut oil. Other foods to avoid include: baked goods (especially from a bakery), pastries, cookies, candy (including chocolate), chili, egg rolls, enchilada sauce, marzipan, mole sauce, and nougat. Some other unexpected sources of peanuts may include: African/Asian/Mexican dishes; sauces—chili, hot, pesto, gravy, mole, salad dressing; pudding, cookies, pie crust and hot chocolate; pancakes; specialty pizzas; vegetarian meat substitutes; glazes and marinades; and pet food (included since young children sometimes consume it).

With FALCPA, the FDA has exempted highly refined peanut oil from being labeled as an allergen. Studies have shown that most individuals can safely consume highly refined peanut oil (but not cold pressed, expelled, or extruded peanut oil—sometimes marketed as "gourmet" oils). However, before proceeding with highly refined peanut oil, confirm it with the physician.

Sunflowers, sunflower seeds, and sunbutter, along with soynuts and soybutter, are sometimes processed on equipment shared with other tree nuts and peanuts. Always be sure to read the labels and check with the manufacturer prior to serving these products. Cross-contact is a main concern for those with peanut allergies. Establishments that pose the highest risk are those that knowingly have peanuts, like African, Asian, Chinese, Indian, Indonesian, Thai, Vietnamese, and Mexican restaurants. Others include bakeries and ice cream shops. (*Source: Food Allergy Research & Education*)

Allergen: Tree Nuts 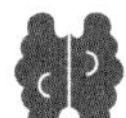

Tree nut allergies are very common in the United States. Tree nut allergies affect about one million people in the U.S. The allergy tends to be lifelong once diagnosed, with only 9% of children outgrowing the allergy. Allergic reactions are usually severe and are potentially life-threatening, leading to anaphylaxis. Like peanut allergies, if a family member is allergic to tree nuts, it increases the risk of an allergy to develop among other family members. If there is an allergy to one type of tree nut, the risk greatly increases the likelihood of being allergic to additional tree nuts. It is advised that shared equipment also poses a risk with tree nuts.

Tree nuts that should be avoided include: almonds, artificial nuts, Brazil nuts, beechnuts, butternut, cashew, chinquapin nut, coconut, filbert, hazelnut, giandjua (chocolate nut mixture), ginkgo nut, hickory nut, litchi/lichee/lychee nut, macadamia nut, marzipan (almond paste), nangai nut, natural nut extracts (almond, walnut), nut butters (cashew butter, Nutella), nut meal, nut meats, nut pastes, pecans, pesto, pili nut, pine nut (aka. Indian, pignoli, pignolia, pignon, pinon, pinyon), pistachio, praline, shea nut, and walnut. Some other foods to avoid are: black walnut hull extract, natural nut extract, nut distillates, alcoholic extracts, nut oils, and walnut hull extract. There are some other unexpected places that tree nuts may be found: cereal and granola, crackers, cookies, candy, chocolates, energy bars, granola bars, flavored coffees, frozen desserts, barbeque sauce, alcoholic beverages, lotions, hair care products, and soaps.

Similar to peanuts, cross-contact is a main concern for those with tree nut allergies. Establishments that pose the highest risk are those that knowingly have tree nuts, like African, Asian, Chinese, Indian, Indonesian, Thai, Vietnamese, and Mexican restaurants. Others include bakeries and ice cream shops.

What about coconuts? A coconut is not a botanical nut; it is classified as a fruit, even though FDA recognizes coconuts as a "tree nut." While no reactions to coconut have been documented, most people who are allergic to tree nuts can safely consume coconut. However, in the nutrition screening and interview, always check to see if there is an allergy to coconut as well. (*Source: Food Allergy Research & Education*)

Allergen: Soy

Soy allergies are common among infants and young children. About 0.4% of the population, approximately 300,000 individuals, have a soy allergy. Allergy to soy is often outgrown by three years of age, with the majority (70%) of children outgrowing the allergy by 10 years of age. Reactions range from mild to severe, including anaphylaxis (which is rare for soy allergy).

Soybeans are also legumes. Those with a soy allergy do not have a greater chance of being allergic to other legumes (including peanuts). In the United States, soy products and soybean oil are widely used in processed foods. This causes the greatest challenge for those who are allergic to soy. Foods to avoid include: edamame, miso, matto, shoyo, soy (soy albumin, soy cheese, soy flour, soy grits, soy ice cream, soy milk, soy nuts, soy sprouts, and soy yogurt), soya, soybean (curd and granules), soy protein (concentrate, hydrolyzed, isolate), soy sauce, tamari, tempeh, textured vegetable protein (TVP), and tofu. Other foods to avoid include Asian cuisine, vegetable gum, vegetable starch, and vegetable broth. Soy can also be found in baked goods, canned tuna and other canned meats, cereals, cookies, crackers, energy/protein bars, infant formula, low-fat peanut butter, processed meats, sauces, canned broth, soups, and vodka. Asian cuisine is considered to be high risk due to the common use of soy as an ingredient. The risk of cross-contact is very high. Therefore, it is recommended that those with a soy allergy avoid Asian cuisine.

With FALCPA, the FDA has exempted highly refined soybean oil from being labeled as an allergen. Studies have shown that many individuals can safely consume highly refined soybean oil (but not cold pressed, expelled, or extruded soybean oil—sometimes identified as "gourmet" oils). However, before proceeding with highly refined soybean oil, confirm it with the physician. (*Source: Food Allergy Research & Education*)

Allergen: Wheat

Wheat allergy is most common in children. Most (65%) children with wheat allergies outgrow the allergy before they reach adulthood, and many prior to age three. Wheat allergy affects 0.4% of children and 0.5% of adults. Symptoms range from mild (hives) to severe (anaphylaxis). Strict avoidance of wheat is essential for managing wheat allergy; however, this can be a difficult task since over 75% of grain products in the United States contain wheat.

Here are the foods that must be avoided with a wheat allergy: bread crumbs, bulgur, cereal extract, club wheat, couscous, cracker meal, durum, einkorn, emmer, farina, flour (all purpose, bread, cake, durum, graham, high gluten, high protein, instant, pastry, self-rising, soft wheat, steel ground, stone ground, and whole wheat), hydrolyzed wheat protein, Kamut, matzoh, matzoh meal, matzo, matzah or matza, pasta, seitan, semolina, spelt, sprouted wheat, triticale, vital wheat gluten, wheat (bran, durum, germ, gluten, grass, malt, sprouts, starch), wheat bran hydrolysate, wheat germ oil, wheat grass, wheat protein isolate, whole wheat berries, wheat berries, and wheat groats. Other foods include: glucose syrup, surimi, soy sauce, and starch (gelatinized starch, modified starch, modified food starch, vegetable starch). There are also unexpected sources of wheat that may be contained in some ice creams, marinara sauce, potato chips, rice cakes, turkey patties, hot dogs, coating on foods, and beer/ale. It is also found in baking mixes, baked products, batter fried foods, breaded foods, breakfast cereals, candy, crackers, processed meats, salad dressings, sauces, and soups.

When thinking about all of the foods that contain wheat, what is left? Encourage lots of fruits, vegetables, lean meats, and dairy foods. There is still a huge variety of foods to choose from.

s a Wheat Allergy the Same as Gluten Intolerance?

No, a wheat allergy is not the same as gluten intolerance. A wheat allergy occurs when a person is allergic to the protein found in a product that causes an IgE mediated response. What is gluten intolerance then? Gluten intolerance, also known as Celiac Disease or Celiac Sprue, is a digestive disease that affects the small intestine. Presence of the wheat gluten in the gastrointestinal tract causes damage to the villi in the small intestine. This damage causes inflammation of the mucosa lining the gut, and a malabsorption of nutrients. It is a cell-mediated allergy, a food intolerance, and an auto-immune disorder all rolled into one.

Gluten intolerance affects about 1% of the population in the United States or about 1 out of 133 people. Gluten intolerance, like other auto-immune diseases such as Type 1 diabetes and arthritis, is linked to genetics and heredity. Gluten intolerance is a life-long disease. Gluten is protein found in wheat products, but it is only found in the endosperm of the grain. Gluten intolerance is triggered by gluten found in wheat, but also in the gluten found in rye, barley, and sometimes oats that are present in the diet. Celiac Disease Foundation website provides lists of food that contain gluten and can be accessed at this URL: https://celiac.org/

Youth onset symptoms for gluten intolerance include: abdominal pain, gas, and distention; chronic diarrhea; vomiting; constipation; pale, foul-smelling or fatty stools; weight loss; failure to thrive; and short stature. Symptoms for adult onset include: unexplained iron deficiency anemia; bone/joint pain; arthritis; bone loss and osteoporosis; depression or anxiety; tingling and numbness; infertility; miscarriages; and dermatitis herpetiformis.

Common sources of gluten in the diet include: bulgar, couscous, durum, einkorn, emmer, farina, triticale, kamut, graham flour, matzo flour and meal, spelt, spelta, wheat germ, wheat starch, barley malt, barley malt extract, semolina, hydrolyzed vegetable protein (HVP), bran, orzo, panko, seitan, udon, and farro. Gluten can also be hidden in processed dairy foods, processed fruits and vegetables, processed meats, fish and poultry, soups and bouillon, matzo and communion wafers, lipstick, toothpaste, gum, mints, licorice, breading, coating mixes, croutons, stuffing, dressing mixes, roux, thickeners, soy sauce, marinades, modified food starch, malt and malt flavoring, supplements, and medications.

In 2014, gluten-free labeling guidelines were released. In order to list gluten-free, no gluten, free of gluten, and without gluten on the label, the food must *not* contain:

- An ingredient that has a gluten-containing grain
- An ingredient that is derived from a gluten-containing grain; unless it has been processed to remove the gluten (threshold: <20 ppm of gluten)

Foods that meet these criteria can carry the gluten-free designation. There are many more gluten-free products in the marketplace to choose from. Most vendors have a gluten-free list of choices that are available to the foodservice operation.

Please refer to the Food Allergy Research & Education "Tips for Avoiding Your Allergen" for a summary of the information provided above.

Treatment and Managing Reactions

Currently, the only way to prevent a food-allergic reaction is to avoid the problem food. Good management starts with a diagnosis of a food allergy, followed by talking to the healthcare team about management of the allergy. In the facility, have a written Food Allergy & Anaphylaxis Emergency Care Plan so that all staff members will know what to do in the event of a reaction.

The only and best way to prevent a food allergy reaction is to avoid the food allergen. For the CDM, CFPP and the foodservice staff, this means having a policy and procedure in place to prevent issues from surfacing.

It starts with getting the right foods. The CDM, CFPP's job is to understand the **Rule of 3** for reading the ingredients:

- Before ordering a product
- When unloading/putting away product
- Before starting a recipe or serving a food

GLOSSARY

Rule of 3
Reading the label/ingredients before ordering a product, when unloading/putting away product, before starting a recipe or serving a food. It is the triple check to make sure you have an allergy-free food

It is the triple check to make sure the food is allergy-free. The labels are to be checked each and every time a food arrives at the door for someone with a food allergy. What if a food was shorted by your distributor and a substitution was made? What if the ingredients in a product change?

The facility should have an established policy for documenting food allergies and procedures for care. The CDM, CFPP will want to clarify the food allergy with the medical staff upon admission. Always consult with the Registered Dietitian Nutritionist about foods and patient care. Be sure to include and gather additional questions in the nutrition assessment.

Work with the distributor to ensure that the right products are ordered. Work with the sales staff and even the nutrition professional on staff with the food vendor to create a menu that will meet the needs of the client. Request and review the food labels and ingredients prior to ordering.

Once the correct products arrive, the CDM, CFPP will need to ensure that there is no cross-contact. Depending on the severity of the food allergy, consider setting up an "allergy-free zone" in the kitchen. Some practices to consider include:

- Assess equipment needs (is there a need for additional equipment to avoid cross-contact).
- Assess food storage area and where allergy-free food will be stored.
- Purchase and store new equipment separately.
- Be aware that rubber, plastic, acrylic, and wooden utensils are porous and can absorb allergens—stainless steel is best.
- Consider a special place to prepare foods in an "allergy-free zone" if you have room.
- Train staff on handling allergy-free foods.

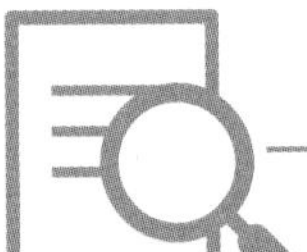

View Supplemental Material for Tips for Avoiding Your Allergen (Food Allergy Research & Education).

Here are some tips to avoid cross-contact:

- Prior to starting, wash hands with soap and water.
- Scrub! Scrubbing is the most effective way to remove allergens. Scrub surfaces and hands prior to starting.
- Always make allergy-free foods first.
- Label foods, cover, and put away to avoid cross-contact.
- If a mistake is made, throw food out and start over.
- Do not share space or equipment if specially designated.
- Separate linens and launder separately.
- Wash dishes, silverware, and cooking equipment separately at the beginning of the shift with the clean water.
- For surfaces use water, soap, and scrubbing! Scrub! Then sanitize.
- Train staff and have lead on each shift responsible for allergy-free food.
- Check each ingredient/food label prior to adding to the recipe.
- Train staff on managing food allergies.

Putting It Into Practice

4. You notice a tray being loaded to take to a patient with a peanut allergy was recently sitting on a table where you know a batch of peanut butter cookies was recently cooling. What should you do?

Food allergy training should include ALL foodservice staff and people that have contact with the client and delivery of food. As the CDM, CFPP working with the RDN, it is important to determine what staff members need to know. Be responsible for the dissemination of information related to the food allergy and policies that assure the right food gets to the right person all of the time. In addition, include food allergy training as a regular part of the in-service schedule and new employee orientation. Train staff to know what to do in the event of an allergic reaction. After an incident, ALWAYS re-evaluate the process and make changes as needed to improve the process. In the organization, the identification of a food allergy should ignite a process to manage the risk of the food allergen. It takes a coordinated, team approach. For more information on food allergies, please visit:

- Food and Drug Administration: www.fda.gov (search for food allergies)
- National Institutes of Health: www.niaid.nih.gov (search for food allergies)
- Food Allergy Research & Education: www.foodallergy.org

SECTION B COMPLEMENTARY AND ALTERNATIVE MEDICINE

Ever been to a chiropractor, a naturopath, or a homeopath? How does this treatment fit into health care? Alternative practices often come up during the provision of nutritional care. It is important to understand complementary and alternative approaches to medical care, how to assess them and promote optimum nutrition for the client. Both terms describe practices that fall outside of conventional medicine in the United States.

The National Center for Complementary and Alternative Medicine (NCCAM) of the National Institutes of Health provides this definition:

> *Complementary and alternative medicine is a group of diverse medical and healthcare systems, practices, and products that are not presently considered to be part of conventional medicine.*

What is meant by **conventional medicine**? This is the science used by physicians (Medical Doctors—MDs and Doctors of Osteopathy—DOs), as well as allied health professionals, as they are trained in the Unites States. Sometimes, conventional medicine is also called mainstream medicine, orthodox medicine, biomedicine, or allopathy.

Any type of intervention that does not fall within this broadly accepted group of practices is **Complementary and Alternative Medicine (CAM). Complementary medicine** is an unconventional medical practice that is used to complement or *add* to conventional medical practice. **Alternative medicine** is an unconventional medical practice that is used *instead of* conventional medicine. CAM therapies may also be called unconventional medicine, simply meaning they are not part of the routine therapeutic approach to treatment.

Integrative medicine is medical practice that combines conventional practice with CAM practices. For example, a physician treating anxiety who prescribes both a drug regimen and meditation is practicing integrative medicine. NCCAM explains: "While scientific evidence exists regarding some CAM therapies, for most there are key questions that are yet to be answered through well-designed scientific studies—questions such as whether these therapies are safe and whether they work for the purposes for which they are used." Figure 4.1 provides information about the more common CAM therapies among adults in the NCCAM survey. Check http://nccam.nih.gov/news/alerts/ for updated information about the safety and effectiveness of CAM therapies.

GLOSSARY

Conventional Medicine
Medicine practiced by physicians (Medical Doctors—MDs and Doctors of Osteopathy—DOs) as well as other trained allied health professionals

Complementary and Alternative Medicine (CAM)
Medicine that does not fall within conventional medicine practice

Complementary Medicine
Using an unconventional medical practice to complement or add to conventional medical practice

Alternative Medicine
Using an unconventional medical practice in place of conventional medicine

Integrative Medicine
Combines conventional medicine with CAM practices

Figure 4.1

CAM Therapy Included in the National Health Interview Survey (NHIS)

CAM Therapy	Definition
Acupuncture	Involves inserting thin needles into specific points on the body to relieve pain or other symptoms.
Ayurveda	A 5,000 year old system of medicine from India aimed to cleanse the body of substances that can cause disease and to balance the body, mind, and spirit.
Biofeedback	Uses electronic devices to teach clients how to consciously regulate bodily functions such as breathing, heart rate, and blood pressure. It is used to reduce stress, eliminate headaches, relieve pain, and recondition injured muscles.
Chelation Therapy	A chemical process used to bind molecules, such as metals or minerals. It has been scientifically proven to rid the body of excess or toxic metals such as lead. This type of therapy is controversial and unproven except for the treatment of mercury and lead poisoning.
Chiropractic or Osteopathic Manipulation	Both are systems of hands-on techniques or adjustments to alleviate pain, restore function, and promote health and well-being.
Deep Breathing Exercises	Involves slow and deep inhalation through the nose followed by slow and complete exhalation.
Diet-Based Therapies	Examples are the South Beach Diet, a vegetarian diet, and the Ornish diet (a high-fiber, low-fat, vegetarian diet: Oils, avocados, nuts and seeds, and all meats are avoided).
Energy Healing Therapy/ Reiki (Ray-Key)	A Japanese word meaning universal life energy. Reiki is based on the belief that when spiritual energy is channeled through Reiki, the patient's spirit is healed, which in turn heals the physical body.
Guided Imagery	Involves relaxation techniques followed by visualizing calm and peaceful images.
Homeopathic Treatment	A belief where "like cures like," meaning that small, highly diluted quantities of medicinal substances are given to cure symptoms. Homeopathic remedies are derived from many natural sources including plants, metals, and minerals.
Hypnosis	An altered state of consciousness used to treat many health conditions including ulcers, chronic pain, respiratory ailments, stress, and headaches.
Massage Therapy	The manipulation of muscle and connective tissue to enhance functions of those tissues to promote relaxation and well-being.
Meditation	Involves techniques from Eastern religious or spiritual traditions where a person learns to focus attention and suspend the stream of thoughts that normally occupy the mind.
Natural Products	Non-vitamins and non-minerals, such as herbs and plant-based products and enzymes.
Naturopathy	Focuses on the healing power in the body that establishes, maintains, and restores health. Treatments include nutrition and lifestyle counseling, dietary supplements, medicinal plants, exercise, homeopathy, and traditional Chinese medicine.
Progressive Relaxation	A system of tensing and relaxing successive muscle groups to relieve tension and stress.
Qi Gong (Chee-Gung)	An ancient Chinese discipline using gentle physical movements, mental focus, and deep breathing directed toward specific parts of the body.
Tai Chi (Ty-Chee)	A mind-body practice that originated as a martial art. Occurs when you move your body slowly and gently while breathing deeply and meditating. It is believed to enhance the flow qi (ancient term meaning vital energy) in the body.
Traditional Healers	An ancient medical practice handed down from generation to generation.
Yoga	An ancient East Indian practice where, in order to be in harmony with oneself and the environment, you must integrate the body, mind, and spirit. This occurs through deep breathing, meditation, and physical postures or poses.

Source: Centers for Disease Control and Prevention, National Center for Health Statistics

The number of people seeking complementary or alternative medicines has increased dramatically in the past decade. A NCCAM report, The Use of Complementary and Alternative Medicine in the United States, indicates "In the U.S., approximately 38 percent of adults (about 4 in 10) and approximately 12 percent of children (about 1 in 9) are using some form of CAM." Figure 4.2 shows the most common CAM therapies among adults from the NCCAM survey. From the NCCAM report, "The most popular natural products are fish oil/omega-3, glucosamine, Echinacea, and flaxseed. Glucosamine is a substance found in the fluid around joints and used by the body to make and repair cartilage. Glucosamine in dietary supplements is made in the laboratory or from the shells of shrimp, lobster, and crabs."

People are willing to pay 11.2 percent of total out-of-pocket expenditures on CAM health care in the U.S. Compare that to the total healthcare expenditures in Figure 4.3.

Figure 4.2

10 Most Common CAM Therapies Among Adults

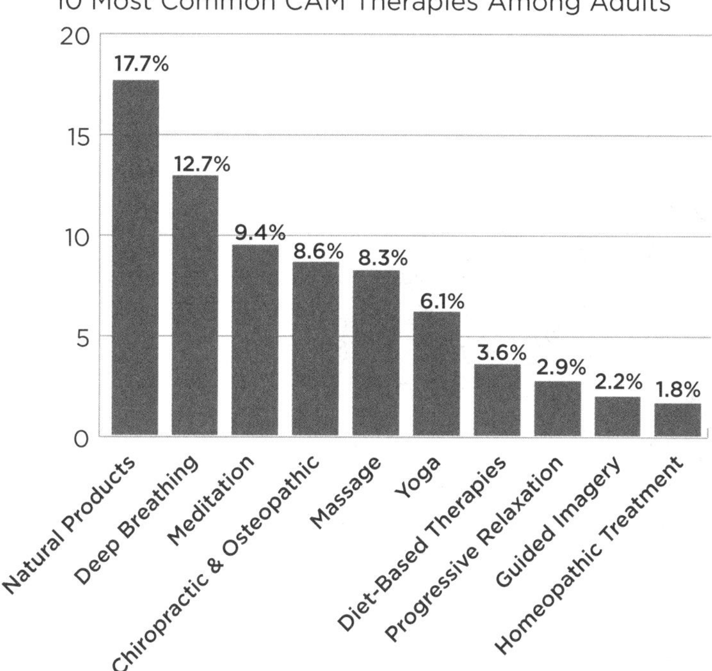

Source: National Center for Complementary and Alternative Medicine

Types of CAM

NCCAM identifies five types of CAM: alternative medical systems, mind-body interventions, biologically-based therapies, manipulative and body-based methods, and energy therapies. Here is a closer look at types of CAM (See Figure 4.1 for explanations and examples). National Institutes of Health (NIH) has a website that you may want to refer to for additional information: https://nccih.nih.gov

Alternative Medical Systems

Represents complete and separate systems for understanding health and illness. Examples include:

- Acupuncture
- Ayureda
- Homeopathic
- Naturopathic

Figure 4.3
CAM Out-of-Pocket Spending

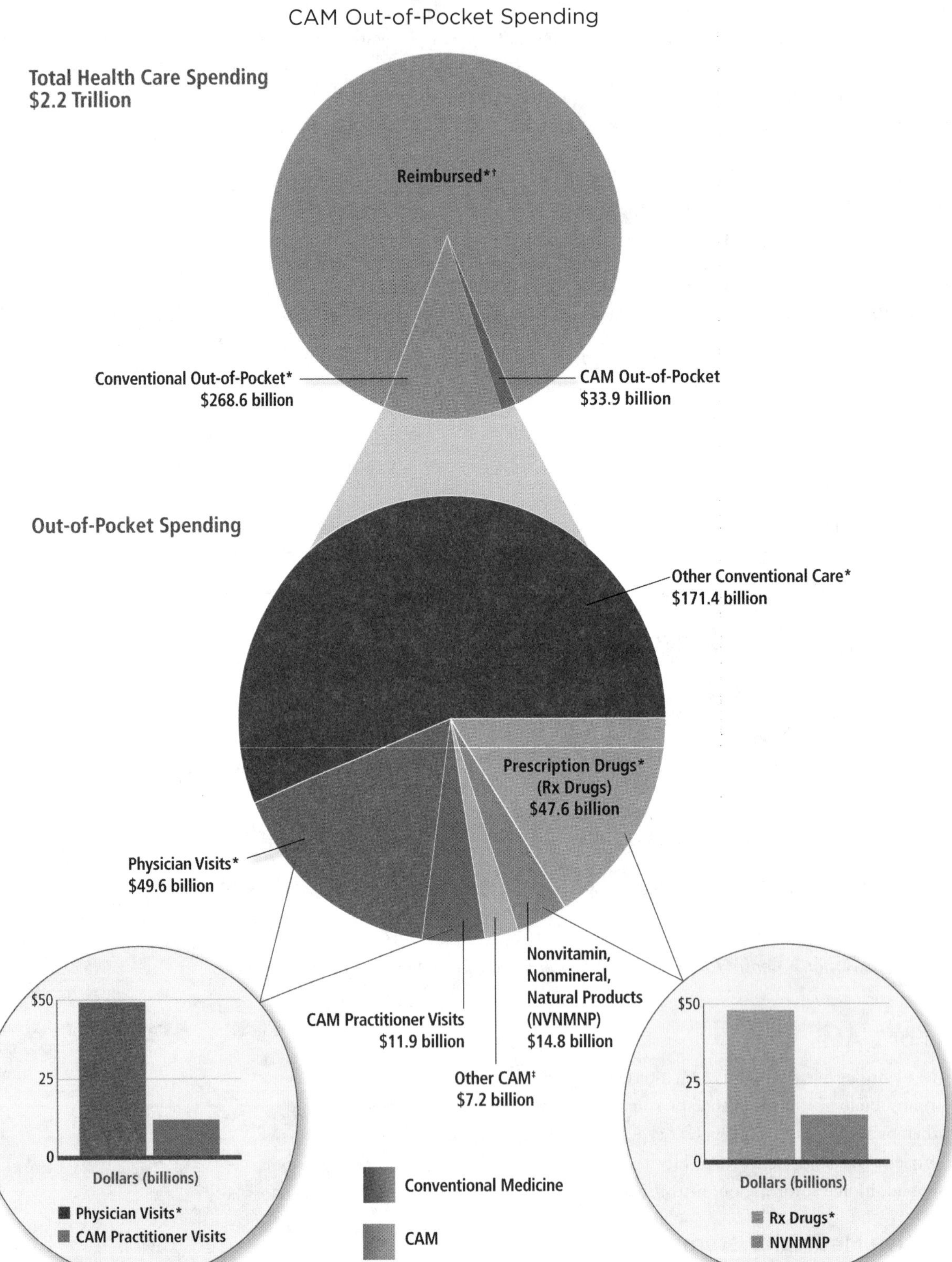

* National Health Expenditure Data for 2007. U.S. Department of Health and Human Services, Centers for Medicare and Medicaid Services Web site. Accessed at: http://www.cms.hhs.gov/NationalHealthExpendData/02_NationalHealthAccountsHistorical.asp#TopOfPage on June 25, 2009.

† Reimbursed spending includes employer and individual private insurance, Medicare, Medicaid, State Children's Health Insurance Program, other private and public spending, and some CAM.

‡ Other CAM includes yoga, tai chi, qi gong classes; homeopathic medicine; and relaxation techniques.

Source: National Center for Complementary and Alternative Medicine

Mind-Body Interventions

Uses the influence of the mind on the body or "mind over matter."

- Biofeedback
- Hypnosis
- Guided imagery
- Traditional healers

Biologically-Based Therapies

Uses biological agents, such as herbs, special foods, or nutritional supplements, to produce therapeutic results.

- Chelation therapy
- Naturopathy
- Natural products
- Probiotics

Manipulative and Body-Based Methods

Involves moving or manipulating parts of the body to promote healing.

- Chiropractic
- Tai Chi
- Massage therapy
- Yoga

Energy Therapies

Uses energy fields believed to surround and penetrate the body.

- Reiki
- Qi Gong

Herbs and Dietary Supplements

Herbs, large doses of vitamins and minerals, and other food components are common forms of CAM. In fact, sales of dietary supplements and foods with added supplements or functional food ingredients total billions of dollars each year. As the role of nutrition in health gains increasing attention from the scientific community, it is easy to believe there is a dietary solution to nearly every condition. This is not exactly true. Dietary practices can become an important component of overall health care, however.

When it comes to herbs and other nutritional supplements, it's important to understand that "natural" does not necessarily mean "safe." Many of nature's poisons are entirely natural—but deadly. Arsenic is an example. Meanwhile, some of today's drug therapies have been derived from plants. An example is digitalis, a medicine for regulating heartbeat. Digitalis comes from the Foxfire plant and was a Native American medicine. Thus, the key point is that any chemical compound that has biological activity—whether derived from natural sources or created in a laboratory—must be evaluated scientifically.

It needs to be proven safe and effective. In addition, the manufacturing practices and dosage need to be controlled.

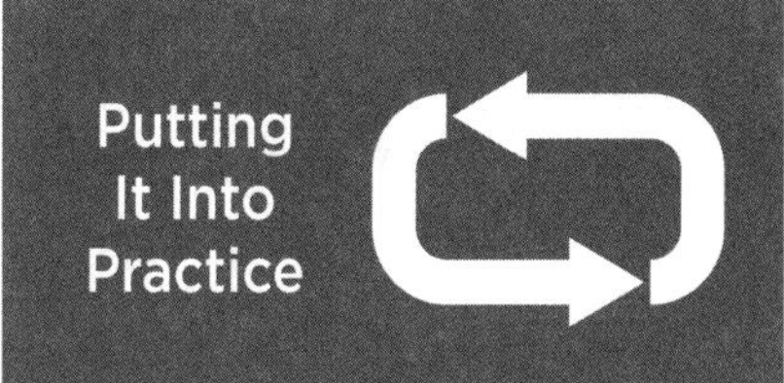

5. A client you are screening mentions he is choosing to use apple cider vinegar to manage his diabetes instead of taking his diabetes medications. Who should you inform of this information?

GLOSSARY

Dietary Supplement
A product that is intended to supplement the diet to increase the total daily intake of a particular substance

U.S. Pharmacopeia (USP)
Model guidelines for prescription drugs

According to the FDA, a **dietary supplement** is:

- A product (other than tobacco) that is intended to supplement the diet that bears or contains one or more of the following dietary ingredients: a vitamin, a mineral, an herb or other botanical, an amino acid, a dietary substance for use by man to supplement the diet by increasing the total daily intake, or a concentrate, metabolite, constituent, extract, or combination of these ingredients.
- Intended for ingestion in pill, capsule, tablet, or liquid form.
- Not represented for use as a conventional food or as the sole item of a meal or diet.
- Labeled as a "dietary supplement."

Under the Dietary Supplement Health and Education Act passed by Congress in 1994, dietary supplements are considered foods, not drugs. It is a manufacturer's responsibility to ensure that their products are safe and properly labeled prior to marketing. This means that dietary supplements are not subject to the same controls as prescription and over-the-counter drugs. For a drug to reach the market, the manufacturer must first prove safety and effectiveness to the FDA. Dietary supplements, in contrast, must be proven unsafe by the FDA to be removed from the market.

In addition, the regulation prohibits dietary supplement manufacturers from making health claims on product labels. For example, a label cannot state that this supplement will "cure cancer" or "treat arthritis." However, manufacturers are allowed to describe the supplement's effects on "structure or function" of the body or "well-being." To use these claims, manufacturers must have substantiation that the statements are truthful and not misleading. A product label must bear the note: "This statement has not been evaluated by the Food and Drug Administration. This product is not intended to diagnose, treat, cure, or prevent any disease." A dietary supplement must have a label identifying its ingredients and must provide nutrition labeling.

Clearly, a dietary supplement package can imply health benefits that may not be well substantiated. What else is not regulated? Controls on product composition, purity and quality, and quantities are minimal. In 2003, the FDA proposed a new rule to control these issues. In short, the contents of a dietary supplement preparation may not be exactly what a consumer thinks. For example, the FDA evaluated a group of soy products on the market and found that some contained as little as half the amount of isoflavones (active ingredients) claimed. Another review found that a supplement of folic acid contained only 35 percent of its declared dose. Conversely, a supplement may contain much larger doses of active ingredients than the label indicates. This can pose risks related to overdosage. In addition, a dietary supplement may contain contaminants such as lead, pesticides, bacteria, or undeclared ingredients. Among other things, the proposed new rule would establish good manufacturing practices for dietary supplements.

In addition, the **U.S. Pharmacopeia (USP)**, which is a research group that is not a part of the government, maintains a certification program for dietary supplements. Based on

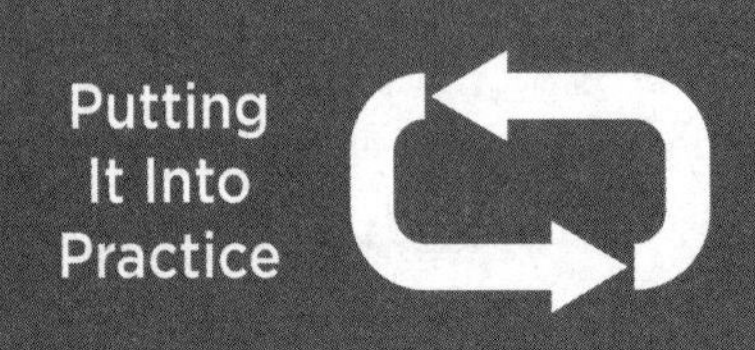

6. Your client mentions his friend suggested he take a zinc supplement because he heard it was good for "men's health." What questions should you ask him?

testing, a supplement can contain a USP certification mark to indicate that ingredients are as claimed. Of course, this mark does not verify that the supplements are effective treatments for specific health conditions nor does it guarantee their safety.

In 2003, the Medicare Prescription Drug Improvement and Modernization Act of 2003 (MMA) was signed into law. As part of that law, U.S. Pharmacopeia (USP) has submitted model guidelines for drug categories and classes that may be used by prescription drug plans to the Centers for Medicare & Medicaid Services (CMS).

It's important to note that safe and effective dosages for herbs and other dietary supplements may not be well established. At least for recognized vitamins and minerals, there are reference standards. Thus, even for an herb that may have beneficial effects, a consumer might not take a dosage that proves beneficial. Or, a consumer may easily overdose. Meanwhile, consumers may mistakenly assume that "more is better" when it comes to supplementation. This can be dangerous. Even a vitamin or mineral known to be essential for life can become toxic in excessive doses. Figure 4.4 identifies overdose risks of several dietary supplements.

Figure 4.4
Risk of Overdose

DIETARY SUPPLEMENT	COMMON USES	EFFECTS OF OVERDOSE
Vitamin B6 > 100 mg/day	A once-popular remedy for carpal tunnel syndrome and premenstrual syndrome (PMS), cardiovascular disease, asthma, autism, and cognition.	Neurological toxicity, nerve injury
Niacin > 500 mg/day	Recommended to help reduce blood cholesterol levels.	Gastrointestinal distress, liver damage, skin flushing and itching, occasionally life-threatening conditions
Vitamin A > 25,000 International Units (IU)/day	Taken to slow the development of macular degeneration, however more research is needed to support supplementation of Vitamin A for this reason.	Liver damage, birth defects, damage to bones and cartilage
Germander	Believed to aid in the treatment for gout. Used in small amounts in the U.S. as a flavoring agent. Banned in France and restricted use in Canada.	Liver disease
Comfrey	Used historically to treat gastrointestinal distress; the oral supplement was banned by the FDA in 2001; may be used topically for sprains, strained muscles.	Liver damage/cirrhosis, sometimes life-threatening
Chaparral	Often consumed as tea for anti-cancer or reducing the effects of radiation or sun damage. It is listed by the FDA as a supplement that should be avoided.	Liver damage

Note: > is the symbol for more than.
Source: Adapted from National Center for Complementary and Alternative Medicine

To avoid overdose of vitamins and minerals, it's helpful to return to basic nutrition science. The body has basic requirements for nutrients. Excesses of many of the water-soluble vitamins are simply excreted in urine. Fat-soluble vitamins and minerals can, in some cases, accumulate in the body. Generally, dietetic professionals recommend that supplementation of vitamins and minerals be used to correct deficiencies, based on an assessment of nutritional status and nutritional needs. A tolerable upper intake level (UL) is the highest level of daily nutrient intake that is likely to pose no risk of adverse health effects for most people. This is different from a recommended level of intake. It provides a reference for evaluating the safety of supplementation.

Drug Interactions

Among the risks of using dietary supplements can be the interactions they present. Herbs, for example, may interact with each other to cause dangerous effects. Herbs may also interact with conventional drugs to modify their action. For instance, the herbal supplement ginkgo has many potential drug interactions. Ginkgo can increase blood levels of antidepressant drugs, accidentally building high drug levels. Used with an antipsychotic medication, ginkgo can cause seizures. Both ginkgo and coenzyme Q10 are supplements that can interfere with the action of anticoagulant medications, such as warfarin or coumadin. The result can be excessive bleeding. Both ginseng and coenzyme Q10 can enhance the action of a drug designed to lower blood sugar. The result can be a crisis with hypoglycemia (very low blood sugar). St. John's Wort may eliminate a number of drugs from the body very quickly. There is concern that taking this supplement may reduce the effectiveness of oral contraceptives. It can also interact with antidepressant drugs to cause headache, upset stomach, and restlessness. Before surgery, it can be dangerous to take certain herbal supplements, including ginseng or goldenseal, which may raise blood pressure. Other herbs can slow down blood clotting and increase the risk of excessive bleeding. These include feverfew, garlic, ginger, and ginkgo.

Because many consumers use dietary supplements as complementary or alternative therapies, they may not choose to discuss these therapies with physicians. Typically, an individual using dietary supplements considers this treatment "separate" from a physician's care. However, it is actually important for a physician to know the complete picture. A CDM, CFPP can facilitate this process by asking patients questions about what dietary supplements they use, reporting this information in the diet history, and discussing it with other members of the healthcare team.

Evaluating CAM Therapies

The following questions can help evaluate any type of medical therapy:

- What research supports the safety of this treatment?
- What are the possible risks and side effects?
- What research indicates this treatment is effective?
- Has research been published in a peer-reviewed journal that is reviewed by trained medical scientists?

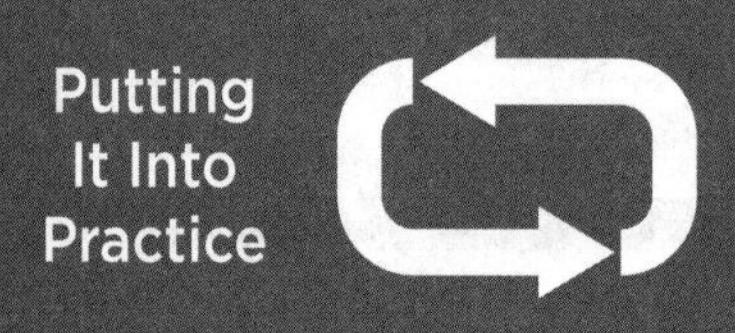

7. A client's family member brought him over-the-counter ginkgo biloba supplements after the client had mentioned he was having difficulty remembering things. What further information would be important to determine safety? Who would you report this information to?

- Has the research been well-controlled, or is the therapy based on anecdotal reports?
- What will the treatment involve?
- What will it cost?
- Is this treatment intended to complement other therapies or replace them (alternative medicine)?
- Has this treatment been discussed with a physician?
- What are the other options and how does this treatment compare?

Figure 4.5 identifies red flags that may indicate fad or fraud in proposed treatments. In addition, the FDA notes that four key assumptions often come into play when consumers are making decisions about therapies. These appear in Figure 4.6.

Healthcare Policy

In 2003, the White House Commission on CAM Policy issued policy suggestions for the healthcare industry. They recommended 10 principles for healthcare policy:

1. A wholeness orientation in healthcare delivery. Health involves all aspects of life—mind, body, spirit, environment—and high-quality health care must support care of the whole person.
2. Evidence of safety and efficacy. The Commission is committed to promoting the use of science and appropriate scientific methods to help identify safe and effective CAM services and products, and to generate evidence that will protect and promote the public health.
3. The healing capacity of the person. The person has a remarkable capacity for recovery and self-healing and a major focus of health care is to support and promote this capacity.
4. Respect for individuality. Every person is unique and has the right to health care that is appropriately responsive to him or her, respecting preferences and preserving dignity.
5. The right to choose treatment. Every person has the right to choose freely among safe and effective care or approaches, as well as among qualified practitioners who are accountable for their claims and actions and responsive to the person's needs.

Figure 4.5
Fads, Frauds, and Quackery

The following claims are cause for caution. Each is a red flag suggesting that the scientific basis for safety and effectiveness may be missing. Based on these red flags, a treatment could be a fad, fraud, or form of quackery. Quackery is a medical treatment that does not perform as claimed and is offered by an untrained or uniformed individual.

Medical Cure:	The treatment is described as a miracle, breakthrough, or cure-all. Few treatments are actually effective!
Anecdotal Evidence: **(Reported Observations)**	Descriptions of the treatment use stories about individual success, rather than citing controlled medical research.
Shaky Terminology:	Some unfounded treatments may claim to purify, energize, or detoxify the body. These terms have little scientific meaning.

Source: Food and Drug Administration

Figure 4.6
Four Questionable Assumptions

1. **"Even if a product may not help me, at least it won't hurt me."**

It's best not to assume that this will always be true. When consumed in high enough amounts, for a long enough time, or in combination with certain other substances, all chemicals can be toxic, including nutrients, plant components, and other biologically active ingredients.

2. **"When I see the term 'natural,' it means that a product is healthful and safe."**

Consumers can be misled if they assume this term assures wholesomeness, or that these food-like substances necessarily have milder effects, which makes them safer to use than drugs. The term "natural" on labels is not well-defined and is sometimes used ambiguously to imply unsubstantiated benefits or safety. For example, many weight-loss products claim to be "natural" or "herbal," but this doesn't necessarily make them safe. Their ingredients may interact with drugs or may be dangerous for people with certain medical conditions.

3. **"A product is safe when there is no cautionary information on the product label."**

Dietary supplement manufacturers may not necessarily include warnings about potential adverse effects on the labels of their products. If consumers want to know about the safety of a specific dietary supplement, they should contact the manufacturer of that brand directly. It is the manufacturer's responsibility to determine that the supplement it produces or distributes is safe, and that there is substantiated evidence that the label claims are truthful and not misleading.

4. **"A recall of a harmful product guarantees that all such harmful products will be immediately and completely removed from the marketplace."**

A product recall of a dietary supplement is voluntary and while many manufacturers do their best, a recall does not necessarily remove all harmful products from the marketplace.

Source: Food and Drug Administration

6. An emphasis on health promotion and self-care. Good health care emphasizes self-care and early intervention for maintaining and promoting health.
7. Partnerships are essential for integrated healthcare. Good health care requires teamwork among clients, healthcare practitioners (conventional and CAM) and researchers committed to creating optimal healing environments, and to respecting the diversity of all healthcare traditions.
8. Education as a fundamental healthcare service. Education about prevention, healthful lifestyles and the power of self-healing should be made an integral part of the curricula of all health care professionals, and should be made available to the public.
9. Dissemination of comprehensive and timely information. The quality of health care can be enhanced by promoting efforts that thoroughly and thoughtfully examine the evidence on which CAM systems, practices, and products are based, and making this evidence widely, rapidly, and easily available.
10. Integral public involvement. The input of informed consumers and other members of the public must be incorporated in setting priorities for health care, healthcare research, and in reaching policy decisions, including those related to CAM, within the public and private sectors.

In its report, the White House Commission on CAM Policy also offered more perspective that is helpful to CDM, CFPPs in evaluating CAM:

> Although most CAM modalities have not yet been proven to be safe and effective, it is likely that some of them eventually will be proven to be safe and effective, whereas others will not...
>
> The question is not, *Should Americans be using complementary and alternative medicine modalities?* Many Americans are already doing so. For the most part, however, they are making these choices in the absence of valid scientific information to guide them in making informed and intelligent choices. (*Source: White House Commission on CAM Policy*)
>
> Many of the commissioners agree with the editors of *The New England Journal of Medicine* who stated in 1998: "There cannot be two kinds of medicine—conventional and alternative. There is only medicine that has been adequately tested and medicine that has not, medicine that works and medicine that may or may not work. Once a treatment has been tested rigorously, it no longer matters whether it was considered alternative at the outset. If it is found to be reasonably safe and effective, it will be accepted." (*Source: White House Commission on CAM Policy*)

A CDM, CFPP's Role

In line with recommended healthcare policy and the state of knowledge on CAM therapies today, CDM, CFPPs and others involved in providing health care can take several approaches to CAM:

- Recognize the individual rights of healthcare consumers to choose their own care.
- Respect individual preferences.
- Facilitate communications with clients about CAM therapies, particularly use of dietary supplements. Have an RDN or a pharmacist review the list of therapies used to prevent drug-nutrient interactions.
- Help communicate information about individuals' CAM therapy choices to the entire healthcare team.
- Inform clients of possible risks; help to educate.
- Keep an open mind and continue to keep abreast of new findings in this fast-growing area of medical science.

Chapter References

RESOURCES	
Centers for Disease Control and Prevention. National Health Interview Survey. National Center for Health Statistics.*	https://www.cdc.gov/nchs/nhis/index.htm
National Council Against Health Fraud.* Updated September 18, 2019.	https://www.ncahf.org
The United States Pharmacopeial Convention*	https://www.usp.org
U.S. Department of Health and Human Services. Food Allergy. National Institute of Allergy and Infectious Diseases.* Updated October 29, 2018.	https://www.niaid.nih.gov/diseases-conditions/food-allergy
U.S. Department of Health and Human Services. National Center for Complementary and Integrative Health.*	https://nccih.nih.gov
U.S. Department of Health and Human Services. Alerts and Advisories. National Center for Complementary and Integrative Health.* Updated March 4, 2019.	https://nccih.nih.gov/news/alerts
U.S. Food and Drug Administration. What You Need to Know About Food Allergies.* Updated September 26, 2018.	https://www.fda.gov/food/buy-store-serve-safe-food/what-you-need-know-about-food-allergies
White House Commission on Complementary and Alternative Medicine Policy Final Report.* Published March 2002.	http://govinfo.library.unt.edu/whccamp/pdfs/fr2002_document.pdf

** Accessed September 18, 2019*

Overview of Body Systems and Medical Nutrition Therapy Interventions

Overview and Objectives

Medical nutrition therapy is important for the prevention and/or treatment of many diseases. A Certified Dietary Manager®, Certified Food Protection Professional® (CDM®, CFPP®) is often responsible for implementing therapeutic diets. Therefore, an understanding of body systems, related health conditions, and diet planning is a cornerstone of the profession. After completing this chapter, you should be able to:

- Identify basic medical nutrition terminology, as related to the gastrointestinal tract, the hepatic and renal systems, and other conditions of the body (Alzheimer's disease and developmental disabilities)
- Define the basic concepts of medical nutrition therapy, as related to the gastrointestinal tract, the hepatic and renal systems, and other conditions of the body (Alzheimer's disease and developmental disabilities)
- Relate basic concepts to nutrition deficiency and excess
- Relate basic concepts of medical nutrition therapy, as related to the gastrointestinal tract, the hepatic and renal systems, and other conditions of the body (Alzheimer's disease and developmental disabilities)
- Compare basic concepts to current diet manual or accepted resource
- Explain utilization of medical nutrition therapy in long-term care and acute care settings

5

GLOSSARY

Chronic Diseases
Degenerative diseases of body organs which may be related to diet

Medical Nutrition Therapy (MNT)
Nutrition assessment and treatment of clients with an illness, disease-related condition or injury, in order to benefit the health of the client

A quote by an unknown author states, "Health is the slowest rate at which you can die." Can what is eaten really affect the risk of disease? *Dietary Guidelines for Americans* reveals what many already suspect: there is a strong correlation between diet and health. A poor diet is related to chronic diseases such as obesity, cardiovascular disease (atherosclerosis, stroke), Type 2 Diabetes, hypertension, hyperlipidemia, some cancers, and osteoporosis. These diseases are classified as problems of nutrient excess. As discussed in previous chapters, in the first part of the twentieth century, nutrition-related problems involved inadequate amounts of nutrients resulting in a deficiency. While those still exist today, **chronic diseases** have increased to epidemic proportions.

The CDM, CFPP and the Nutrition Care Team will be responsible for providing nutrition intervention to protect the health of the client. The need for nutrition intervention is determined and accounts for the actual needs of an individual or group, adjusting nutrient levels and fine-tuning the balance of nutrients to promote wellness. What exactly needs to be done can vary based on an individual's medical condition and how body systems are functioning. At times, a diet helps to compensate for unhealthy shifts in the body's metabolism and functioning. This chapter will explore these ideas in detail. This chapter is divided into three sections that address the following:

- **Section A**—Gastrointestinal System, Medical Nutrition Therapy, and Modified Consistency Diets
- **Section B**—Organs That Impact Digestion: Liver, Gallbladder, Pancreas, and Kidneys
- **Section C**—Additional Medical Nutrition Therapy for Alzheimer's Disease, Immobility, and Developmental Disabilities

Medical Nutrition Therapy (MNT)

Sometimes dietary changes are dictated by health conditions. As a group, these changes are called therapeutic or modified diets. Medical nutrition therapy is a broader term. **Medical nutrition therapy (MNT)** is the nutritional assessment and treatment of a condition, illness, or injury that places an individual at risk. It involves two components: assessment of the client's nutritional status and treatment/intervention. MNT generally focuses on individuals at risk for nutritional problems. Nutrition screening is part of the healthcare process to identify individuals at risk.

Treatment may include therapeutic diets, counseling, and/or the use of nutrition support and goes hand-in-hand with other therapies, such as medication, surgery, physical therapy, radiation, and many others. Foodservice professionals work with others on the healthcare team to address the medical therapeutic needs of clients. All MNT intervention must be done in consultation with the Registered Dietitian Nutritionist.

A therapeutic diet is a regular diet that has been modified to meet a client's special nutrient needs. Diets may be adjusted to control specific nutrients. Examples include calorie-controlled diets for weight loss, fat and cholesterol-controlled diets for treatment of cardiovascular disease, and sodium-controlled diets used in hypertension or renal (kidney) disease. Even water or fluid may need to be limited—or increased—based on medical conditions. Protein needs to be limited during renal failure. Furthermore, some therapeutic diets accommodate difficulties in chewing or swallowing—such as pureed diets or dysphagia diets. Others are used in treatment of problems in the digestive system. These include clear liquid diets, very low-fat diets, and gluten-free diets. As can be seen, medical nutrition therapy is critical in the treatment of many diseases, and is directed by the Registered Dietitian Nutritionist and the other members of the Nutrition Care Team.

SECTION A GASTROINTESTINAL SYSTEM, MNT, AND MODIFIED CONSISTENCY DIETS

The gastrointestinal (GI) tract involves several organs and runs through the center of the body, starting with the mouth and ending with the anus. A number of dietary disorders, chronic illnesses, or simple GI upsets can affect the GI tract. This chapter provides a brief introduction to the most common GI conditions and medical nutrition therapy, starting with the mouth. Review Figure 3.1 (Chapter 3) to see the GI tract organs.

Dentition and Tooth Decay

Dentition is the development of teeth in the gums of a human, their arrangement, and the function of those teeth in the process of digestion. The teeth (mechanical breakdown) and mouth (chemical breakdown—saliva) provide the beginning of the digestive process. Dental caries or cavities are a major health issue caused by eating sugary and starchy foods. The more often these foods—even small amounts—are eaten and the longer they are in the mouth before teeth are brushed, the greater the risk for tooth decay. This is because every time we eat something containing sugar or starch, the bacteria that naturally live on teeth produce acid for 20 to 30 minutes. This acid eats away at the teeth, and cavities may eventually develop. Eating sugary or starchy foods as frequent between-meal snacks may be more harmful to teeth than having them at meals. Foods such as dried fruits, candies, soda pop, breads, cereals, cookies, and crackers increase chances of dental caries when eaten frequently. Fruit chews and chewy candies are particularly troublesome. Foods that do not seem to cause cavities include some vegetables, meats, fish, aged cheeses, and nuts. To prevent cavities, it is important to brush teeth frequently and floss daily.

Tooth decay leads to tooth loss and dentures or dental bridges later in life. If a person is **edentulous**—having no teeth or toothless—it can cause significant issues with eating properly. Approximately 50 percent of Americans have lost their teeth by age 65. Despite widespread use of dentures, chewing still presents problems for many elderly people who may require a modified consistency diet.

> **GLOSSARY**
>
> **Dentition**
> The development of teeth in the gums of a human, their arrangement, and the function of those teeth in the process of digestion
>
> **Edentulous**
> Absence of teeth (i.e., toothless)

Modified Consistency Diets

Some clients have difficulty chewing or swallowing due to surgery, loose-fitting dentures, missing teeth, inadequate saliva production (this commonly occurs in aging), mouth injury or infection, surgery of the head and neck, or stroke. Depending on the nature and severity of the problem, any of the following diets that are modified in consistency may be needed: pureed diet, mechanical soft, or dysphagia diet. Each is described below.

Pureed Diet

A pureed diet includes foods that require very little (if any) chewing and may be recommended for alert clients with impaired ability to chew or swallow. Pureed foods typically do not look very appetizing, thus, many foodservice operators are making efforts to improve the appearance of pureed foods. For example, thickeners may be used to make pureed foods cohesive and shaped into forms like their original food source. There are several commercial thickeners that use different types of starches, vegetable gums, pectin, and proteins. Some facilities use cornstarch or dry mashed potato flakes instead of commercial thickeners. Many commercial food thickeners are powdered and can be mixed with liquids and pureed foods. Pre-formed frozen products are also available.

Mechanical Soft Diet

A mechanical soft diet is a modification of the regular diet, and consists of foods that are easy to chew. Figure 5.1 lists guidelines for a mechanical soft diet and includes foods on a regular diet that are modified for consistency. Because each client's need for chopped or ground foods varies, this diet should be individualized to each client, and reassessed as needed.

Dysphagia Diet

Dysphagia means difficulty swallowing. A number of signs may suggest a problem with dysphagia:

- Oral leaking or drooling
- Choking or gagging
- Pocketing food (capturing it in the cheeks)
- Taking longer than two to ten seconds to swallow
- Weakness, poor motivation
- Poor chewing ability, which may lead to choking on food

GLOSSARY

Dysphagia
Difficulty swallowing

Figure 5.1
Guidelines for a Mechanical Soft Diet

- Meat and poultry may be ground or chopped (as specified in the diet order), or moistened to become tender. Ground meats can be used in soups, stews, and casseroles. Cooked dried beans and peas, soft cheeses, and eggs are additional softer protein sources. Fish must be flaked.
- Dice or chop vegetables if needed and cook thoroughly without skins.
- Serve mashed potatoes or rice with gravy, if desired.
- Salads are possible if chopped and tolerated by the client.
- Soft, ripe fruits such as fresh bananas, berries, or melon; canned peaches, pears, or applesauce are some possible choices.
- Soft breads can be made even softer by removing the crust, if needed.
- Puddings and custard are good dessert choices.
- No nuts or seeds are allowed, as they are hard to chew.

Source: Adapted from Nutrition 411

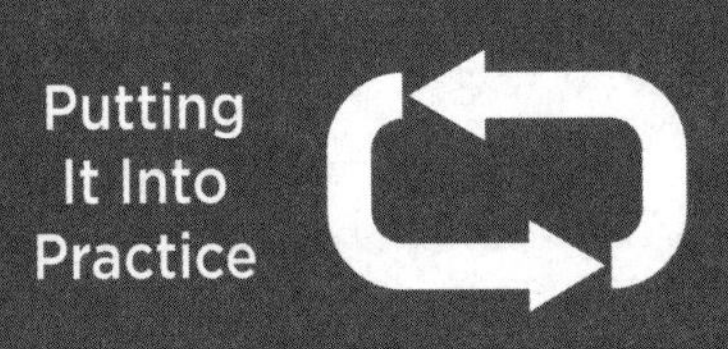

1. You notice on the trayline that a client has a mechanical soft diet, but the tray contains a lettuce salad with crackers. Can the patient have these foods?

If these signs are present, the client may need further evaluation to avoid severe choking or aspiration. This information should be referred to the Registered Dietitian Nutritionist or nursing supervisor so the speech pathologist can be notified. In all, up to 14 percent of hospitalized patients and up to 50 percent of residents in nursing homes may be experiencing some form of dysphagia. Dysphagia may be caused by stroke, neurological disease, dementia, or other factors. It poses the danger of aspiration and choking, while also increasing the likelihood of dehydration and malnutrition. There are many variations of dysphagia; it's a very individualized condition. A speech pathologist can perform an indepth evaluation of swallowing, and recommend the type of dietary treatment required.

There is no universal diet for clients with dysphagia. One misconception about dysphagia is that foods need to be thin and liquid in order to be swallowed. On the contrary, liquids (especially thin liquids) are usually harder to swallow than solid foods.

A number of experts collaborated over three years to develop a way for dysphagia diets to use standardized language worldwide, thus creating the International Dysphagia Diet Standardisation Initiative (IDDSI) in 2013. IDDSI was created to reduce confusion for the different dysphagia diet textures and liquids for healthcare professionals and caregivers, and to reduce occurrences of choking and aspiration. Figure 5.2a demonstrates the IDDSI framework. The IDDSI framework will be the standard starting in 2021. Please check the Supplemental Material for further details and announcements on IDDSI.

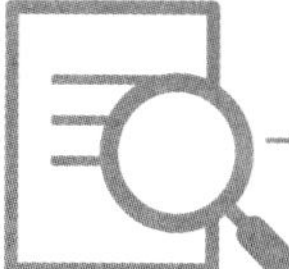

There is also an International Dysphagia Diet that is a global standard with definitions to describe textured-modified foods. Learn more at www.iddsi.org.

More details on the International Dysphagia Diet Standardisation Initiative can be found in the Supplemental Materials.

The National Dysphagia Diet (NDD), now the national standard for dietary treatment of dysphagia, accounts for modifications in food textures, as well as liquids. Based on evaluation, a customized dysphagia diet recommendation contains two specifications: one for food texture, and a second one for liquids. Thus, a dysphagia diet may be specified as: NDD 3 or Dysphagia Advanced with thin liquids, or NDD Level 1 or Dysphagia Pureed with honey-thick liquids. Figure 5.2a and 5.2b describe IDDSI and NDD guidelines. Additional lists of food may be accessed at the Ohio State University Wexner Medical Center website: https://patienteducation.osumc.edu/Pages/search.aspx?k=dysphagia+

When clients have swallowing problems, the speech pathologist may encourage special positioning and other suggestions to help ease swallowing during meals. In general, positioning residents as close to a 90-degree angle as possible makes swallowing both easier and safer. If clients are in bed, they may need support for their heads, backs, necks, and sides. It may also be helpful to wait for the client to swallow prior to placing any more food in the mouth, and alternate solids and liquids.

Nausea and Vomiting

Nausea is an unpleasant feeling in the stomach, accompanied by an urge to vomit. A number of medical conditions and medications can prompt nausea. Because nauseous clients do not feel like eating, nausea that lasts for more than a few days can create nutrition concerns.

Whereas a muscular process called peristalsis normally moves foods down the gastrointestinal tract, vomiting occurs when the waves of peristalsis reverse direction. Vomiting is often seen as a symptom of a disease or of the body's equilibrium being upset (i.e. motion sickness). Vomiting is often seen as a symptom of a disease or of the body's equilibrium being upset (i.e. motion sickness). Vomiting is the body's way to get rid of an irritating substance, and is not dangerous unless large amounts of fluids are

Figure 5.2a
The IDDSI Framework

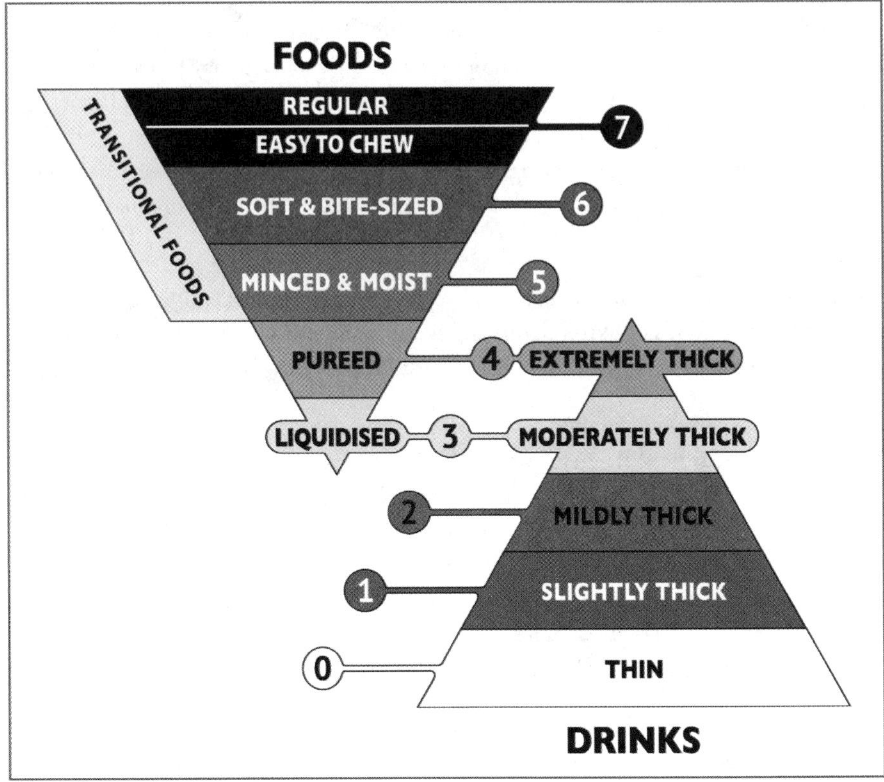

Figure 5.2b
National Dysphagia Diet Liquid Levels

1. THIN	3. HONEY-LIKE
Thin liquids include clear liquids, milk, commercial nutritional supplements, water, tea, coffee, soda, beer, wine, broth, and clear juice. Individuals tolerating thin liquids will also be able to tolerate foods containing thin liquids, such as watermelon, grapefruit, or oranges. Foods like ice cream, frozen yogurt, or plain gelatin which turn to liquid in the mouth are also considered thin liquids.	Honey-like resembles the consistency of honey at room temperature. Commercial thickeners can be added to bring liquids to this level of thickness or purchased commercially pre-thickened to honey-like thickness.
2. NECTAR-LIKE	**4. SPOON-THICK**
Medium thickened liquids include nectars, vegetable juices, and handmade milkshakes or shakes made with thickeners. Thin liquids can be thickened with commercial thickeners or purchased pre-thickened to nectar-like thickness.	This includes high viscosity liquids too thick for a straw. Commercial thickeners can be added to any beverage to obtain this level of thickness or purchased commercially pre-thickened to spoon-thick.

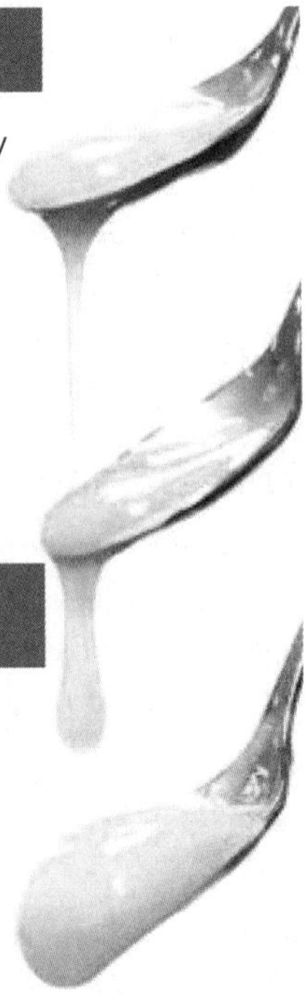

Source: Nutrition 411.

lost. In simple cases of vomiting it's recommended to refrain from eating or drinking for at least four hours followed by intake of a small amount of liquid as tolerated. When vomiting is prolonged, medical care to replace lost fluids and restore electrolyte balance is essential. Medical nutrition therapy for nausea and vomiting frequently calls for using the **BRAT diet**. BRAT is an acronym for:

- Bananas
- Rice
- Applesauce
- Toast

Consuming these more bland foods may give the stomach a rest because they are easier to digest. In the past, the BRAT diet was often given to children when they had nausea and vomiting. The research now suggests that children should return to a normal diet as quickly as possible in order to assure adequate nutrition. Ginger has been shown to alleviate nausea and vomiting in some patients.

Gastroesophageal Reflux Disease (GERD)

Gastroesophageal reflux disease (GERD) or reflux esophagitis is the medical term for acid indigestion or heartburn. Normally, the lower esophageal sphincter muscle relaxes to let food into the stomach, and then closes immediately so the acidic stomach contents won't go back up the esophagus. When this muscle doesn't close tightly, the acidic stomach contents splash up into the esophagus, causing irritation. This irritation is often described as acid indigestion or heartburn. Reflux esophagitis frequently develops in aging. It can also be caused by a condition called a hiatal hernia. Normally, the lower esophageal sphincter sits right in the diaphragm (a strong muscle that separates the abdominal cavity from the chest cavity). The esophagus sits above the diaphragm and the stomach is below it. In the case of a hiatal hernia, part of the stomach extends up through the diaphragm into the chest cavity. Because the diaphragm no longer reinforces the esophageal sphincter, stomach contents reflux into the esophagus.

Unfortunately, reflux esophagitis causes more harm than just a burning sensation. Chronic heartburn can result in inflamed and scarred tissue in the esophagus, which can reduce its inner diameter. This is known as esophageal stricture, and this condition can eventually become cancerous.

MNT goals include reducing gastric acidity and preventing esophageal reflux. Treatment for reflux esophagitis often includes the following:

- Avoid/limit foods that irritate the esophagus: citrus fruits and juice, tomatoes, spicy foods (i.e., chili powder and black pepper), and coffee.
- Avoid/limit foods that relax the lower esophageal sphincter: alcohol; caffeinated drinks such as coffee, tea, and cola soft drinks; chocolate, peppermint, spearmint, and fat.
- Eat smaller amounts of food at meals and drink most fluids between meals.
- Reduce fat intake. High-fat meals empty from the stomach slowly.
- Wait two to three hours after eating a meal to lie down or exercise.
- Wear clothing that does not constrict the waist or abdomen, so as not to increase the upward pressure on the lower esophageal sphincter.
- Refrain from stooping over; instead bend from the knees.

GLOSSARY

BRAT Diet
Diet commonly recommended for nausea and vomiting that contains bananas, rice, applesauce, and toast. They are easier to digest and give the GI tract a rest

Gastroesophageal Reflux Disease (GERD)
Acid indigestion or heartburn

- Elevate the head of the bed.
- If overweight, lose weight, since obesity increases pressure on the stomach leading to gastroesophageal reflux.
- Avoid smoking.

In addition, physicians may prescribe any of a variety of medications to help control GERD, including antacids and drugs that prevent acid production in the stomach.

Gastritis and Peptic Ulcer Disease

GLOSSARY

Gastritis
Inflammation of the stomach lining

Peptic Ulcer Disease (PUD)
Term used to describe chronic inflammation of the stomach and duodenum

Gastritis is a painful inflammation of the mucosal lining of the stomach. The top layer of cells lining the stomach, called the mucosa, protects the stomach lining from the acidic gastric juices. Gastritis symptoms may include nausea, vomiting, anorexia, pain, bleeding, and belching.

Gastritis may be either acute (meaning it has a relatively short duration) or chronic (meaning it lasts a long time). Causes of acute gastritis include: H. pyloric infection, chronic use of aspirin or other NSAIDS, steroid use, alcohol abuse, ingestion of erosive substances, tobacco, or a combination of these. Nutrition care generally includes withholding food for one to two days to let the stomach rest and heal.

Ulcerative colitis is often seen in the elderly. As this type of gastritis progresses, stomach cells become smaller in size, stomach secretions decrease, and production of intrinsic factor (needed for vitamin B12 absorption) decreases. MNT for chronic gastritis involves an individualized diet that avoids foods causing discomfort.

According to the National Institutes of Health, ulcers affect more than 25 million Americans at some point in their lives. Those who suffer an ulcer describe it as a burning, cramping, gnawing, or aching in the abdomen that comes in waves, for three to four days at a time, but may subside completely for weeks or months. Pain is worst before meals and at bedtime, when the stomach is usually empty.

Mention "ulcer" and most people envision a stressed-out, workaholic, junk food-gobbling worrier. But that image is substantially incorrect. Now, the medical community views painful ulcers in a new light—as an easily treatable bacterial infection. The name of the bacteria is Helicobacter pylori. The ulcer itself in an open sore in the lining of the stomach (called a gastric ulcer) or in the first few centimeters of the duodenum (called a duodenal ulcer). The mucosa is eroded away, exposing the underlying submucosa, which is rich in nerves and blood vessels. Ulcers therefore cause pain and possibly bleeding. Regardless of location, **peptic ulcer disease (PUD)** is the term used to describe chronic inflammation of the stomach and duodenum.

Treatment for PUD generally includes anti-secretory drugs (drugs that reduce the amount of acid secreted in the stomach), antibiotics, antacids, and MNT. Examples of

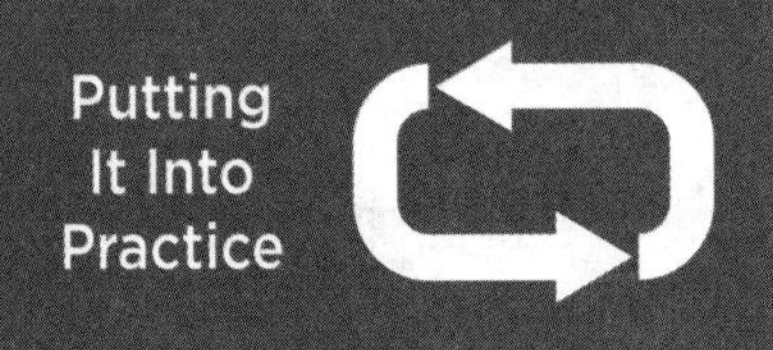

2. Often after meals, you notice a client has to clear his throat frequently. He also seems to have a raspy, almost gurgling, voice when you are chatting with him. What should you do?

antisecretory drugs used in peptic ulcer disease include Tagamet® (cimetidine), Pepcid® (famotidine), and Zantac® (ranitidine hydrochloride). The use of antibiotics to remove Helicobacter pylori prevents most peptic ulcers from recurring.

The MNT goals for PUD revolve around reducing and neutralizing stomach acid secretion and limiting discomfort. These goals can be met by:

- Avoiding any foods or beverages that cause indigestion (dyspepsia)
- Eating small, frequent meals and avoiding large meals that cause stomach distention

The foods allowed on the soft/bland diet have changed over the years, and now the diet is much more liberal. Because of the success of drugs and antacids in reducing gastric acid levels, this diet is not recommended often, and may be nearly obsolete. The soft/bland diet usually excludes the following gastric stimulants:

- Alcohol
- Regular and decaffeinated coffee
- Red and black pepper

Like many other diets, the soft/bland diet should be individualized to meet each client's needs.

Gastroparesis

Gastroparesis means gastro (stomach) paresis (paralysis). For people with diabetes, it may also be called diabetic enteropathy. Gastroparesis is seen more frequently in those with diabetes and occurs when the vagus nerve in the stomach ceases to function. There are two types of digestion action in the stomach: chemical, from the hydrochloric acid; and mechanical, from the stomach pulsing to break up the food. That pulsing action is driven by the vagus nerve. When the vagus nerve is damaged from diabetes, the pulsing, churning action in the stomach does not occur. The food is not broken down and the stomach empties too slowly into the small intestine.

Medical nutrition therapy for gastroparesis involves reducing the amount of food eaten at one time and limiting those foods that are harder to digest such as high-fiber and high-fat foods. Additional nutrition strategies include:

- Consume more foods in liquid form.
- Eat smaller, more frequent meals (6-8 or more if necessary).
- Consume solid food early in the day and switch to liquids for the evening meal.
- Restrict high fiber and high-fat foods.
- Chew foods extremely well so some mechanical breakdown of the food occurs before it enters the stomach.

GLOSSARY

Gastroparesis
Paralysis of the stomach caused by damage to the vagus nerve, causing slow emptying of the stomach. Also referred to as diabetic enteropathy

Inflammatory Bowel Disease (IBD)
Ulceration of the mucosa lining in both the large and small intestine. Two types of IBD are ulcerative colitis and Crohn's disease

Inflammatory Bowel Disease

Inflammatory bowel disease (IBD) includes two conditions with similar symptoms and clinical management: Crohn's disease and ulcerative colitis. The causes for either disease are not known, and there is no cure. They often present for the first time between 15 and 30 years of age, but may continue for a lifetime.

Crohn's disease, also called regional enteritis, is characterized by long-term, progressive inflammation of sections of the intestinal tract and lesions in the mucosal wall of the small intestine, large intestine, and/or rectum. The lesions often go through the entire intestinal wall. Chronic inflammation can cause fistulas (abnormal passages from an internal organ to a body surface or to another internal organ), abscesses (localized inflammation), and obstruction. Symptoms include persistent diarrhea, abdominal pain, fatigue, malabsorption, weight loss, anemia, fever, and anorexia.

During acute phases of Crohn's disease, enteral and parenteral nutrition may be used, particularly if the client has part of the intestines surgically removed. Once the acute phase closes, medical nutrition therapy often includes a diet high in protein (due to the protein losses from the mucosal lesions and poor dietary intake) and calories (due to weight loss commonly seen). Fiber is generally limited if intestines are inflamed, and fat is limited if it is not being absorbed properly. Any other offending foods, such as milk in the case of lactose intolerance, should be omitted. Supplemental vitamins and minerals are often used.

Ulcerative colitis is a disease that causes inflammation and sores, called ulcers, in the lining of the large intestine. Ulcerative colitis usually affects the lower part of the colon. Inflammation destroys intestinal cells, resulting in ulcers. Intestinal mucosa become so fragile that they bleed easily. Symptoms include painful diarrhea (often bloody), rectal bleeding, dehydration, anorexia, and malnutrition.

During active phases of ulcerative colitis, bowel rest is often necessary, meaning the client cannot eat or drink anything by mouth. Once the client resumes eating, the same guidelines are used for ulcerative colitis as for Crohn's disease.

A high-protein diet is one in which high-protein snacks or supplements, from the dairy and protein groups, are given in addition to the regular diet. The diet consists of approximately 1.5 grams of protein/kilogram of body weight per day for an adult. An effective diet is also high in calories.

Diverticular Disease

Diverticulosis is a disease of the intestine in which the intestinal walls become weakened and bulge out into pockets called *diverticula*. (A single one of these pockets is called a *diverticulum*.) About 10 percent of Americans over 40, and half of Americans over 60, have diverticula. Most don't know it. There are no symptoms unless these pouches become infected or inflamed due to fecal matter collecting in the pockets. This condition develops in about one or two out of every 10 people who have diverticula, and is called **diverticulitis**. If the terminology seems confusing, consider this rule of medical terminology using the Greek roots:

- The word ending *osis* or *asis* means "presence of."
- Diverticulosis means "presence of diverticula."
- The word ending *itis* means "inflammation of."
- Diverticulitis means "inflammation of diverticula."

Understanding the roots of the word will help with understanding and remembering many other medical terms, such as gastritis (inflammation of the stomach), arthritis (inflammation of the joints), and others.

A low-fiber diet, along with decreased strength of intestinal muscle walls that occurs during aging, probably explain why diverticula develop. Increased fiber is recommended to decrease the pressure in the intestine that causes the pockets to form. A high-fiber diet (20-35 grams per day) is often prescribed.

GLOSSARY

Diverticulosis
A disease of the intestine where the intestinal walls become weakened and bulge into pockets called diverticula

Diverticulitis
A disease where the diverticula (found in the colon) become inflamed or infected

While an individual with diverticulosis will benefit from a high-fiber diet, this is not true for the acute, temporary condition of diverticulitis. Dietary treatment of diverticulitis often restricts fiber so that it doesn't add to the inflammation. Typically, this diet eliminates most fresh fruit (except ripe bananas) and raisins, substituting canned or cooked fruits without seeds. Fruit juices are allowed. A lower fiber diet is recommended during an acute bout of diverticulitis; however, no evidence supports that seeds or nuts get "trapped" in the diverticula. Cooked or canned vegetables without skins or seeds are permitted. Dried beans (legumes), peas, sauerkraut, and winter squash are not permitted. During this treatment, a patient may receive antibiotics. When the problem has resolved, an individual can usually return to a high-fiber diet.

Diarrhea and Irritable Bowel Syndrome

Diarrhea, frequent watery bowel movements, may be the result of emotional upset, food allergies, lactose intolerance, foodborne illness, gastrointestinal disease, medications, radiation therapy, or other conditions. Prolonged diarrhea can be serious, causing dehydration, weight loss, and malnutrition.

Diarrhea is often treated with a mixture of water, salts, and sugar, called oral rehydration therapy (ORT). In serious cases of diarrhea, bowel rest may be necessary. This allows the gastrointestinal tract to heal. Fluid and electrolytes are given intravenously in these cases. After adequate bowel rest, the client may start on a clear liquid diet and slowly progress back to a regular diet. Lactose and any irritating foods are omitted from the diet.

Diarrhea alternating with constipation may be a sign of **irritable bowel syndrome (IBS)**, a condition of unknown cause that first presents itself around age 20. Other symptoms of irritable bowel syndrome are abdominal pain, bloating, gas, indigestion, nausea, and rectal pain. The National Institute of Diabetes and Digestive and Kidney Diseases (NIDDK) estimates one in five adults (or 20 percent) suffers from irritable bowel syndrome. The good news, though, is that this condition does not lead to any serious harm, but may disrupt work and social interaction. It really describes a cluster of gastrointestinal symptoms that are, unfortunately, common.

The National Institute of Diabetes and Digestive and Kidney Diseases says the following have been associated with a worsening of IBS symptoms:

- Large meals
- Bloating from gas in the colon
- Medicines
- Wheat, rye, barley, chocolate, milk products, or alcohol
- Drinks with caffeine, such as coffee, tea, or colas
- Stress, conflict, or emotional upsets

Symptoms occur due to stress and, for women, to phases in the menstrual cycle. Dietary recommendations include a high-fiber diet (unless diarrhea is present), adequate fluid intake, and smaller meals.

GLOSSARY

Irritable Bowel Syndrome (IBS)
Common disorder that affects the large intestine that can cause abdominal pain, bloating, nausea, and diarrhea

Constipation

GLOSSARY

Constipation
Passage of small amounts of hard, dry bowel movements (stool)—usually fewer than three times per week

Constipation is one of the most common gastrointestinal problems in the United States. It accounts for two million visits to the doctor every year, according to the National Institutes of Health. Constipation is the passage of small amounts of hard, dry bowel movements, usually fewer than three times a week. Bowel movements may be difficult and/or painful. Some people also experience bloating. Avoiding foods known to aggravate symptoms may provide relief. These foods include excess dietary fat, caffeine, sugars such as lactose, fructose, and sorbitol, plus alcohol.

Because the gastrointestinal system tends to slow down with aging, constipation is common in older Americans. It is also common among individuals with limited mobility, as imposed by an injury, disability, or medical condition. Constipation can be an after-effect of stroke, or a side effect of various neurological disorders. It may also occur in certain hormonal disorders, gastrointestinal disorders, and other conditions. Lifestyle habits can contribute to constipation, such as infrequent exercise, low dietary fiber intake, high intake of fat, and low intake of fluids.

Constipation can be triggered by many factors including laxative use, enema use, and can be a side effect from taking certain medications. Laxative abuse can trigger constipation. Laxatives are considered habit-forming, can damage nerve cells in the colon, thus, interfering with the colon's natural ability to contract. Likewise, frequent use of enemas can diminish normal bowel functioning. As stated above, many medications can cause constipation; it's a common side effect of drugs such as narcotics, antacids, antidepressants, blood pressure medications, antispasmodics, and even iron (dietary) supplements. Individuals who change the consistency of their diets because of chewing or swallowing problems may also inadvertently reduce dietary fiber intake.

Treatments for constipation include MNT, laxatives, stool softeners, and drugs that stimulate bowel contractions, such as Correctol®, Dulcolax®, Purge®, and Senokot®. Exercise may also be a component of treatment. A diet that helps to correct constipation includes 20-35 grams of fiber daily and adequate fluid intake.

Gastrointestinal Progression Diets

A clear liquid diet allows foods that are clear liquid foods or become clear liquid at room temperature. Figure 5.3 lists foods included in a clear liquid diet, and Figure 5.4 shows a sample menu. The clear liquid diet may be used:

- After surgery (Usually it's the first diet because it is easily digested and absorbed.)
- Before surgery (Starting about eight hours before surgery, all foods and fluids are usually withheld. This is to prevent vomiting while under anesthesia, which could lead to aspiration—when food, vomit, or other foreign substances accidentally enter the lungs.)
- Before various diagnostic tests (such as tests involving the intestinal tract, because the clear liquid diet helps keep the intestines clear)

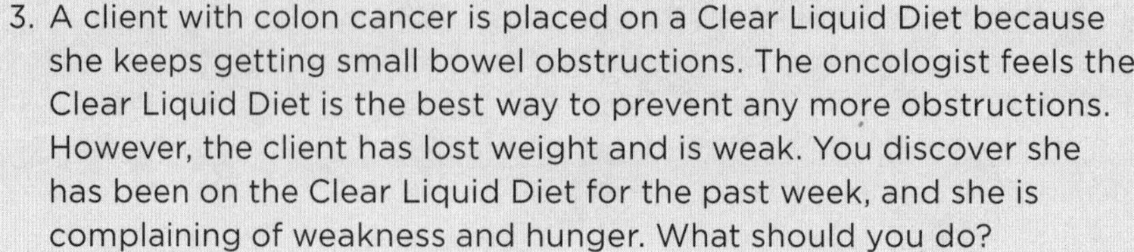

3. A client with colon cancer is placed on a Clear Liquid Diet because she keeps getting small bowel obstructions. The oncologist feels the Clear Liquid Diet is the best way to prevent any more obstructions. However, the client has lost weight and is weak. You discover she has been on the Clear Liquid Diet for the past week, and she is complaining of weakness and hunger. What should you do?

Figure 5.3
Foods Included in a Clear Liquid Diet

- Apple, grape, cranberry, or cranapple juice
- Strained orange or grapefruit juice
- Fruit punch, lemonade, limeade
- Carbonated beverages
- Clear broth, bouillon, or consommé
- Flavored gelatin
- Tea and coffee
- Sugar and salt

Source: Adapted from Nutrition 411

- Following periods of vomiting, diarrhea, or other upset of the digestive tract
- In the acute stages of many illnesses, such as fever, when only the clear liquid diet may be tolerated
- To test the ability to tolerate oral feedings

A clear liquid diet is intended to provide fluids, electrolytes, and some calories (however, limited), with minimal stimulation of the digestive tract and minimal development of fecal material (also called residue). It is useful in preventing dehydration and relieving thirst. This diet is inadequate in all nutrients except vitamin C and should not be used for more than three days without supplementation. Be sure to reference the Diet Manual approved by the facility for clarification and additional details.

Full Liquid Diet

The full liquid diet contains foods that are either liquid at room temperature or become liquid at room temperature. It differs from the clear liquid diet mostly by the addition of milk products and other opaque liquids. Figure 5.5 lists foods included in a full liquid diet, and Figure 5.6 shows a sample menu.

The full liquid diet is indicated in postoperative situations when the client has not fully recovered the ability to consume and tolerate solid food. In this case, a full liquid diet often acts as a transition between a clear liquid and soft or regular diet. It may also be indicated for clients who have esophageal or stomach disorders that interfere with the normal handling of solid foods.

The full liquid diet may be adequate in calories, protein, vitamin C, calcium, sodium, and potassium, depending on what foods are consumed. It is inadequate in iron, niacin, and folate, and other nutrients. However, due to the limited selection of foods, a multivitamin and mineral supplement may be necessary if this diet is to be used for more than two weeks and a commercial liquid formula is not used. Be sure to refer to the Diet Manual approved by the facility for clarification and additional details.

4. You see a family member bring in a fruit smoothie from the cafeteria to give her father, your client. He is on a Full Liquid Diet. What do you tell the family member?

Figure 5.4
Sample Menu for a Clear Liquid Diet

BREAKFAST	LUNCH	DINNER
1 cup strained orange juice	1 cup apple juice	1 cup cranberry juice
1/2 cup gelatin	3/4 cup clear broth	3/4 cup consommé
2 tsp. sugar	1/2 cup fruit ice	1/2 cup gelatin
1 cup coffee	2 tsp. sugar	1 cup tea
12 oz. ginger ale	1 cup tea	12 oz. lemon-lime flavored soda
	12 oz. lemon-lime flavored soda	

Source: Adapted from Nutrition 411

Figure 5.5
Foods Included in a Full Liquid Diet

- Carbonated beverages, coffee and tea (regular and decaffeinated), fruit drinks
- Milk and milk drinks, yogurt without seeds or nuts
- Puréed meat added to broth or cream soup (if allowed by physician)
- Custard, gelatin desserts, smooth ice cream, sherbet, puddings, popsicle, frozen yogurt
- Cooked, refined cereal (if allowed by physician)
- All vegetable juices
- All fruit juices and fruit ice
- Sugar, honey, syrup
- Butter, margarine, cream, vegetable oils
- Consommé, broth, bouillon, strained soup made from allowed foods—no solids
- Salt
- Commercial liquid formulas that are nutritionally complete

Figure 5.6
Sample Menu for a Full Liquid Diet

BREAKFAST	LUNCH	DINNER
1 cup whole milk	1 cup whole milk	1 cup whole milk
1 cup eggnog	1 cup vanilla milkshake	1 cup chocolate milkshake
1 cup orange juice	1 cup apple juice	1/2 cup egg custard
1/2 cup frozen yogurt	non-dairy creamer	1 cup cranberry juice
non-dairy creamer	3/4 cup beef broth	non-dairy creamer
2 tsp. sugar	1 tsp. sugar	3/4 cup chicken broth
1 Tbsp. honey	1/2 cup sherbet	1 tsp. sugar
salt	salt, pepper	salt, pepper
coffee	tea	tea

Source: Adapted from Nutrition 411

Soft Diet (or "GI Soft Diet")

The soft diet is designed for use during transition from liquid (either clear or full) to regular diet after surgery. It provides a modified consistency, but is also intended to be easy on the gastrointestinal tract during a sensitive time. Foods in a soft diet are:

- Soft in consistency (but not ground or chopped)—unless otherwise indicated on the diet order
- Mildly spiced
- Moderately low in fiber content

Cooked vegetables (with the exception of corn) and fruits without seeds or peels are allowed. Raw vegetables, highly seasoned or fried foods, and nuts and seeds are not allowed. This diet must be individualized to each client.

SECTION B ORGANS THAT IMPACT DIGESTION

Liver, Gallbladder, Pancreas, and Kidneys

In the discussion about gastrointestinal progression diets, it is important to consider the other organs involved in digestion: the liver, the gallbladder, pancreas, and kidneys.

The liver, the largest organ in the body, has many important roles. The following are some of its functions:

- The liver converts blood glucose to fat and glycogen.
- The liver makes glucose.
- The liver has an important role in regulating blood glucose levels.
- The liver makes triglycerides and cholesterol.
- The liver also excretes cholesterol in bile.
- The liver makes many of the proteins found in the blood, such as the proteins necessary for blood to clot after an injury.
- The liver removes drugs, hormones, and other molecules by excreting them in the bile.

Fatty liver, a condition in which triglycerides build up in the liver and cause it to swell, is often an early sign of more liver problems to come. Fatty liver most often occurs due to excessive alcohol intake, infection, or malignant disease. It can also be caused by certain drugs or by extremely low protein intake (to the point of protein malnutrition). Treatment for fatty liver centers on removing its cause, whether it be alcohol, drugs, or a poor diet. The effects of fatty liver can be reversed when the cause is eliminated.

Hepatitis is more serious than fatty liver, and refers to inflammation of the liver due to alcohol, drugs, toxins, or viral infection. Symptoms include low fever, fatigue, nausea, anorexia, vomiting, constipation, or diarrhea. Symptoms cause malnutrition in some instances, particularly in cases of alcohol abuse. A high-calorie, high-protein diet is appropriate for malnourished clients, and fat-soluble vitamins in water-soluble form are often prescribed.

Cirrhosis is a term used for advanced stages of liver disease that occurs when fatty liver or hepatitis are not reversed. At this point, liver cells harden and die. The damage can't be reversed. The liver shrinks and is not able to complete all of its vital functions.

Cirrhosis due to alcohol abuse is called Laennec's cirrhosis. It is the most common type of cirrhosis.

GLOSSARY

Ascites
Abnormal accumulation of fluid in the abdomen

Hepatic
Relating to the liver

Jaundice
Yellowing of the skin associated with liver disease

Symptoms of cirrhosis include nausea, anorexia, weight loss, weakness, iron-deficiency anemia, stomach pain, esophageal varices (blood vessels that project into the esophagus), steatorrhea (fat is malabsorbed and is found in the stool, this can affect nutrient absorption especially fat-soluble vitamins.), and **ascites** is the abnormal accumulation of fluid in the abdomen. The level of ammonia in the blood, which is toxic to the brain and nervous system, also increases. Edema is the overall term for abnormal water retention. When patients have edema, the degree of fluid accumulation should be assessed. Additional fluid retained will affect the body weight; therefore, patient's body weight need to be used with caution as an assessment tool.

When cirrhosis progresses to the point where the liver function has decreased to 25 percent or less, **hepatic** failure occurs. Liver failure is characterized by **jaundice**, a yellowing of the skin. Over time, liver failure results in portal systemic encephalopathy (PSE), which affects the brain and is a life-threatening complication of liver failure. Symptoms range from confusion and poor coordination to flapping of the hands (called asterixis), and finally to loss of consciousness and coma.

Several laboratory tests help in evaluation of liver function. Elevated liver enzymes mean the liver cells are being destroyed and the enzymes are released into the blood. This suggests liver failure. Blood ammonia tests are also used as a measurement of the degree of liver failure. The liver turns over proteins and amino acids. Ammonia is a byproduct. The liver converts ammonia into urea. Urea is excreted by the kidneys. When the liver is failing, it cannot convert ammonia to urea. Thus, a high blood ammonia level is an early sign of liver failure. It may be accompanied by symptoms of confusion. A low protein diet may be part of the therapy at this point, because this minimizes the production of ammonia. In cases of hepatic coma, hepatic formulas that are low in a type of amino acid called aromatic amino acids, and high in branched-chain amino acids may be used. Figure 5.7 shows the MNT for cirrhosis.

Gallbladder Disease

The liver also makes and secretes bile, a substance that aids in the digestion and absorption of fats. Bile is carried by ducts from the liver to the gallbladder. The gallbladder stores and concentrates bile until food is in the stomach and duodenum. Then the gallbladder contracts and bile travels to the duodenum.

There are various diseases of the gallbladder, such as cholelithiasis (gallstones) or cholecystitis (inflammation of the gallbladder, which is usually caused by gallstones). A

Figure 5.7
Medical Nutrition Therapy for Cirrhosis

- High calories, 35-45 Kcal/kg body weight
- High protein, 1.0-1.5g/kg body weight
- Moderate fat
- Vitamin and mineral supplementation
- Fluid and sodium restrictions if ascites and edema are present

Source: Adapted from Nutrition 411

low-fat diet, usually interpreted to mean no more than 40 grams of fat per day, may be used to treat these diseases in the hospital. Clients with chronic cholecystitis may need a long-term diet with 25 to 30 percent of total energy (Kcal) consumed from fat. Less fat in the diet results in fewer gallbladder contractions and less pain. A client who has the gallbladder removed can progress as tolerated to a regular diet.

Pancreatitis

Pancreatitis is an inflammation of the pancreas in which pancreatic enzymes are blocked from emptying, causing some of these strong enzymes to digest the pancreas itself. Pancreatitis can be either acute or chronic. Gallstones are the most common cause of acute pancreatitis, while alcohol abuse is a common cause of chronic pancreatitis. Symptoms include tender abdomen, nausea, vomiting, fever, and rapid pulse. Pancreatitis causes fat malabsorption and **steatorrhea** (fatty stools). When fat is lost in the stool, so are calories and fat-soluble vitamins.

During acute pancreatitis, oral feedings are usually withheld until the acute phase subsides to give the pancreas a rest, at which time the client may slowly progress as tolerated to a low-fat diet. For clients with chronic pancreatitis, MNT includes pancreatic enzyme replacements (taken orally with meals), a low-fat diet, vitamin and mineral supplements, and MCT oil if steatorrhea is present.

GLOSSARY

Steatorrhea
Fatty stool

Renal Failure
When the kidneys fail to function normally

Renal Disease

The kidneys perform the vital function of maintaining the proper balance of water, electrolytes (sodium, potassium, and chloride), and acids in body fluids. This is done by secreting some substances into the urine and holding back others in the bloodstream for use in the body. In addition to forming urine, the kidneys also have an endocrine function, meaning they produce hormones. The kidneys secrete renin (a substance that is important in maintaining normal blood pressure), erythropoietin (a hormone that regulates the production of red blood cells), and a form of vitamin D.

Certain conditions damage the cells of the kidneys, making it difficult for the kidneys to perform their jobs. **Renal failure** occurs when the kidneys fail to maintain normal fluid and electrolyte balance and to excrete waste products within normal limits. It may strike at any age, due to a variety of causes. Renal failure may occur over a period of time (chronic renal failure) or suddenly (acute renal failure). Acute renal failure may result from shock, burns, or severe injuries. It is often reversible.

Chronic renal failure (CRF) is not reversible, due to the progressive destruction of kidney tissue. Many diseases can damage the kidneys, such as nephritis (inflammation of the kidneys), high blood pressure, and complications of diabetes. Clients who suffer from chronic renal failure may eventually require dialysis, in which waste materials such as urea (a byproduct of protein metabolism that can be toxic at high levels) are separated from the bloodstream. Dialysis removes excess wastes and fluids but can't perform any of the hormonal functions of the kidney. When the client is to the point

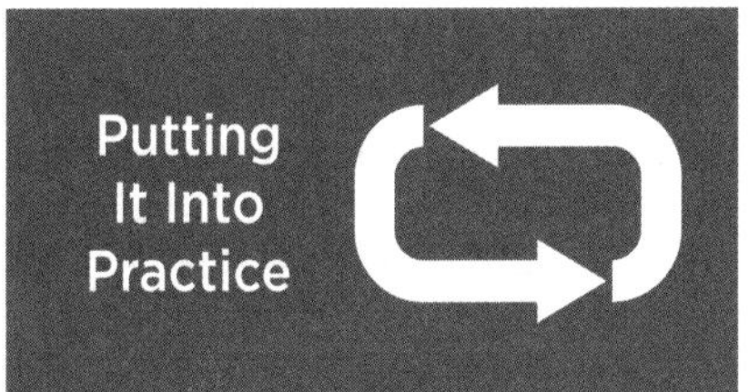

5. How would you modify the following meal to be appropriate for a renal (hemodialysis) diet?
    - Peanut butter & jelly sandwich on whole grain bread
    - 8 oz 2% milk
    - 1/2 a banana

Figure 5.8a
Dietary Guidelines for Adults Starting Hemodialysis

NUTRIENT	DIETARY GUIDELINES
Salt & Sodium	• Use less salt and eat fewer salty foods. • Use herbs, spices, and low-salt flavor enhancers. • Avoid salt substitutes made with potassium.
Meats/ Protein	• Eat a high protein food at every meal or 8-10 oz. every day. • 3 oz. = size of a deck of cards: a medium pork chop, a 1/4 lb. hamburger, 1/2 chicken breast, a medium fish fillet. • 1 oz. = 1 egg or 1/4 cup egg substitute, 1/4 cup tuna, 1/4 cup ricotta cheese, 1 slice of low-sodium lunchmeat. • Note: Peanut butter, nuts, seeds, dried beans, peas, and lentils have protein but are not recommended because they are high in both potassium and phosphorus.
Grains, Cereals, and Breads	• Unless one needs to limit calorie intake for weight loss and/or manage carbohydrate intake for diabetes, 6-11 servings from this group may be eaten daily. • Avoid "whole grain" and "high fiber" foods to help limit the intake of phosphorus.
Milk, Yogurt, and Cheese	• Limit the intake of milk, yogurt, and cheese to 1/2 cup milk or 1/2 cup yogurt or 1 oz. cheese per day. • The phosphorus content is the same for all types of milk—skim, low-fat, and whole. • If any high phosphorus foods are consumed, take a phosphate binder with that meal. • Certain brands of non-dairy creams and "milk" (such as rice milk) are low in phosphorus and potassium. • Dairy foods "low" in phosphorus.
Fruits and Juice	• Eat 2-3 servings of low potassium fruits each day. • Always avoid star fruit (carambola). • Limit oranges, orange juice, kiwis, nectarines, prunes, prune juice, raisins and dried fruits, bananas, melons (cantaloupe and honeydew).
Vegetables and Salads	• Eat 2-3 servings of low-potassium vegetables each day. • Avoid potatoes, tomatoes, winter squash, pumpkin, asparagus, avocado, beets, beet greens, cooked spinach, parsnips, and rutabaga.
Dessert	• Depending on calorie needs, the Registered Dietitian Nutritionist may recommend high-calorie desserts. • Limit dairy-based desserts and those made with chocolate, nuts, and bananas. • If diabetes is present, discuss low carbohydrate dessert choices with the Registered Dietitian Nutritionist.

Source: National Kidney Foundation

Figure 5.8b
Nutrition for Chronic Kidney Disease in Adults

NUTRIENT	NUTRITION GUIDELINES
Salt & Sodium	• Limit sodium intake to 1500 mg per day. • Choose sodium-free or low-sodium foods. • Use lemon juice, salt-free seasoning mixes, or hot pepper sauce. • Avoid salt substitutes made with potassium.
Meats/Protein	• Reduce daily protein intake by 0.2 g/kg of body weight (e.g. a 154 lb. man would reduce protein from 56 grams to 42 grams/day). • Limit meat to two 3-oz. servings daily.
Grains, Cereals, and Breads	• No specific recommendation.
Milk, Yogurt, and Cheese	• Limit high-potassium foods including dairy foods.
Fruits and Juice	• Limit high-potassium foods including oranges, orange juice, melons, apricots, bananas, and kiwi.
Vegetables and Salads	• Limit high-potassium foods including potatoes, tomatoes, sweet potatoes, cooked spinach, beans (baked, kidney, lima, pinto).
Dessert	• No specific recommendation.

Source: National Institute of Diabetes and Digestive and Kidney Diseases

of requiring dialysis or a kidney transplant, the disease is referred to as end-stage renal disease (ESRD).

Part of the treatment for ESRD may be dialysis. There are two types of dialysis: hemodialysis and peritoneal dialysis. In hemodialysis, the client's blood is routed through a dialysis machine, which performs many of the kidney's functions. Then, the blood is returned to the body. In peritoneal dialysis, fluid is introduced into the abdominal cavity by a catheter or tube permanently placed into the abdomen.

The goals of the renal diet are as follows:

- To provide normal growth in children
- To achieve and maintain an optimal nutritional status through adequate protein, energy, vitamin, and mineral intake
- To attain and maintain a desirable body weight
- To lighten the work of a diseased kidney by reducing the amount of waste products, such as urea made from protein, that have to be excreted
- To control edema and electrolyte imbalance by controlling sodium, potassium, and fluid intake
- To replace proteins that are lost in hemodialysis
- To prevent or slow down the development of bone disease (called renal osteodystrophy) by controlling phosphorus (the blood level of which increases during renal failure, leading to bone disease) and increasing calcium intake
- To provide a palatable diet

Of all the modified diets and MNT, the renal diet is probably the most complex. The intake of protein, sodium, potassium, phosphorus, and fluid are carefully regulated from day-to-day. Actual nutrient restrictions vary based on many factors, such as:

- Degree of kidney failure
- Age of the client
- Mode of treatment and/or dialysis
- Need to maintain or achieve an ideal or desired weight
- Other medical conditions: diabetes, high blood pressure, hyperlipidemia, or malnutrition

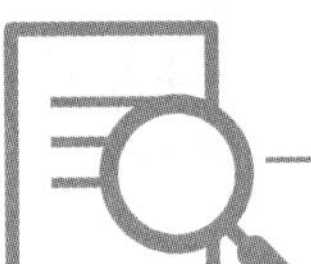
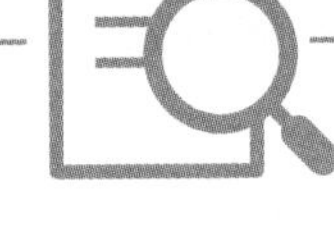

View the Supplemental Material for Figure 5.9, Sample Menu for a Client on Hemodialysis.

The National Kidney Foundation has established Dietary Guidelines for Adults starting on hemodialysis. As stated before, the renal diet looks at protein, sodium, potassium, phosphorus, and fluid. In general, adults on hemodialysis should:

- Increase the consumption of high-protein foods
- Decrease the consumption of high-salt, high-potassium, and high-phosphorus foods
- Learn how much fluid to safely drink (including coffee, tea, and water)

See Figure 5.8a for the Dietary Guidelines for Adults starting on hemodialysis and Figure 5.8b for additional nutritional information for chronic kidney disease. Figure 5.9 shows a sample menu for a client on hemodialysis.

SECTION C ADDITIONAL MNT FOR ALZHEIMER'S DISEASE, IMMOBILITY, AND DEVELOPMENTAL DISABILITIES

Alzheimer's Disease

GLOSSARY

Alzheimer's Disease
Most common form of dementia marked by a loss of cognitive ability

Alzheimer's disease is the most common form of dementia (impairment of mental functioning), although it is not part of normal aging. It proceeds in stages over months or years and gradually destroys memory, reason, judgment, language, and eventually the ability to carry out even simple tasks. About half of individuals over age 85 have Alzheimer's disease, but it can also appear as early as middle age (Source: www.ncbi.nlm.nih.gov). It accounts for 60 percent of admissions to nursing homes. Managing the nutritional well-being of a resident with Alzheimer's disease is challenging and ever-changing, as no two individuals' needs and abilities are the same. Techniques that successfully maintain food intake and weight in some residents may not work for others. Nutrition management of a resident with Alzheimer's must be individualized according to the person's ability and current stage of the disease.

Understanding the progression of the disease is the first step toward nutrition management. There are basically three stages of Alzheimer's:

- **Early Stage.** This stage is characterized by forgetfulness, a tendency to misplace things, and some withdrawal from usual interests. Individuals may have trouble finding the right words to communicate their thoughts. Initially, they may not have problems eating their meals, but environmental surroundings may cause a problem. They may not want to eat in public or in a noisy environment. This stage of Alzheimer's may go unnoticed.
- **Intermediate Stage.** Persons with Alzheimer's usually cannot initiate a specific

movement or course of action without assistance during this stage. There is confusion and difficulty carrying out usual routines. Individuals may begin to need redirection at mealtime as they forget how to use flatware or are unaware of what to do with the food in front of them. Some individuals also wander at mealtimes and therefore require constant supervision. Partial to total feeding is usually required. At times, they may refuse to open their mouths, making the dining experience a conflict situation between client and caregiver. Situations like this can promote violent behavior in some individuals. Also, clients become disoriented with respect to their surroundings, time, and place. This may explain why they become lost walking to the dining room or forget if they have eaten meals. Losing the ability to remember whether they have eaten not only can lead to weight loss, but also to weight gain.

- **Late Stage.** At this stage, the person's motor skills deteriorate. Patients lose the ability to chew and swallow, and often to speak. Their sensitivity to seizures, aspiration, and pneumonia increases, making it difficult for caregivers to provide them with fluids and food orally. Food and fluid textures have to be modified to promote oral intake as long as possible. Correct feeding and positioning techniques must be exhibited by the caregiver during mealtimes. Decisions by families and medical staff must be made regarding enteral nutrition support.

Compiling a comprehensive nutrition assessment upon admission of each client with Alzheimer's is a key aspect in MNT. Continuous assessment is necessary due to the disease progression. During the initial three to five days after admission, the client must be closely monitored at mealtimes for changes in eating/feeding ability. Depending on the severity of the eating skill deficiency, close monitoring should be done weekly to monthly.

Nutritional care strategies must be individualized to patients and their current stages of the disease. All techniques do not work for all clients with Alzheimer's. The old saying, "If at first you don't succeed, try, try again," is never more true than for this population. MNT for Alzheimer's requires implementing techniques appropriate for specific problems, as outlined below.

To maintain weight and appetite:

- Serve the larger meals at breakfast when the resident is more alert and his/her appetite is larger. Even clients with good appetites will consume smaller evening meals due in part to the "**sundowning**" effect (increased restlessness and anxiety as evening approaches).
- Provide nutrient-dense foods routinely in the diet, such as whole milk with meals, fortified cereal at breakfast, and additional juices and whole-grain breads.
- Offer nutritious snacks between meals, such as juice and graham crackers, sandwich halves, fruit and cheese.
- Implement a weekly weight program for all clients. Close monitoring is a must.
- Involve all facility staff during mealtimes to assist residents in the dining rooms and those who receive room service.

GLOSSARY

Sundowning
When confusion or disorientation worsens at the end of the day. Common with Alzheimer's disease

Observe for changes in a client's eating habits, such as decreased use of utensils, playing with food, or using fingers. If observed, make appropriate changes in meal service to maintain their independence. There are some considerations to maintain feeding independence:

- If there is a decreased use of utensils: offer utensils only as needed, use "hand-overhand" techniques in promoting self-feeding, and provide verbal cues for client, e.g., "Mrs. Jones, pick up your fork."
- If the client is playing with or mixing food: offer one food at a time, place foods in individual bowls, put condiments on food before serving, and have staff provide constant redirection and verbal cues at mealtimes.
- If the client is using fingers to eat, maximize the situation. Offer finger foods to allow resident to maintain independence, yet eat in a dignified manner.

If the client experiences confusion at meal times:

- Offer meals at the same time, same place, and same seating arrangement every day.
- Serve the meal immediately after the resident is in the dining room.
- Allow adequate time for meals.
- Make the physical environment pleasant and calming.
- Limit the use of intercoms.
- Play soft background music.
- Seat residents in groups of four to six.
- Use square rather than round tables.
- Set the table with solid, contrasting colors between the china and the tablecloth.
- Limit the centerpieces at mealtimes.
- Maintain a high staff-to-resident ratio at mealtime.

If the client has difficulty chewing and/or swallowing:

- Check fit of dentures, if applicable.
- Position the resident correctly (at 90-degree angle) in chair, wheelchair, or bed.
- Provide verbal cues in a soft, gentle manner to remind residents to chew food, eat slowly, and swallow.
- Evaluate need for a texture-modified diet. Offer soft or ground meat first, then go to pureed consistency.
- Use gravies and sauces to moisten food.
- Ensure that food temperatures are safe.
- Avoid offering a food with a combination of textures, e.g. vegetable soup.
- Consult a speech therapist for swallowing evaluation.
- Learn techniques to overcome problems of refusing to open mouth or of pocketing food.

Finger Food Diet

The Finger Food Diet has existed for many years. However, the increased attention to this diet is due to the emphasis on maintaining quality of life by providing additional rehabilitation services. Finger foods are useful for clients with physical or functional impairments who have lost their ability to eat with utensils. They allow a client to maintain independent eating ability, e.g., in the case of Alzheimer's disease.

The biggest obstacle with this diet may be family members who feel it is socially unacceptable to eat with fingers and beneath the dignity of the client. If the family is not aware of the need to maintain independence in eating, they may believe it is more acceptable to eat with a spoon and/or be fed by staff. A team effort among the client, family, foodservice staff, speech therapy, and nursing staff will help make this diet a successful intervention.

The characteristics of finger foods include:

- Bite-size pieces—not too large or too small, but this varies with the client
- Not too soft, squishy, slippery, or crumbly
- No thick, gooey sauces or gravy poured on the food

A finger food diet may include foods such as: pudding in an ice cream cone, chicken nuggets, sandwiches cut into quarters, cold cereals formed in large pieces (e.g. shredded wheat), bar cookies, donuts, turnovers, peanut butter on crackers, tater tots or baked potatoes cut into pieces, batter-dipped vegetables, corn on the cob, thin soup served in a mug, popcorn, bite-sized fruit or vegetable pieces.

Immobilization

Long periods of immobilization, such as following an injury or being bedridden, can result in pressure ulcers. **Pressure ulcers/injury**, pressure sores, or **decubitus ulcers** are lesions caused by unrelieved pressure resulting in damage to underlying tissue. Over one million clients in hospitals and nursing homes suffer from pressure ulcers. The first preventive step is to identify clients at high risk (see Figure 5.10). Clients with pressure ulcers need to be monitored closely, using a staging system (see Figure 5.11).

MNT plays a vital role in preventing and treating pressure ulcer/injury. Clients who are malnourished and/or eating and drinking poorly have a greater chance of developing pressure ulcers. Medical nutrition therapy for this condition commonly includes a high energy, high-protein diet along with adequate fluids.

The nutritional needs for energy, protein, and fluid increase with the stage of the ulcer, as shown in Figure 5.11. Multivitamin/mineral supplements are frequently given for Stages II-IV. Additional vitamin C and zinc may be given for Stage IV, but the research

GLOSSARY

Pressure Injury/ Decubitus Ulcers
Lesions caused by unrelieved pressure resulting in damage to the underlying tissue

Figure 5.10
Risk Factors for Pressure Ulcers

- Impaired transfer or bed mobility
- Bedridden, hemiplegia, quadriplegia
- Loss of bowel or bladder control
- Peripheral vascular disease
- Diabetes mellitus
- Hip fracture
- Weight loss/poor nutrition
- Pressure ulcer history
- Impaired tactile sensory perception
- Medications
- Restraints
- Severe chronic obstructive pulmonary disease
- Sepsis
- Terminal cancer
- Chronic or end-stage renal, liver, and/or heart disease
- Disease or drug-related immunosuppression
- Full-body cast
- Steroid, radiation, or chemotherapy
- Renal dialysis
- Head of bed elevated the majority of the day

Source: Adapted from Nutrition 411 and National Institutes of Health

Figure 5.11

Pressure Ulcer/Injury Staging and Nutritional Needs

A staging system describes the extent of tissue damage in pressure ulcers. Stages also influence nutritional recommendations. The stages and related nutritional advice follow:

STAGE	NEEDS	CALORIES	PROTEIN	FLUID
STAGE 1	Intact skin with non-blanchable redness of a localized area usually over a bony prominence. Darkly pigmented skin may not have visible blanching; its color may differ from the surrounding area.	30 Cal/kg	1.0-1/1 gm/kg	30 ml/kg
STAGE 2	Partial thickness, loss of dermis presenting as a shallow open ulcer with a red/pink wound bed, without slough. May also present as an intact or open/ruptured serum-filled blister.	30 Cal/kg	1.2 gm/kg	30 ml/kg
STAGE 3	Full thickness tissue loss. Subcutaneous fat may be visible but bone, tendon, or muscle are not exposed. Slough may be present but does not obscure the depth of tissue loss. May include undermining and tunneling.	35 Cal/kg	1.3-1.4 gm/kg	30-35 ml/kg
STAGE 4	Full thickness tissue loss with exposed bone, tendon, or muscle. Slough or eschar may be present on some parts of the wound bed. Often includes undermining and tunneling.	35 Cal/kg	1.5-1.6 gm/kg	35 ml/kg

Source: National Pressure Injury Advisory Panel

to support this is not substantiated. More aggressive calorie, protein, and vitamin/mineral supplementation is needed for a client with multiple pressure ulcers/injury.

Developmentally Disabled and Handicapped Clients

The term *developmental disability* refers to a severe, chronic disability that:

- Is attributable to a mental or physical impairment, or a combination of mental and physical impairments.
- Is manifested before the person reaches the age of 22 years.
- Is likely to continue indefinitely.
- Results in substantial functional limitations in three or more of the following areas of major life activity: self-care, receptive and expressive language, learning, mobility, selfdirection, capacity for independent living, and economic self-sufficiency.
- Reflects the person's need for a combination and sequence of special interdisciplinary or generic care, treatment, or other services that are lifelong or of extended duration and individually planned and coordinated (Developmental Disabilities Assistance and Bill of Rights Act, 1978).

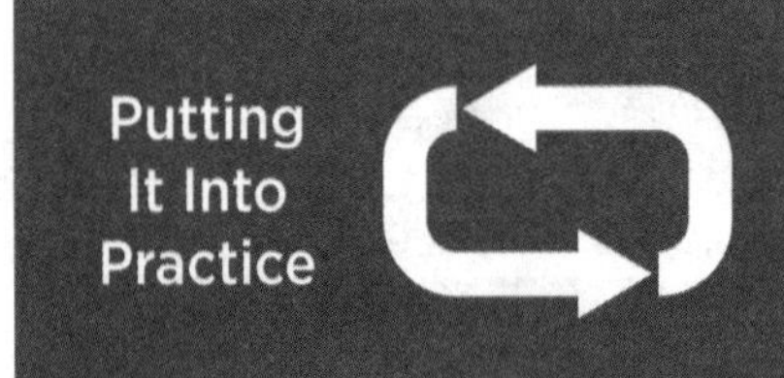

6. A client's family member suggests the client restrict what he is eating so he can lose some weight. However, the client was recently discovered to have a pressure injury. How do you address the situation?

Examples of developmental disabilities are mental retardation, cerebral palsy (partial paralysis and lack of muscular coordination), muscular dystrophy (progressive weakness and deterioration of muscles), epilepsy (sudden, passing disturbances of brain function), genetic disorders such as Down Syndrome, Prader-Willi Syndrome, and autism (withdrawal and lack of responsiveness to others). Developmentally disabled children are at high risk for nutritional problems and deficiencies. Frequent nutrition-related problems that contribute to nutritional risk include the following:

- **Feeding problems.** There may be either physical or psychological factors that cause feeding problems. For example, in children with cerebral palsy, the muscles involved in chewing and swallowing may not function normally.
- **Drug-nutrient interactions.** Many individuals with developmental disabilities are on long-term medications to treat chronic problems such as epilepsy and infections. Nutrition counseling may be needed as well as vitamin or mineral supplements.
- **Obesity.** Some developmentally disabled are more prone to obesity due to limited activity, poor muscle tone, small stature, and/or overeating. Nutrition counseling and regular exercise may be useful.
- **Constipation.** Constipation is common due to decreased activity and certain medications.
- **Dehydration.** Some developmentally disabled individuals are not able to feel or express thirst. Others need extra fluids because of drooling or to prevent frequent urinary infections. Fluid intake should be encouraged, and individuals assisted when necessary.

MNT is more effective with an interdisciplinary team approach that includes other professionals such as nurses, occupational therapists, physical therapists, social workers, physicians, psychologists, and dentists. Nutrition intervention is also more effective when the traditional nutrition assessment process has been modified for this population. For example, it is necessary to overcome difficulties in weighing and measuring clients and in selecting appropriate standards (such as weight) for comparison. Nutrition programs for the developmentally disabled can greatly benefit these individuals by improving their health and their capacity to socialize and function in an educational, work, or home environment.

A physical handicap can be caused by a variety of illnesses or accidents. Some of the common causes are arthritis, amputations, spinal cord injuries, stroke, Parkinson's disease, or multiple sclerosis. These illnesses can result in feeding problems for either emotional or physical reasons. Depression, which can occur with any illness, can result in a loss of appetite leading to weight loss, or in increased consumption of high-energy (Kcal), easily consumed foods, leading to obesity. Parents of a child with developmental disability may feel the need to reward and compensate with food leading to obesity in the child. Depressed clients may be extremely demanding and very selective in their food preferences. Demands requiring many substitutions can be very frustrating to the foodservice staff. Tremors or paralysis may make it difficult for a client to use utensils. Use of adapted utensils may help the patients eat by themselves. Dysphagia may make eating certain consistencies of food difficult.

With all of these body systems that require MNT, all nutrition care should be completed in consultation with the Registered Dietitian Nutritionist.

Chapter References

RESOURCES	
Academy of Nutrition and Dietetics*	https://www.eatright.org
Alzheimer's Foundation of America*	https://alzfdn.org
American Speech-Language-Hearing Association. Dysphagia Diets. Clinical Topics and Disorders.*	https://www.asha.org/SLP/clinical/dysphagia/Dysphagia-Diets/
International Dysphagia Diet Standardisation Initiative. What is the IDDSI Framework.*	https://iddsi.org/framework/
Mayo Clinic*	https://www.mayoclinic.org
National Kidney Foundation*	https://www.kidney.org
National Pressure Injury Advisory Panel*	https://npuap.org
National Pressure Injury Advisory Panel. NPIAP Pressure Injury Stages. Accessed September 16, 2020.	https://cdn.ymaws.com/npiap.com/resource/resmgr/online_store/npiap_pressure_injury_stages.pdf
Nutrition 411—Dysphagia Diets	https://www.consultant360.com/nutrition411
U.S. Department of Agriculture. Scientific Report of the 2015 Dietary Guidelines Advisory Committee.* Published February 2015.	https://health.gov/dietaryguidelines/2015-scientific-report/pdfs/scientific-report-of-the-2015-dietary-guidelines-advisory-committee.pdf
U.S. Department of Health and Human Services. National Institute of Diabetes and Digestive and Kidney Diseases.*	https://www.niddk.nih.gov

* Accessed September 18, 2019.

Fundamentals of Medical Nutrition Therapy for the CDM, CFPP

Overview and Objectives

Medical nutrition therapy is important for the prevention and/or treatment of many diseases. A Certified Dietary Manager®, Certified Foodservice Protection Professional® (CDM®, CFPP®) is often responsible for implementing therapeutic diets. Therefore, an understanding of body systems, related health conditions, and diet planning is a cornerstone of the profession. After completing this chapter, you should be able to:

- Identify basic medical nutrition terminology, as related to obesity, weight management, cardiovascular disease, diabetes, cancer, and HIV/AIDS
- Define the basic concepts of medical nutrition therapy, as related to obesity, weight management, cardiovascular disease, diabetes, cancer, and HIV/AIDS
- Relate basic concepts to nutritional deficiencies and excesses
- Relate basic concepts of medical nutrition therapy, as related to obesity, weight management, cardiovascular disease, diabetes, cancer, and HIV/AIDS
- Compare basic concepts to current diet manual or other accepted resources
- Explain utilization of medical nutrition therapy in long-term care and acute care settings

6

As noted, there is a strong correlation between diet and health. A poor diet increases the risk of certain chronic diseases such as obesity, cardiovascular disease (atherosclerosis, stroke), Type 2 Diabetes, hypertension, hyperlipidemia, some cancers, and osteoporosis. In the first part of the 20th century, nutrition-related problems involved inadequate amounts of nutrients resulting in a deficiency. Today, however, there have been dramatic increases in obesity-related chronic diseases due to energy (calorie) excesses (see Figure 6.1).

Research is now showing many risk factors that contribute to disease development resulting in death in the United States. However, knowledge can be used to modify risk factors to prevent disease. Figures 6.2a, 6.2b, and 6.2c describe the preventable causes of death, their contribution to the development of chronic disease, and the leading causes of death in the United States.

Smoking, high blood pressure, obesity, physical inactivity, high blood glucose, high blood lipid levels, and inadequate diet are the major risk factors for developing chronic diseases. This chapter will discuss the development of these chronic diseases (obesity, cardiovascular disease, diabetes, and cancer) and the medical nutrition therapy that is used to treat these diseases.

CDM, CFPPs and other health professionals can provide help in dietary planning; they can also serve as good role models. Dietary planning takes into account the actual needs of an individual or group, adjusting nutrient levels and fine-tuning the balance of nutrients to promote wellness. Individual needs can vary based on one's medical condition and how body systems are functioning. At times, a diet helps to compensate

Figure 6.1
Leading Causes of Death—United States

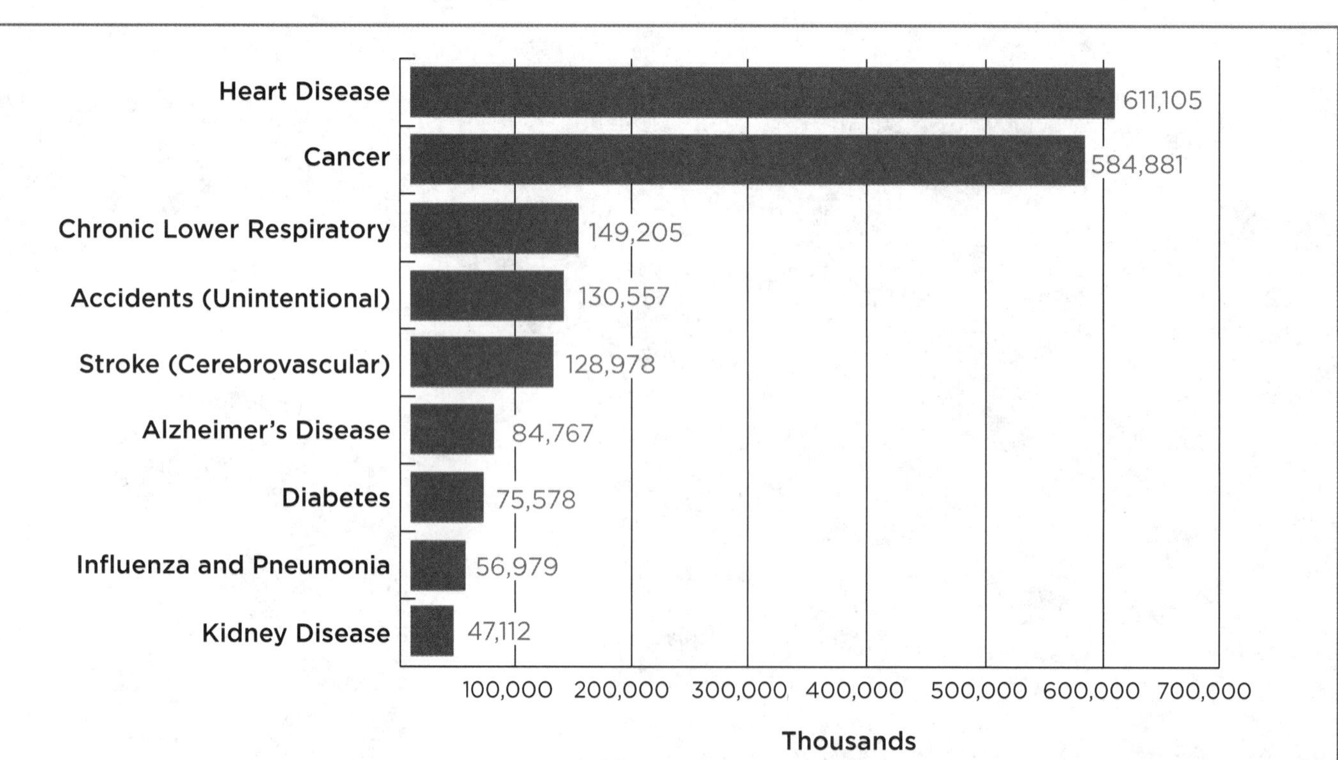

Source: National Vital Statistics System, National Center for Health Statistics, Centers for Disease Control and Prevention.

Figure 6.2a
Deaths Attributable to Individual Risks: Men & Women

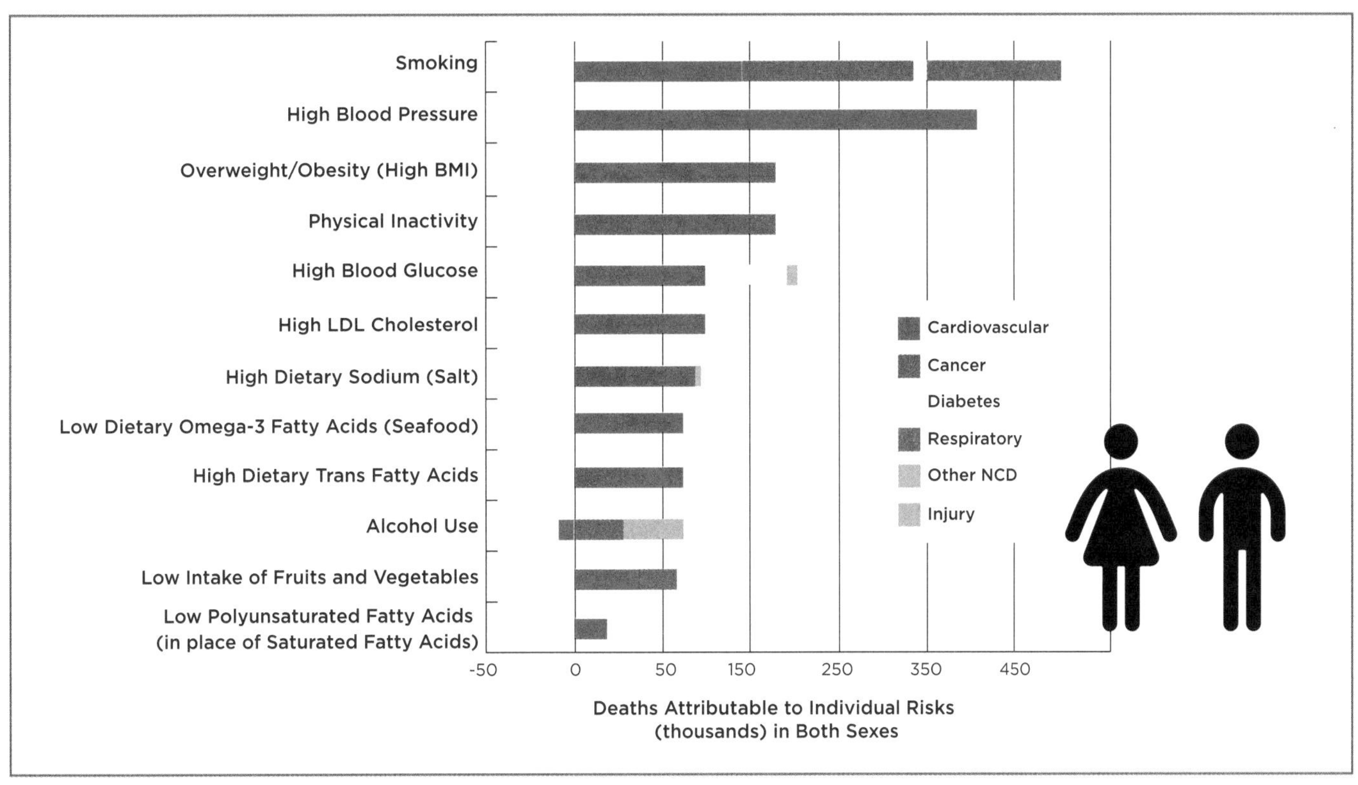

Figure 6.2b
Deaths Attributable to Individual Risks: Men

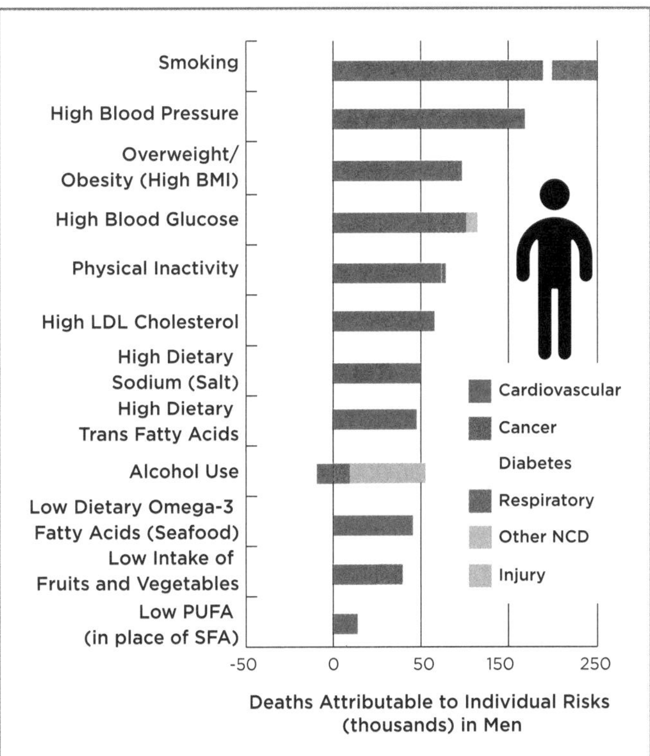

Figure 6.2c
Deaths Attributable to Individual Risks: Women

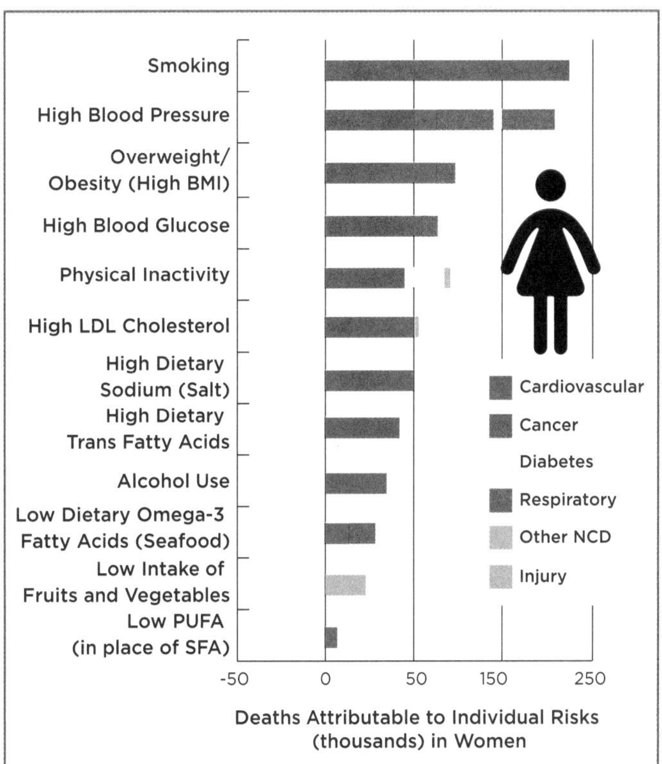

Danaei G, Ding EL, Mozaffarian D, et al. The preventable causes of death in the United States: comparative risk assessment of dietary, lifestyle, and metabolic risk factors. PLoS Med. 2011;6(4): e1000058. doi:10.1371/journal.pmed.1000058.

for unhealthy shifts in the body's metabolism and functioning. This chapter will explore these ideas in detail. This chapter is divided into four sections:

- **Section A**—Medical Nutrition Therapy and Obesity/Weight Management
- **Section B**—Medical Nutrition Therapy and Cardiovascular Disease Management
- **Section C**—Medical Nutrition Therapy and Diabetes Management
- **Section D**—Medical Nutrition Therapy and the Treatment of Cancer and HIV/ AIDS

Medical Nutrition Therapy (MNT)

Sometimes dietary changes are dictated by health conditions. As a group, these changes are called therapeutic or modified diets. *Medical Nutrition Therapy* (MNT) is a broader term referring to the nutritional assessment and treatment of a condition, illness, or injury that places an individual at risk. It involves two components: assessment of the client's nutritional status and treatment intervention. MNT generally focuses on individuals at risk for nutritional problems. Part of the healthcare process is to identify individuals at risk using a process known as nutrition screening.

Treatment may include therapeutic diets, counseling, and/or the use of nutrition support. This dietary treatment goes hand-in-hand with many other therapies, such as medication, surgery, physical therapy, and radiation. Thus, nutrition professionals work with others on the healthcare team to address the MNT needs of each patient.

A therapeutic diet is a regular diet that has been adjusted to meet a client's specific nutrient needs. Examples include calorie-controlled diets for weight loss; fat and cholesterol-controlled diets for treatment of cardiovascular disease; sodium-controlled diets used in hypertension or renal (kidney) disease; or protein-controlled diets for patients in kidney failure. Other types of therapeutic diets might include limiting or increasing water or fluids. Additionally, some therapeutic diets accommodate difficulties in chewing or swallowing, such as pureed diets or dysphagia diets. Still other therapeutic diets are used in treatment of digestive system-related problems. As an example, these could include clear liquid diets, very low-fat diets, or gluten-free diets. Thus, medical nutrition therapy is critical in the treatment of many diseases. The Nutrition Care Team is responsible for the daily management of nutrition interventions. The CDM, CFPP plays a key role in implementing the nutrition care plan as written by the Registered Dietitian Nutritionist.

SECTION A MEDICAL NUTRITION THERAPY AND OBESITY/WEIGHT MANAGEMENT

Medical Nutrition Therapy of Overweight and Obesity

Obesity poses a major health problem among children, teens, and adults. There is no single cause for obesity, and therefore no single cure. Obesity results when energy (calorie) intake exceeds the amount of energy expended. Over time, every 3500 excess calories becomes one extra pound of body weight. Figure 6.3 shows how energy intake has increased over time, and the sources of those added calories. Major calorie contributors include carbonated sweetened beverages (sodas), as well as other high-calorie beverages (e.g. sports drinks, juice drinks, smoothies, shakes, and creamy coffee drinks).

Figure 6.3

Average Daily Per Capita Calories from the U.S. Food Availability in 1970, 1990 and 2008 Adjusted for Spoilage and Other Waste

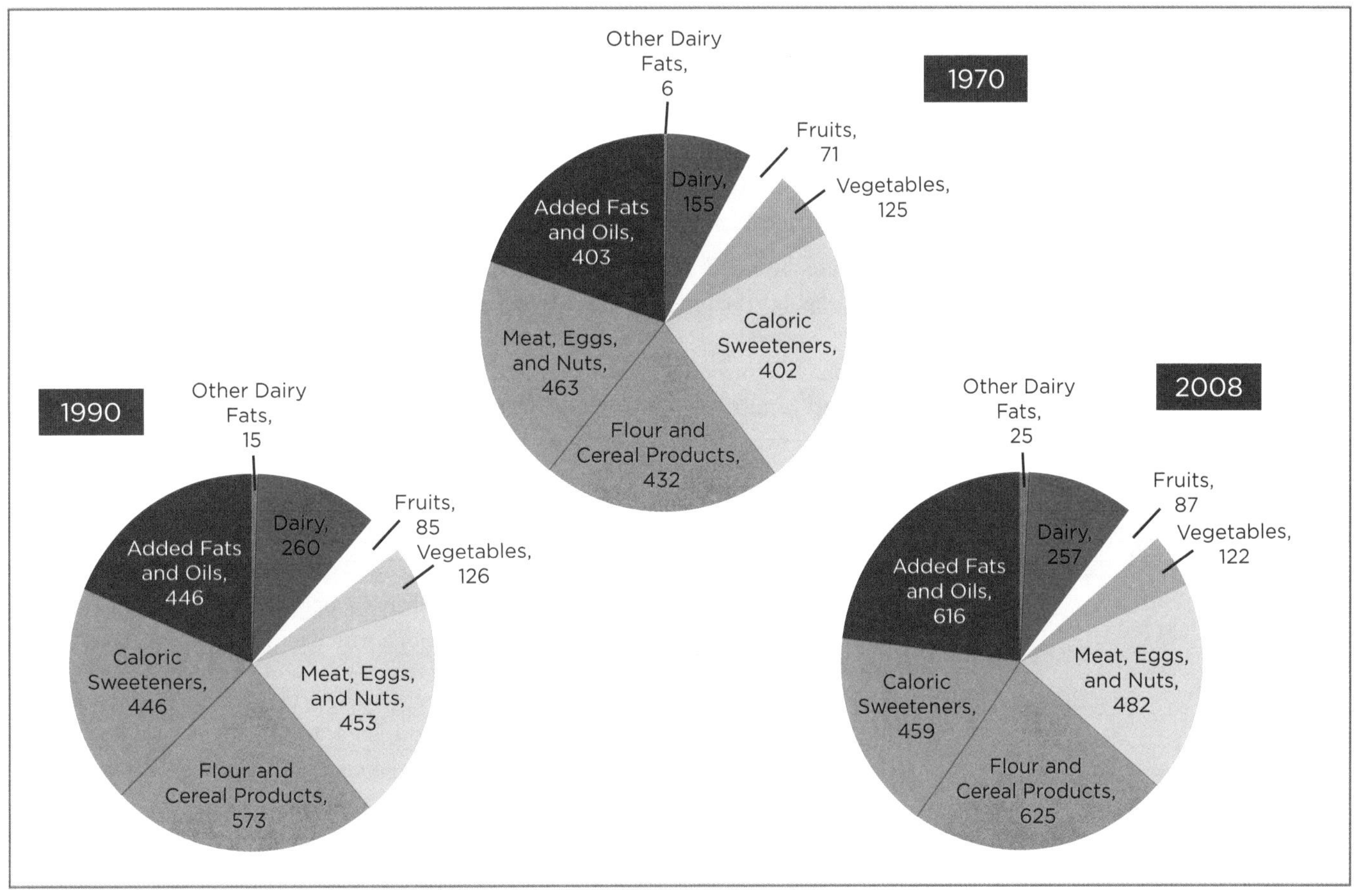

ERS Food Availability (Per Capita) Data System, Report of the DGAC on the Dietary Guidelines for Americans, 2010, D-1, pg. 10. http://www.cnpp.usda.gov/Publications/DietaryGuidelines/2010/DGAC/Report/D-1-EnergyBalance.pdf

The causes and effects of obesity are multifactorial. According to the *Dietary Guidelines for Americans*, the number of restaurants increased by 89 percent between 1972 to 1998; during that same period, the number of fast food restaurants grew by 147 percent and the amount of time spent in food preparation at home decreased from 91 minutes to 51 minutes per day. At that same time, serving sizes and total caloric intake have also increased.

Research suggests that the location of body fat is an important factor in health risks for adults. Excess fat around the waistline, along with low High Density Lipoproteins (HDL), high blood triglycerides, high blood pressure, and high fasting blood sugar, are linked to Type 2 diabetes and heart disease. Waist circumference and BMI are interrelated. Waist circumference measurement is particularly useful in clients who are normal or overweight on the BMI scale. Men with a waist circumference of > 40 inches and women with a waist circumference of > 35 inches are at increased risk of developing chronic disease. Smoking and excessive alcohol intake have been shown to increase abdominal fat and the risk for diseases related to obesity. Vigorous exercise and dietary efforts to reduce abdominal fat help to reduce the risk for these diseases.

Overweight people who lose even small amounts (10 percent) of weight are likely to:

- Lower their blood pressure
- Reduce abnormally high levels of blood glucose
- Bring blood levels of cholesterol and triglycerides down to more desirable levels
- Reduce sleep apnea or irregular breathing during sleep
- Decrease the risk of osteoarthritis
- Decrease depression

Treatment of Obesity

Because the causes of and contributors to obesity are multifactorial, treatment is challenging. The prospect of attaining and maintaining normal weight is very low—about 5 percent. A comprehensive approach to treating obesity focuses on the whole person. Treatment success is measured not only by the number of pounds lost, but also by other factors, such as reduction in medication, improved laboratory results, etc. Components of this approach typically include nutrition education, exercise, behavior modification, attitude modification, social support, maintenance support and, when indicated, drugs/medication and/or surgery.

An increasing number of health professionals are incorporating a non-dieting approach to obesity. This approach emphasizes helping clients adopt a healthier lifestyle that includes exercise and behavior modification, along with a nutritionally balanced diet.

In fact, problems can emerge from an excessive restriction of food intake. These can include unmanageable hunger and obsession with food, which may in turn lead to binge eating. Those who follow extremely low-calorie regimens essentially starve their bodies. The body may also respond by reducing basal energy expenditure. The result is that the body begins to require fewer calories. Generally, increased weight is caused by taking in more calories than one uses. There is evidence that a decrease in calories (regardless of the macronutrient restricted, i.e., fat, protein, or carbohydrate) can result in meaningful weight loss.

Nutrition Education

Anyone who wants to lose weight needs to understand several basic concepts of nutrition before planning a diet:

- Calories should not be overly restricted. A progressive weight loss of one to two pounds per week is considered safe.
- No foods should be forbidden. This only makes them more attractive.
- Portion control is vital. Measuring and weighing foods is helpful because "eyeballing" is not always accurate. Comparisons to common objects can also be helpful. For example, a 3 oz. portion of meat is the size of a deck of cards or a computer mouse.

1. How would you describe the controllable versus uncontrollable factors associated with the leading causes of death?

- Variety, balance, and moderation are key to satisfying all nutrient needs.
- Weighing oneself is important, but should not be done every day because minor weight gains and losses can occur on a daily basis due to fluid shifts. Weekly weigh-ins are more meaningful.
- Food journaling helps one be aware of the foods being consumed, trends in eating habits, and reasons for eating. In addition, food journals can be a helpful tool for nutrition education.

Exercising

Exercise is a vital component of any weight loss program. Physical activity alone has a modest impact on weight loss. However, physical activity does have an impact on other health indicators. Regular physical activity:

- Burns off calories to help lose extra pounds or maintain desirable weight
- Tones muscles
- Helps control appetite
- Helps in coping with stress
- Reduces fatigue; energizes the body
- Helps improve mental health and mood
- Promotes relaxation
- Reduces risk of cardiovascular disease
- Reduces risk of osteoporosis

Source: www.cdc.gov

Besides burning calories, an added bonus of a regular exercise regimen is that it helps shift the body's balance to include proportionally more muscle and less fat. In turn, this change in body composition increases the basal energy expenditure. Even at rest, a person with more lean muscle mass needs more calories. See Figure 6.4 for calories burned with exercise.

Figure 6.4
Calories and Exercise

Activity (by a 150 lb. person)	Calories Burned Per Hour
Bicycling, 6 mph	240
Bicycling, 12 mph	410
Jogging, 5-1/2 mph	740
Jogging, 7 mph	920
Jumping Rope	750
Running in Place	650
Running, 10 mph	1,280
Swimming, 25 yards per minute	275
Swimming, 50 yards per minute	500
Tennis, Singles	400
Walking, 2 mph	240
Walking, 3 mph	320
Walking, 4-12 mph	440

Source: National Heart, Lung, and Blood Institute

Behavior Modification

Behavior modification deals with identifying and changing behaviors that affect weight gain. Keeping a food diary helps to identify eating habits. A food diary is a daily record that includes things like the types and amounts of foods and beverages consumed, time and place of eating, with whom a person eats a meal, mood at the time, and degree of hunger. A diary can increase awareness about how and why a person eats. Once harmful patterns that encourage overeating are identified, the behavior can be changed to become more positive.

For example, overeating may occur as a reaction to stressful situations, emotions, or cravings. A client can learn to handle these situations in new ways. Solutions might include exercising or using relaxation techniques to relieve stress; or switching to a new activity such as taking a walk, knitting, or reading. A delay in food consumption can also be effective. A client could simply wait five minutes before eating, and the urge to eat could dissipate during this time. Positive self-talk is also important for good control. Instead of saying, "I cannot resist that cookie," a client could say, "I will resist that cookie." An understanding of causes of unhealthy eating, if applicable, forms a crucial basis for long-term weight management. Clients can use behavior modification to make long-lasting lifestyle changes.

Attitude Modification

A common problem people have is thinking that they are either "on or off" a diet. Being "on a diet" implies that, at some point, the diet will be over, resulting in weight gain if old habits are resumed. Dieting should not be so restrictive and with such unrealistic goals that the person cannot wait to get "off the diet." Remember, the original Greek meaning of *diet* is "manner of living." When combined with exercise, behavior and attitude modification, social support, and a maintenance plan, dieting is really a plan of sensible eating that allows for periodic indulgences.

Setting realistic and measurable goals, followed by monitoring and self-reward when appropriate, is critical to the success of any weight loss program. Through goal setting, goals involving complex behavior changes can be broken down into a series of small, successive steps. Goals need to be reasonable, positive, measurable, and behavior-oriented. For example, if a problem behavior is buying a chocolate bar every afternoon at work, a goal may be to bring an appropriate afternoon snack from home (instead of buying the chocolate bar) at least three days per week. This gives the client flexibility (since it's not every day) in working toward a healthier goal.

Even with reasonable goals, occasional lapses in behavior occur. Knowing that this can happen and having a constructive attitude are critical. Rather than having feelings of guilt and failure, it is better to accept the situation, then resume working toward the healthier behavior.

Hunger and food categorization (i.e. categorizing food that is "good for you" or "bad for you") should also be discussed. *Hunger* is a physiological need for food, whereas *appetite* is a psychological need. Eating should be in response to hunger, not to appetite. Obese people frequently think certain foods are "good" for them and certain foods are "bad." No food is inherently good or bad; some foods do contain more nutrients per calorie (are more nutrient-dense), and other foods provide few nutrients per calorie and provide less nutrition. The message should be that no food is so bad that it can never be eaten.

Social Support

A supportive environment may assist in weight loss for many people. When possible, clients need to enlist the support of someone who is easy to talk to, understanding, and genuinely interested in helping. Partners can model good eating habits and give praise and encouragement. The client needs to tell the partner exactly how to be supportive; and requests of the partner need to be specific and positive. As an example, the client could ask the partner to help by not offering high-calorie snacks.

Social media can be used as an effective way of providing social support. Many physicians, exercise professionals, Registered Dietitian Nutritionists, and weight loss companies use social networking sites to connect with individuals with whom they are working. Programs have been designed so that the client can input data to help track food intake, exercise, and other health habits. One can personalize a diet and fitness plan, connect with Registered Dietitian Nutritionists and trainers, and join a support group. Little research has been done to determine the long-term effects of these activities in maintaining weight loss.

Drugs and Surgery

In some situations, obesity becomes so severe that it threatens health, even in the immediate short-term. Or, it may be so difficult to manage that a physician feels that more aggressive treatment is in order, and a physician may prescribe drugs for weight loss. Researchers have developed some drugs that may alter appetite, feelings of fullness, and body metabolism. So far, experts agree that there is no perfect diet drug. Common weight loss medications include Xenical®, Qsymia®, and Belvig®. All of these medications should be used in conjunction with lifestyle intervention and therapies.

With the increased incidence of moderate-to-severe obesity, there has been a rise in the number of bariatric surgical procedures performed. One procedure, the gastric bypass, actually reduces the size of the stomach. This makes it difficult to eat much food at one time because the smaller stomach becomes full more easily. After surgery, some clients experience gastric upset and/or vomiting, and decreased absorption. Clients may require supplementation with calcium, iron, and/or vitamin B12. About 80 percent of clients lose weight following gastric bypass, but less than half attain a desirable weight; and over time, many patients regain weight. This dramatic procedure requires long-term behavior change, and a team approach to weight management.

Other types of weight loss surgery include gastroplasty, gastric banding, and gastric sleeve. These restrict the amount of food that can be taken into the stomach. Like gastric bypass surgery, the success of the surgery depends upon personal motivation, a commitment to a new lifestyle, and healthy eating habits.

Menu Planning for Weight Loss and Maintenance

A gradual approach to dietary change can have lasting effects on weight control. This is a big advantage over dramatic treatments, many of which tend to produce only

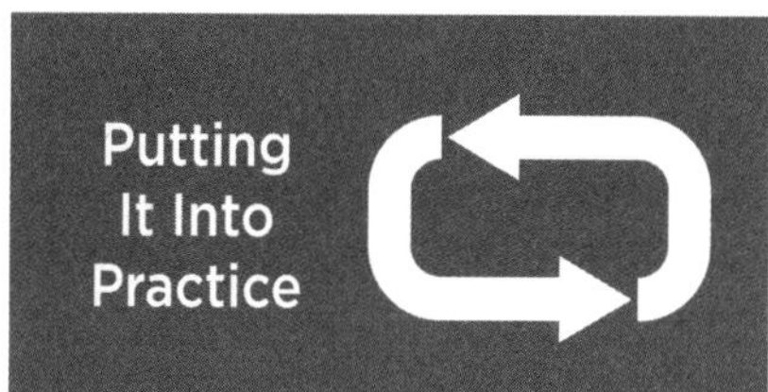

2. What suggestions could you make to a client who has "tried every diet that exists" but cannot seem to lose weight or keep it off? She lives alone, and mentions that she does not buy any "bad" foods.

temporary results. A commonsense approach combines regular exercise with reduced caloric intake to shift the balance of calories and achieve weight loss. As was previously stated, there are many diet options where one or more macronutrients are restricted (i.e. fat, carbohydrates, and protein), and each of them can provide meaningful weight loss. Overall, decreasing calorie intake can lead to increased weight loss and improved weight maintenance. *The Dietary Guidelines for Americans 2015-2020* generally recommends the following:

- Protein: 10-35 percent of total calories
- Carbohydrate: 45-65 percent of total calories
- Fat: 20-35 percent of total calories

According to the *Dietary Guidelines for Americans 2015-2020*, "A moderate amount of evidence demonstrates that intake of dietary patterns with less than 45% calories from carbohydrate or more than 35% calories from protein are not more effective than other diets for weight loss or weight maintenance, are difficult to maintain over the longterm, and may be less safe. One tool for nutritional planning is MyPlate, described in Chapter 1. The following advice can be useful:

- Everything you eat and drink over time matters. The right mix can help you be healthier now and in the future. Start with small changes to make healthier choices you can enjoy.
- Find your healthy eating style and maintain it for a lifetime. This means:
  - Make half your plate fruits and vegetables.
  - Focus on whole fruits.
  - Vary your veggies.
  - Make half your grains whole grains.
  - Move to low-fat and fat-free milk or yogurt.
  - Vary your protein routine.
  - Drink and eat less sodium, saturated fat, and added sugars.

Maintenance Support

Only recently has weight maintenance support started to receive the attention it deserves as a crucial component of a weight loss program. Unfortunately, little is known about factors associated with weight maintenance success or what support is needed during the first few months of weight maintenance, when a majority of people begin to relapse. Once a goal weight has been achieved, maintaining that weight can bring about stress, because adjustments in previous lifestyle behaviors are needed. Food is no longer a focal point, and old friends and activities may not fit very well into the new regime. Support and encouragement from significant others may diminish. A formal maintenance program can help deal with those issues as well as others.

SECTION B MEDICAL NUTRITION THERAPY AND CARDIOVASCULAR DISEASE MANAGEMENT

Medical Nutrition Therapy of Cardiovascular Disease

Cardiovascular disease (CVD) is a general term that refers to diseases of the heart and blood vessels. It is the number one cause of death in the U.S. About one in five Americans dies of heart disease, and one in four Americans has one or more of these forms of cardiovascular disease:

- Coronary artery disease (CAD)
- Stroke
- High blood pressure
- Chronic obstructive pulmonary disease (COPD)

Coronary Artery Disease (CAD)

Most heart disease is the result of **atherosclerosis**, a process in which deposits of cholesterol, fat, calcium, and other substances accumulate on the inside of arteries. Atherosclerosis is also called hardening of the arteries. This process gradually reduces the amount of blood that can flow through an artery and also makes the artery less elastic and stretchy. Sometimes the buildup, also called *plaque*, can even close off an artery and stop blood flow completely (see Figure 6.5—Atherosclerosis).

Figure 6.5
Atherosclerosis

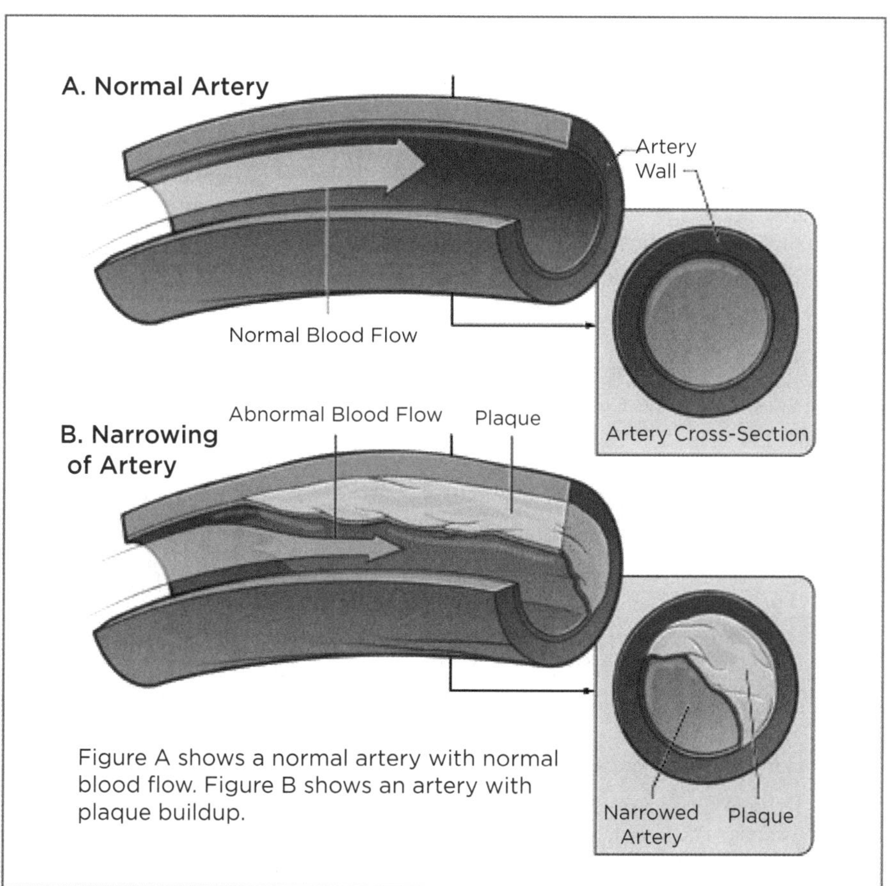

Figure A shows a normal artery with normal blood flow. Figure B shows an artery with plaque buildup.

Source: National Heart, Lung, and Blood Institute: www.nhlbi.nih.gov

GLOSSARY

Cardiovascular Disease (CVD)
General term that refers to the diseases of the heart and blood vessels

Atherosclerosis
Development of plaque in the coronary arteries

GLOSSARY

Coronary Artery Disease (CAD)
When the coronary arteries (which supply blood to the heart) are clogged with atherosclerotic deposits

Myocardial Infarction (MI)
Heart attack

Hyperlipidemia
High blood cholesterol

Low-Density Lipoproteins (LDL)
The lipoprotein that carries most of the cholesterol in the blood—"lousy" (bad) cholesterol

High-Density Lipoproteins (HDL)
The lipoprotein that carries cholesterol away from the body organs to the liver—"healthy" (good) cholesterol

Coronary artery disease (CAD) occurs when the coronary arteries, which supply blood to the heart, are clogged with atherosclerotic deposits. A heart attack occurs when the arteries that feed the heart muscle are blocked. A heart attack is called a **myocardial infarction (MI)**. If part of the heart muscle is denied oxygen, it dies. A piece of the heart is damaged and no longer contracts, so the heart works less efficiently. A heart attack may develop slowly or suddenly. Major symptoms and warning signs are:

- Chest discomfort that lasts several minutes or longer. This may feel like pressure, squeezing, fullness, or pain.
- Discomfort in other areas of the upper body, such as one or both arms, the back, neck, jaw, or stomach.
- Shortness of breath.
- Breaking out in a cold sweat.
- Nausea or light-headedness.

Many of the risk factors for coronary heart disease have nutrition connections. Let's look more closely at one of these factors—**hyperlipidemia** (high blood cholesterol). Cholesterol travels through the bloodstream in little clusters of proteins and lipids called *lipoproteins*. Usually, blood cholesterol measurements are divided into two types: Low-Density Lipoproteins (LDL) and High-Density Lipoproteins (HDL).

Low-Density Lipoproteins (LDL), or "bad cholesterol," carries most of the cholesterol in the blood. Cholesterol and fat from LDLs are the main source of dangerous buildup and blockage in the arteries. Thus, the higher the LDL cholesterol level, the greater the risk of heart disease. As a memory aid, think of LDL as "L=lousy" cholesterol.

High-Density Lipoproteins (HDL), or "good cholesterol," carries cholesterol away from body organs and takes it to the liver for destruction. Think of HDL as cholesterol that is on its way out of the body. A high level of HDL is a favorable health indicator. As a memory aid, think of HDL as "H=healthy" cholesterol.

Triglyceride is the most common type of fat in the body and in food. Triglycerides are made up of three (think tri=three) fatty acid units and one unit of glycerol. Triglyceride levels can increase from excess carbohydrates or excess alcohol in the diet. A high triglyceride level combined with low HDL cholesterol or high LDL cholesterol increases the risk of atherosclerosis.

For HDL, high numbers are better. A level less than 40 mg/dl is low and is considered a major risk factor because it increases the risk of developing heart disease. HDL levels of 60 mg/dl or more help to lower the risk. Triglyceride levels are borderline high at 150-199 mg/dl or high at over 200 mg/dl.

More than 90 million Americans have blood cholesterol levels that present risks for heart disease. Reaching and/or maintaining a normal weight, exercising, and limiting fat and cholesterol in the diet can all help adjust LDL and HDL levels to a healthier profile. Drugs are also used for this purpose. Keep in mind that the preventive goal is to reduce LDL and raise HDL. The National Cholesterol Education Program provides guidelines for cholesterol levels, shown in Figure 6.6.

Relationship between Saturated Fats, Trans-fats, and Cardiovascular Disease. To control risk factors for heart disease, the critical issue is the type of fat in the American diet. The consumption of fats, specifically saturated fat and trans-fat, increases the risk of cardiovascular disease. Conversely, unsaturated fats, specifically as monounsaturated

Figure 6.6
Cholesterol Guidelines

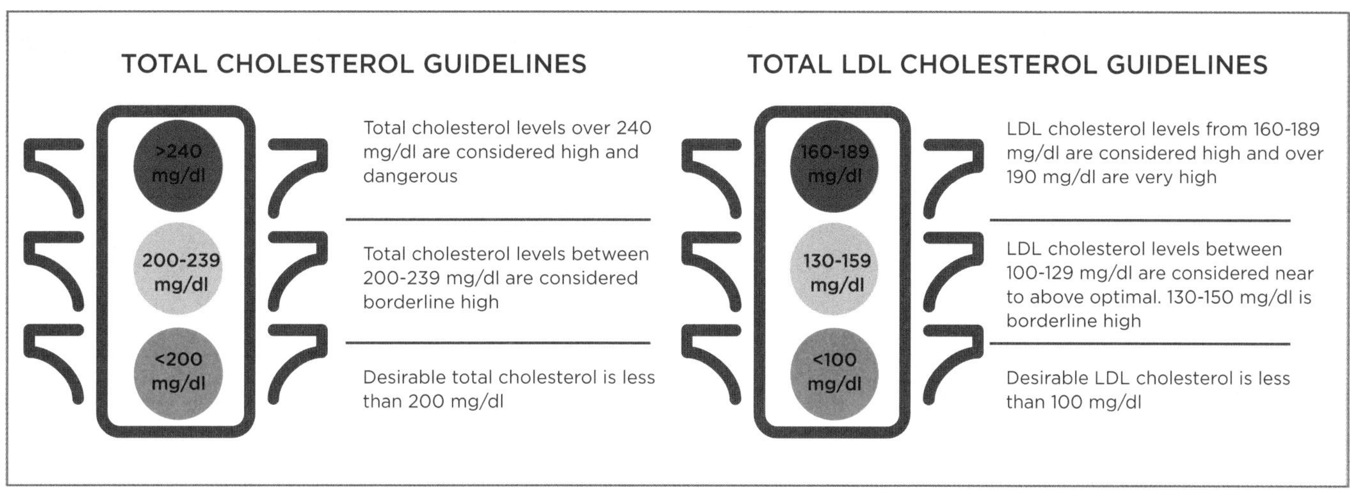

Source: National Cholesterol Education Program

and polyunsaturated fatty acids, promote heart health. In the past, recommendations have been made to limit the total amount of fat in the diet. Today, there is more evidence to indicate that decreasing saturated fat and trans-fat are more effective at decreasing CVD than limiting total fat intake. Moreover, it is important to note that each person may not react to decreases in dietary fat in a uniform way. The effects of dietary fat are dependent on many factors such as physical activity, lifestyle habits, and genetics.

To lower LDL cholesterol with MNT, it is important to choose foods low in saturated fat and trans-fat. Saturated fat is found in greater amounts from animal sources and tends to remain solid at room temperature. Decreasing foods high in saturated fats and using lower fat choices (overall) will help reduce saturated fat in the diet. In 2015, based on a review of the literature, the U.S. Food and Drug Administration (FDA) finalized its determination of partially hydrogenated oils (PHOs), which are the primary source of artificial trans-fats in processed foods. PHOs are not generally recognized as safe (GRAS) for use in food. Removing PHOs from processed foods could prevent heart attacks and deaths. As of June 18, 2018, the FDA prohibits manufacturers to use PHOs in foods.

Whenever possible, it is best to substitute unsaturated fat for saturated fat. Unsaturated fat is usually liquid at room temperature and can be either monounsaturated or polyunsaturated. Examples of foods high in monounsaturated fat are olive oil and canola oil. Those high in polyunsaturated fat include safflower, sunflower, corn, and soybean oils. Saturated fat should be limited to no more than 7 percent of the diet. Figure 6.7 compares saturated fat in some common food choices. Trans-fats should be limited or omitted in the diet since they raise total cholesterol and LDL cholesterol. Trans-fats are produced when oils are partially hydrogenated (partially solidified) to make margarine, shortening, and other products that need to be more "solid" at room temperature. Trans-fats appear in many types of stick margarines, and are also ingredients in snack foods, purchased frosting, and some commercial baked goods.

Foods rich in complex carbohydrates (high in starch and fiber) are excellent substitutes for foods high in saturated and trans-fats. Foods such as breads, cereals, pasta, grain, fruits, and vegetables—are naturally low in saturated fat and cholesterol, and

Figure 6.7
Comparison of Saturated Fat in Common Foods

LOW SATURATED FAT FOOD CHOICES		SATURATED FAT IN COMMON FOODS	
Low Fat Cheddar	1.2 g	Cheddar Cheese	6.0 g
Frozen Yogurt	2.5 g	Ice Cream	4.5 g
Extra Lean Ground Beef	5.3 g	Ground Beef	7.2 g
Bagel	0.1 g	Croissant	6.6 g
1% Milk	1.6 g	Whole Milk	5.1 g
Soft Margarine	0.7 g	Butter	2.4 g

Source: U.S. Department of Agriculture

are usually lower in calories. Research indicates that some forms of fiber may help reduce blood cholesterol (LDL) levels. Specifically using plant-based foods, such as beans, peas, and lentils, for much of the dietary protein is beneficial in reducing LDL cholesterol. In addition, some research indicates that meat-based protein, even aside from its fat content, may stimulate LDL cholesterol levels. So, reducing meat-based protein is a good idea.

Other nutritional factors that can favorably influence blood cholesterol include omega-3 fatty acids (found primarily in fish), garlic, and green tea. That is why according to MyPlate, it is recommended that Americans consume fish at least twice a week.

Relationship between Cholesterol and Cardiovascular Disease (CVD). Decreasing saturated fat and trans-fat has been shown to be more effective in combating CVD than decreasing dietary cholesterol intake. Figure 6.8 offers suggestions for choosing foods low in saturated fat and cholesterol. However, the recommendation is to reduce the intake of both.

High cholesterol foods include egg yolks, liver, the fat in meats and poultry, shellfish, and dairy fat (cream, whole milk, regular cheeses, etc.). Remember, cholesterol is found only in foods of animal origin. The recommendation is to limit dietary cholesterol intake to less than 300 mg per day.

Experts also advise maintaining a healthy weight. People who are overweight tend to have higher blood cholesterol levels than people of a healthy weight. Overweight adults with an "apple" shape—bigger (pot) belly—tend to have a higher risk for heart disease than those with a "pear" shape—bigger hips and thighs. For anyone who is overweight, losing even a little weight can help to lower LDL and raise HDL. Being physically active and controlling caloric intake helps with weight management, while lowering LDL.

Drug Treatment. Drug treatment is considered appropriate for adults who have a high LDL level, especially if they also have other CAD risk factors. Drugs referred to as *bile acid sequestrants*, such as cholestyramine, are approved for use in clients with high LDL levels who don't respond to MNT alone. Constipation is the most common side effect.

Statin drugs, along with MNT, are effective in lowering total and LDL cholesterol. Examples of statin drugs are atorvastatin (Lipitor®), simvastatin (Zocor®), lovastatin (Mevacor®), pravastatin (Pravachol®), and rosuvastatin (Crestor®). The most common

Figure 6.8
Tips for Foods Low in Saturated Fat and Cholesterol

MEAT, POULTRY, FISH, AND SHELLFISH

Buying Tips

- Choose lean cuts of meat. Look for meats labeled "lean" or "extra lean." Eat moderate portions—no more than about 6 ounces per day (a 3 ounce portion is about the size of a deck of cards).
- Limit organ meats like liver, sweetbreads, and kidneys. Organ meats are high in dietary cholesterol, even though they are fairly low in fat.
- Limit high-fat processed meats like bacon, bologna, salami, hot dogs, and sausage. Some chicken and turkey hot dogs are lower in saturated fat and total fat than pork and beef hot dogs. There are also "lean" beef hot dogs that are low in fat and saturated fat. Usually, processed poultry products have more fat and dietary cholesterol than fresh poultry. To be sure, check the nutrition label on deli products to find those that are lowest in fat and saturated fat.
- Try fresh ground turkey or chicken made from white meat (the breast).
- Limit use of goose and duck. They are higher in saturated fat, even with the skin removed.
- Choose fish wisely. Squid, shrimp, and oysters are fairly high in dietary cholesterol, whereas scallops, mussels, and clams are low in dietary cholesterol. Finned fish is usually low in cholesterol. The recommendation is to eat fish twice a week. Consider baking, poaching, or grilling, as opposed to frying.
- Buy canned fish packed in water, not oil.

Preparation Tips

- Trim fat from meat and remove skin from poultry before eating.
- Bake, broil, microwave, poach, or roast instead of frying. If frying, use a nonstick pan and nonstick cooking spray or a small amount of vegetable oil to reduce the fat.
- When roasting meat, place the meat on a rack so the fat can drip away.
- Brown ground meat and drain well before adding other ingredients.
- Use fat-free ingredients like fruit juice, wine, or defatted broth to baste meats and poultry.

DAIRY FOODS

Buying Tips

- Choose skim or 1 percent milk, rather than 2 percent or whole milk.
- When looking for hard cheese, select versions that are labeled fat-free, reduced-fat, low-fat, light, or part skim.
- When shopping for soft cheeses, choose low-fat (1 percent or skim) or nonfat cottage cheese and mozzarella, farmer cheese, pot cheese; or part skim or light ricotta.
- Use low-fat or nonfat yogurt; try it in recipes or as a topping, in place of cream or whipping cream.
- Try low-fat or fat-free sour cream or cream cheese blends for spreads, toppings, or in recipes.

Preparation Tips

- Try low-fat cheese in casseroles, or try a sharp-flavored regular cheese and use less than the recipe calls for. Save most of the cheese for the top.
- Use skim, 1 percent, or evaporated skim milk for cream soups or white sauces.

Source: U.S. Department of Agriculture and U.S. Department of Health and Human Services

Continued...

Figure 6.8

Tips for Foods Low in Saturated Fat and Cholesterol *(Continued)*

EGGS

Buying Tips

- Eggs are included in many processed foods and baked goods. Look at the nutrition label to check the cholesterol content.
- Try egg substitutes.

Preparation Tips

- Substitute two egg whites for one whole egg in recipes (egg whites have no saturated fat) or use egg substitutes.

FRUITS AND VEGETABLES

Buying Tips

Buy fruits and vegetables often—fresh, frozen, or canned. They have no cholesterol and most are low in saturated fat. Also, most fruits and vegetables, except avocados, coconut, and olives, are low in total fat.

Preparation Tips

- Use fruits as snacks or desserts.
- Prepare vegetables as snacks, side dishes, and salads. Season with herbs, spices, lemon juice, or fat-free or low-fat mayonnaise. Limit use of regular mayonnaise, salad dressings, and cream cheese, or other fatty sauces.

BREADS, CEREALS, PASTA, RICE, AND DRY PEAS AND BEANS

Buying Tips

- Use more whole grain breads, rolls, and cereals.
- Limit baked goods made with large amounts of fat, especially saturated fat (e.g., croissants, biscuits, doughnuts, butter rolls, muffins, coffee cake, Danish pastry). Avoid baked goods listing palm, palm kernel, and coconut oils as ingredients. These oils are high in saturated fats, even though they are vegetable oils.
- Choose ready-to-eat cereals often. Most are low in saturated fat. (Exceptions would be if they are the types made with coconut or coconut oil.)
- Buy dry peas and beans often.
- Serve beans or peas at least once a week. Try a "meatless Monday" (or another day of the week), where beans and peas are the main entrée instead of meat.

Preparation Tips

- Try using whole grain pasta or brown/wild rice in soups, or with low-fat sauces as main dishes or casseroles.
- Stretch meat dishes with pasta, beans, peas, or vegetables for hearty meals.
- Bake homemade muffins and quick breads using unsaturated vegetable oils; substitute two egg whites for each egg yolk, or use egg substitutes. Experiment with substituting applesauce for oil or cut back the amount of oil in the recipe. For every two cups of flour in a recipe, try using just a 1/2 cup of vegetable oil. Also, use whole wheat flour as a substitute for 1/2 of the all-purpose flour.
- Use dry peas and beans as the main ingredient in casseroles, soups, or other one-dish meals.

Source: U.S. Department of Agriculture and U.S. Department of Health and Human Services

side effect is muscle or joint pain although nausea, constipation, and diarrhea may occur. There may be potentially serious side effects if you have liver or kidney disease. If statins are effective at lowering LDL cholesterol, a person may be on one for life.

Selective cholesterol absorption inhibitors are another class of cholesterol-lowering drugs. They are most effective at lowering LDL cholesterol, have a modest effect on lowering triglycerides, and raise HDL cholesterol. An example is ezetimibe (Zetia®).

Stroke

Stroke is the fifth leading cause of death in the U.S. About 795,000 Americans have a stroke each year. Of these, 129,000 people die from a stroke. A **stroke** occurs when blood-rich vessels bringing oxygen to the brain burst or become clogged. The interruption of blood flow to the brain stops body functions and damages nerve cells. The brain must have a continuous supply of blood rich in oxygen and nutrients for energy. If deprived of blood flow for more than a few minutes, brain cells die. These brain cells control speech, muscle movement, and comprehension. When the brain cells die, sometimes these functions die too.

GLOSSARY

Stroke
Occurs when the blood vessels bringing oxygen to the brain become clogged or burst, causing damage to the brain and nerve cells

The majority of strokes are also linked to atherosclerosis, a result of blockages in the arteries that supply blood to the brain. The blockages may be caused by a *thrombus* (a clot) that forms on the inner lining of a brain or neck artery that is already partly clogged by atherosclerotic plaque. A blood clot formed in another part of the body may also cause a stroke. Usually a wandering clot like this—called an *embolus*—breaks off from plaque in an artery wall, or originates in the heart. The most serious kinds of stroke occur not from blockage, but from hemorrhage. A hemorrhage occurs when a spot in a brain artery weakened by disease—usually high blood pressure or atherosclerosis—ruptures and leaks blood. If an artery inside the brain ruptures, it is called a *cerebral hemorrhage*. Sometimes, hemorrhage may be caused by an *aneurysm*, a section of the artery wall so thin that it may balloon out and burst, especially when high blood pressure is present.

An incident involving physical symptoms that last less than 24 hours and leaves no permanent disability is called a *transient ischemic attack* (TIA) or "mini-stroke." Some individuals have repeated attacks of TIAs without any serious consequences, but these symptoms should not be ignored and need immediate medical attention.

The kind of disability after a stroke depends on the location and extent of brain damage. The brain can be resourceful. After brain swelling goes down following a stroke, small blood vessels around the blocked area can sometimes enlarge to allow more blood flow to the damaged section. Some incapacitated cells may recover partially or completely. In many cases, other brain cells can assume the functions of the damaged ones.

Relationship between Stroke and Diet. A stroke can lead to a loss of nutrition-related functions, such as the ability to chew and/or swallow foods. This places a person at risk for malnutrition. It is important to properly manage dietary intake so that nutritional

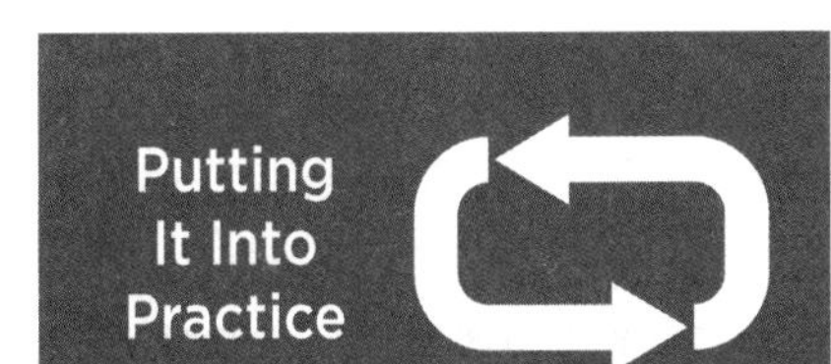

3. Which would be a better choice in terms of saturated fat content, and overall nutrition: a sausage, egg, and cheese croissant sandwich, or two eggs scrambled with peppers and onions and a teaspoon of butter?

balance is maintained. MNT is effective in treating atherosclerosis. Increasing dietary intake of fruits, vegetables, and whole grains, while decreasing intake of dietary fats, particularly saturated and trans-fats, can help reduce the risk of atherosclerosis, thus reducing the risk of strokes.

Hypertension (High Blood Pressure)

Hypertension (HTN) is a medical condition resulting in chronic high blood pressure. Hypertension, or high blood pressure, causes the heart to pump harder than it should to get blood to all the parts of the body. Because high blood pressure usually doesn't have early warning signs, it is known as the "silent killer." Hypertension increases the risk of stroke, heart attack, and kidney disease. The higher the blood pressure, the greater the risk. An estimated 80 million people, more than half of the adult population, have either prehypertension or hypertension. Each year, half a million strokes and over a million heart attacks result from hypertension.

With the *Dietary Guidelines for Americans* comes a heightened concern about increasing blood pressure levels that is being seen in children and teens. Studies have shown that high blood pressure in youth increases the development of atherosclerosis. Blood pressure rises with age as a normal part of growth. With the increase in blood pressure levels in children, an increase in the number of adults with hypertension is probable in future generations.

Blood pressure is expressed as a fraction, such as 120/80 millimeters of mercury (abbreviated as "mmHg"). The numerator (120) is the **systolic pressure**—the pressure of blood within arteries when the heart is pumping. The denominator (80) is the **diastolic pressure**—the pressure in the arteries when the heart is resting between beats. An easy way to remember which number goes on top is to think about "sky" and "dirt." The "s" (sky=systolic) is the top number; the "d" (dirt=distolic) is the bottom number. A typical blood pressure for a young adult might be 120/80 mmHg. Hypertension Stage 1 (see Figure 6.9) is the most common form of high blood pressure. To be diagnosed as hypertensive, a person has had at least two to three readings performed on each of three separate visits.

Secondary hypertension occurs when elevated blood pressure persists due to a medical problem, such as hormonal abnormality or an inherited narrowing of the aorta. This means the high blood pressure is "secondary" to another condition. The causes of most

GLOSSARY

Hypertension (HTN)
Medical condition resulting in chronic high blood pressure

Systolic Pressure
The top number ("s") of the blood pressure reading—pressure when the heart is pumping

Diastolic Pressure
The bottom number or the denominator ("d") of the blood pressure reading—pressure when the heart is at rest/ between beats

Figure 6.9

Categories for Blood Pressure Levels in Adults

Expressed in mmHg or millimeters of mercury

CATEGORY	Systolic (top number)		Diastolic (bottom number)
Normal	Less than 120	*And*	Less than 80
Prehypertension	120-139	*Or*	80-89
High Blood Pressure			
Stage 1	140-159	*Or*	90-99
Stage 2	160 or higher	*Or*	100 or higher

Source: National Heart, Lung, and Blood Institute

cases of hypertension are unknown; this is referred to as *essential hypertension*. Because the cause is a mystery, essential hypertension cannot be cured, but it can be controlled. Treatment is long-term and includes lifestyle modifications and possibly medications. Lifestyle modifications include weight reduction, increased physical activity, medical nutrition therapy, reducing intake of alcohol, and avoiding tobacco.

When lifestyle modifications do not succeed in lowering blood pressure to within normal limits, adding medication is the next step. Reducing blood pressure with medication decreases the incidence of cardiovascular death and disease. Two classes of antihypertensive drugs—*diuretics* and *beta blockers*—are common for initial drug therapy. Diuretics are a class of blood pressure medications that cause increased urine output. Some diuretics can cause an increased excretion of potassium in the urine, thereby requiring an increase in the consumption of high potassium foods. Beta blockers reduce the heart rate so that the heart puts out less blood.

Medical Nutrition Therapy (MNT). MNT for hypertension often includes a reduction in sodium intake. Sodium is one of the main minerals in salt; the other mineral is chloride. (The symbol for table salt is NaCl: Na stands for sodium and Cl stands for chloride.) The current recommendation from the American Heart Association (AHA) is to reduce sodium intake to less than 1,500 mg of sodium daily. Unfortunately, reducing dietary sodium intake is not effective for everyone who has hypertension. It is estimated that about half of people with hypertension are sensitive to sodium and half are not. For some (we refer to those as *sodium-sensitive hypertensives*), reducing dietary sodium may be very effective. For others with hypertension, there may have to be other approaches to control hypertension. Individuals ages 14 and older should limit sodium to less than 2300 mg/day; for children ages 1-3 less than 1500 mg/day; for children ages 4-8 less than 1900 mg/day, and for children ages 9-13 less than 2200 mg/day.

To give a perspective, note that just one level teaspoon of salt provides about 2,300 milligrams of sodium. However, most people do not obtain the majority of their sodium by adding salt to foods. In fact, about 75 percent of our dietary sodium is added to food during processing and manufacturing. Figure 6.10 illustrates sodium content of many foods. Besides salt, common sources of sodium in the diet include:

- Processed foods with salt or other sodium compounds added.
- Other sodium-containing compounds, such as baking soda (hint: *sod*-ium), mono*sodium* glutamate (MSG), and soy sauce.
- Foods in which sodium is naturally present. Milk and milk products are somewhat high in sodium.
- In some areas, the water supply provides 10 percent of an individual's daily sodium consumption. Sodium is often present in water that has gone through a water softening process.
- Some medications, such as some antacids.

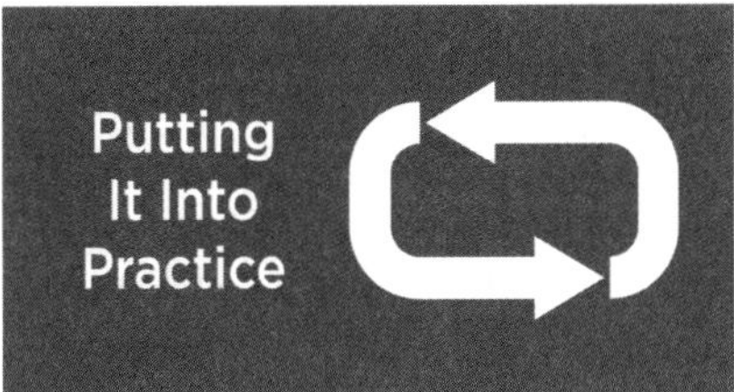

4. Which of the following low-sodium foods would you recommend, considering overall nutrition value?
    - No-salt-added canned green beans
    - Unsalted potato chips
    - Unsalted almonds
    - Low sodium vegetable juice
    - Unsalted pretzels

Figure 6.10
Food Sources of Sodium

FOOD	PERCENT	FOOD	PERCENT
Yeast Breads	7.3%	Chicken and Chicken Mixed Dishes	6.8%
Pizza	6.3%	Pasta and Pasta Dishes	5.1%
Cold Cuts	4.5%	Condiments	4.4%
Mexican Mixed Dishes	4.1%	Sausage, Franks, Bacon, and Ribs	4.1%
Grain-Based Desserts	3.4%	Regular Cheese	3.3%
Soups	3.3%	Beef and Beef Mixed Dishes	3.3%
Rice and Rice Mixed Dishes	2.6%	Eggs and Egg Mixed Dishes	2.6%
Burgers	2.4%	Salad Dressing	2.4%
Ready-to-Eat Cereals	2.0%	Potato, Corn, and Other Chips	1.8%
Pork and Pork Mixed Dishes	1.8%	Quick Breads	1.7%
Other White Potatoes	1.6%	Other Fish and Fish Mixed Dishes	1.5%
Reduced Fat Milk	1.3%	Pancakes, Waffles, French Toast	1.1%
Crackers	1.1%	Whole Milk	0.7%

Sources of Sodium Among the US Population. Risk Factor Monitoring and Methods Branch. Applied Research Program. National Cancer Institute. Printed in the Report of the DGAC Dietary Guidelines for Americans, 2010, Part D. Section 6, pg. 19 http://www.cnpp.usda.gov/DGAs2010-DGACReport.htm

The *Dietary Guidelines for Americans* recommends a significant change in dietary sodium consumption. In the past, a typical sodium-restricted diet was described as a "No Added Salt" diet or a "4 Gram (4000 mg) Sodium" diet. This typically eliminated adding salt at the table and restricting some very high-sodium foods. Another type of therapeutic diet was a "2 Gram (2000 mg) Sodium" diet or a "Sodium Controlled" diet, which recommended also limiting milk, regular bread, and starch foods. Current nutrient label claims for sodium are shown in Figure 6.11.

Both sodium (NA or NA+) and potassium (K or K+) are frequently listed on a diet order. A 2-gram sodium diet might also be written as a "2 gram NA diet." An increased potassium diet might be listed as an "increased K diet." See Figure 6.12 for tips on reducing sodium intake.

Another factor that may impact medical nutrition therapy for cardiac disease management is potassium intake. Today, the average intake of dietary potassium is below the recommended levels of 4700 mg per day. In contrast to recommendations about reducing sodium intake, the recommendation is to increase potassium intake. Dietary potassium has been shown to lower blood pressure. Therapeutic diets should emphasize both a lower sodium intake and an increased potassium intake. Figure 6.13 shows a few good to excellent food sources of potassium.

One diet that addresses both reducing sodium and increasing potassium is the DASH (Dietary Approaches to Stop Hypertension) diet. The DASH diet emerged as part of the National High Blood Pressure Education Program from the National Institutes of Health, and was designed to help treat hypertension. There are several versions of the DASH diet. The version selected for this chapter is the one that best addresses the

Figure 6.11
Nutrient Label Claims for Sodium

Label	Claim
Sodium Free	Less than 5 mg of sodium
Very Low Sodium	35 mg or less of sodium
Low Sodium	140 mg or less of sodium
Reduced or Less Sodium	At least 25 percent less sodium than the usual food product
Light in Sodium	At least 50 percent less sodium than the usual food product

Source: Food and Drug Administration

Figure 6.12
Tips for Reducing Sodium Intake

- Choose low- or reduced-sodium, or no-salt-added versions of foods and condiments when available.
- Buy vegetables fresh, frozen, or canned with no salt added.
- Use fresh poultry, fish, and lean meat, rather than canned, smoked, or processed types.
- Choose ready-to-eat breakfast cereals that are lower in sodium.
- Limit cured foods (such as bacon and ham), foods packed in brine (such as pickles, pickled vegetables, olives, and sauerkraut), and condiments (such as MSG, mustard, horseradish, catsup, and barbecue sauce). Even limit intake of the lower sodium versions of soy sauce and teriyaki sauce. Treat these condiments like table salt. Replace pickles and olives with fresh lettuce, greens, or tomatoes.
- Replace high-sodium cheeses and peanut butter with low-sodium varieties.
- Use spices instead of salt. In cooking and at the table flavor foods with herbs, spices, lemon, lime, vinegar, or salt-free seasoning blends.
- Cook rice, pasta, and hot cereals without salt. Cut back on instant or flavored rice, pasta, and cereal mixes, which usually have added salt.
- Choose convenience foods that are lower in sodium. Cut back on frozen dinners, mixed dishes such as pizza, packaged mixes, canned soups or broths, and salad dressings, as these often have a lot of sodium.
- Rinse canned foods, such as tuna and canned legumes (beans and peas), to remove some sodium before eating them.
- Use unsalted pretzels or crackers, or fresh fruits and vegetables to replace salty snack foods.
- Use fresh or frozen vegetables instead of canned, or choose low-sodium canned foods.

Compiled from National Heart, Lung, and Blood Institute and other sources

Dietary Guidelines for Americans. Figure 6.14 shows a comparison of the DASH diet guidelines to the usual U.S. intake and the USDA Base Pattern. As can be seen, the usual United States intake is considerably higher in sodium and lower in potassium than the DASH diet. The DASH diet emphasizes potassium-rich vegetables, fruits, and low-fat milk products. It includes whole grains, poultry, fish, and nuts, and limits red meats, sweets, and sugar-containing beverages.

The National Institutes of Health also suggests limiting alcohol consumption to no more than 1 ounce of ethanol (e.g., 24 ounce beer, 10 ounce wine, or 2 ounce 100-proof whiskey) per day for most men, and no more than 0.5 ounce per day for

Figure 6.13
Food Sources of Potassium

FOOD	AMOUNT (in mg)	FOOD	AMOUNT (in mg)
Baked Potato, 1 small	738	White Beans, 1/2 cup	595
Tomato Juice, 1 cup	556	Plain, Low-Fat Yogurt, 8 oz.	531
Sweet Potato, 1 medium	542	Fresh Orange Juice, 1 cup	496
Low-Fat Chocolate Milk, 1 cup	425	Banana, 1 medium	422
Spinach, cooked, 1/2 cup	400	Pork Loin, 3 oz.	371

Source: U.S. Department of Agriculture

women. Very much in accordance with other dietary guidance for health, a DASH diet includes plenty of whole grains, fresh fruits and vegetables, as well as low-fat or fat-free dairy products. Note that dairy products are rich sources of calcium. Calcium appears to have a protective role in managing hypertension, so maintaining adequate calcium intake is important.

Limiting sodium does not mean sacrificing flavor. Often, reducing sodium intake requires some adjustment and adaptation. People who have become accustomed to reduced sodium intake may find they enjoy other flavors in foods more. Search the Internet for ideas to create herb blends to replace salt. Many cookbooks provide advice for seasoning foods with herbs and spices, instead of salt.

Congestive Heart Failure. Another common disease of the circulatory system is called congestive heart failure (CHF). Atherosclerosis and hypertension both contribute to this condition in which the heart itself weakens. In an effort to provide adequate circulation throughout the body, the heart works harder and harder, but is not highly effective. The heart beats faster and becomes enlarged. This can lead to fluid retention in the body. According to the National Institutes of Health (NIH), CHF is a major health concern that affects at least 5 million Americans. Newest evidence does *not* support 2 gram sodium diet for CHF (Academy of Nutrition and Dietetics, 2017). Fluid restriction may also be necessary. MNT for the underlying conditions of atherosclerosis and hypertension are also recommended. If a client is overweight, effective weight management may also help to reduce the burden on the heart.

GLOSSARY

Congestive Heart Failure (CHF)
Inability of the heart to effectively pump blood to the body's organs—can be due to coronary artery disease

Chronic Obstructive Pulmonary Disease (COPD)
A group of lung diseases that include chronic bronchitis, emphysema, and asthmatic bronchitis

Chronic Obstructive Pulmonary Disease (COPD)

Chronic obstructive pulmonary disease (COPD) is the name of a group of diseases that includes chronic bronchitis, emphysema, and asthmatic bronchitis. These afflictions reduce the airflow out of the lungs. The most common symptom is shortness of breath. COPD is a leading cause of disability and death in the U.S., and at least 75 percent of the cases result from smoking. COPD can cause malnutrition due to loss of

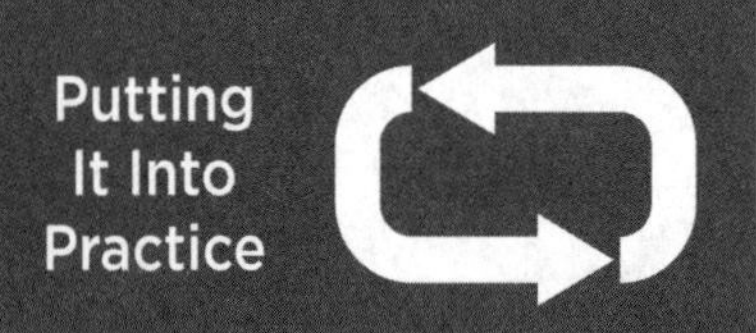

5. If a diet order is written as 2 gm NA, what does this mean?

Figure 6.14
Dietary Pattern Comparison (Adjusted to 2,000 Calories)

DIETARY PATTERN	Usual US Intake	DASH with Reduced Sodium	USDA Base Pattern
	NHANES 2001-04; 2005-06; Ages 19+	Karanja et al, 1999 and Lin et al., 2003	Britten et al., 2006
NUTRIENTS			
Calories	2000	2000	2000
Carbohydrates (% total kcal)	48.4%	58%	56.7%
Protein (% total kcal)	15.2%	18%	15.2%
Total Fat (% total kcal)	33.5%	27%	32%
Saturated Fat (% total kcal)	10.9%	6%	8.4%
Monounsaturated (% total kcal)	12.5%	10%	12.0%
Polyunsaturated (% total kcal)	6.8%	8%	9.0%
Cholesterol (mg)	269	143	229
Fiber (g)	15	29	30
Potassium (mg)	2909	4371	3478
Sodium (mg)	2846	1095	1722
FOOD GROUPS			
Vegetables total (cup)	1.6	2.1	2.5
Fruits and Juices (cup)	1.0	2.5	2
Grains total (oz.)	6.4	7.3	6
Whole Grains (oz.)	0.6	3.9	3
Milk and Milk Products (cup)	1.5	0.7	—
Low-Fat Milk (cup)	Not Described	1.9	3
ANIMAL PROTEINS			
Meat (oz.)	2.5	1.4	2.5
Poultry (oz.)	1.2	1.7	1.5
Eggs (oz.)	0.4	Not Described	0.4
Fish (total oz.)	0.5	1.4	0.5
PLANT PROTEINS			
Legumes (oz.)	Not Described	0.4	See Vegetables
Nuts and Seeds (oz.)	0.5	0.9	0.6
Oils (g)	17.7	24.8	27
Solid Fats (g)	43.2	Not Described	16
Added Sugar (g)	79.0	12 (Snacks/Sweets)	32
Alcohol (g)	9.9	No Recommendation	No Recommendation

Usual US Intakes—WWEIA, NHANES 2001-2004 and WWEIA, NHANES 2005-2006, one-day mean intakes consumed per individual. Male and female intakes adjusted to 2000 calories, averaged, and rounded to one decimal point. Adapted from the Report of the DGAC on the Dietary Guidelines, 2010, Section B, Table B2.4, pg. B2-22

appetite, changes in taste, or gastrointestinal distress. In addition, COPD makes the body work harder to breathe, thus increasing energy (calorie) needs from day-to-day. In some cases, protein-calorie malnutrition occurs as the body breaks down muscle to provide energy. Body wasting and decreased resistance to infection can result.

Relationship between COPD and Diet. The goal of MNT for a client with COPD is to maintain adequate nutritional status without overfeeding. This is important because too much food causes the body to produce excess carbon dioxide (CO2), making it more difficult for the lungs to exhale. In the case of acute breathing problems, or when a client is on a ventilator (breathing machine), the Registered Dietitian Nutritionist sometimes increases the percentage of calories from fat and decreases the percentage of calories from carbohydrates. When the body uses fat, it needs less oxygen, thus producing less (CO2), and reducing the load on the lungs. For a client with COPD, it is also important to maintain an adequate intake of foods rich in nutrients such as vitamins A and C, as these help to guard against infection. Fluid retention around the lungs may also be a problem. If so, dietary fluid restriction may be needed. Clients who experience difficulties in eating comfortably require common-sense support, which may include small, frequent meals and a diet planned around foods the client enjoys and tolerates well.

SECTION C MEDICAL NUTRITION THERAPY AND DIABETES MANAGEMENT

Diabetes Mellitus

Diabetes Mellitus (DM) is a metabolic disorder in which the body cannot use glucose properly, so blood glucose levels are high. This manifests as **hyperglycemia**. (Hint: hyper=high; gly=glucose; emia=blood). There is either an insufficient level of *insulin* or the insulin is ineffective. Insulin is a hormone (a chemical messenger) made by the pancreas, an organ located near the liver. Insulin is supposed to enable glucose in the blood to enter the body's cells, where it is used as energy. Without glucose, the cells are deprived of energy. The kidneys remove the extra glucose from the blood by dumping it into the urine, a condition called **glycosuria**. Some early symptoms of diabetes can include weight loss, insatiable hunger (called polyphagia), unquenchable thirst (called polydipsia), frequent urination (called polyuria), dehydration, weakness, and fatigue.

Diabetes is a serious disease. It is the seventh leading cause of death in the United States, and its prevalence is on the rise. More than 9 percent of the U.S. population has diabetes—about 29.1 million people. The American Diabetes Association estimates that about one-third of people with diabetes have not had the condition diagnosed. See Figure 6.15 for the prevalence of diabetes in the United States.

The life expectancy for people with diabetes is only two-thirds that of the general population. Poorly controlled diabetes can, over time, result in extensive damage throughout the body, affecting kidneys, heart, blood vessels, nerves, and eyes. Diabetes is the nation's leading cause of kidney failure and adult blindness. And, because of its damaging effect on blood vessels and nerves of the lower limbs, it can lead to amputations of toes, feet, or legs. Having diabetes increases the risk of having a stroke or heart disease by two to four times. It is hardly surprising that this is a very expensive disease that costs the nation over $245 billion each year in healthcare costs, time lost from work, and Social Security disability payments.

GLOSSARY

Diabetes Mellitus
A metabolic disorder marked by high levels of blood glucose resulting from defects in insulin production, insulin action, or both

Hyperglycemia
High blood sugar

Glycosuria
Condition where the kidneys remove the extra glucose by dumping it into the urine for removal by the body

Diagnosis and Classification of Diabetes

Diabetes may be diagnosed based on A1C criteria, or plasma glucose criteria, either fasting plasma glucose (FPG) or the 2-hour plasma glucose value after a 75 g oral glucose tolerance test (OGTT). Using the FPG, the glucose concentration in the blood is measured after an eight to twelve-hour overnight fast. A diagnosis of diabetes is generally made after testing on two occasions has revealed concentrations over 126 mg/dl (see Figure 6.16). Physicians may also perform an oral glucose tolerance test (OGTT) to better understand how the body handles glucose. This begins with a fasting blood glucose measurement. Then the patient receives a concentrated glucose drink (75 g carbohydrate). At intervals afterwards, a technician keeps re-testing blood glucose for 2 hours. This provides a pattern of glucose levels that demonstrates the body's response. When using an A1C, blood will be drawn and measured in a lab. An A1C > 6.5% indicates a diagnosis of diabetes.

Finally, if a client presents with classic symptoms or in hyperglycemic crisis, or random plasma glucose of > 200 mg/dl and symptoms, this prompts a diagnosis as well.

There are three categories of diabetes: Type 1, Type 2, and gestational diabetes. Each one will be discussed in this section as well as a condition called prediabetes.

Figure 6.15

Age-Adjusted Estimates of Percentages of Adults* With Diagnosed Diabetes

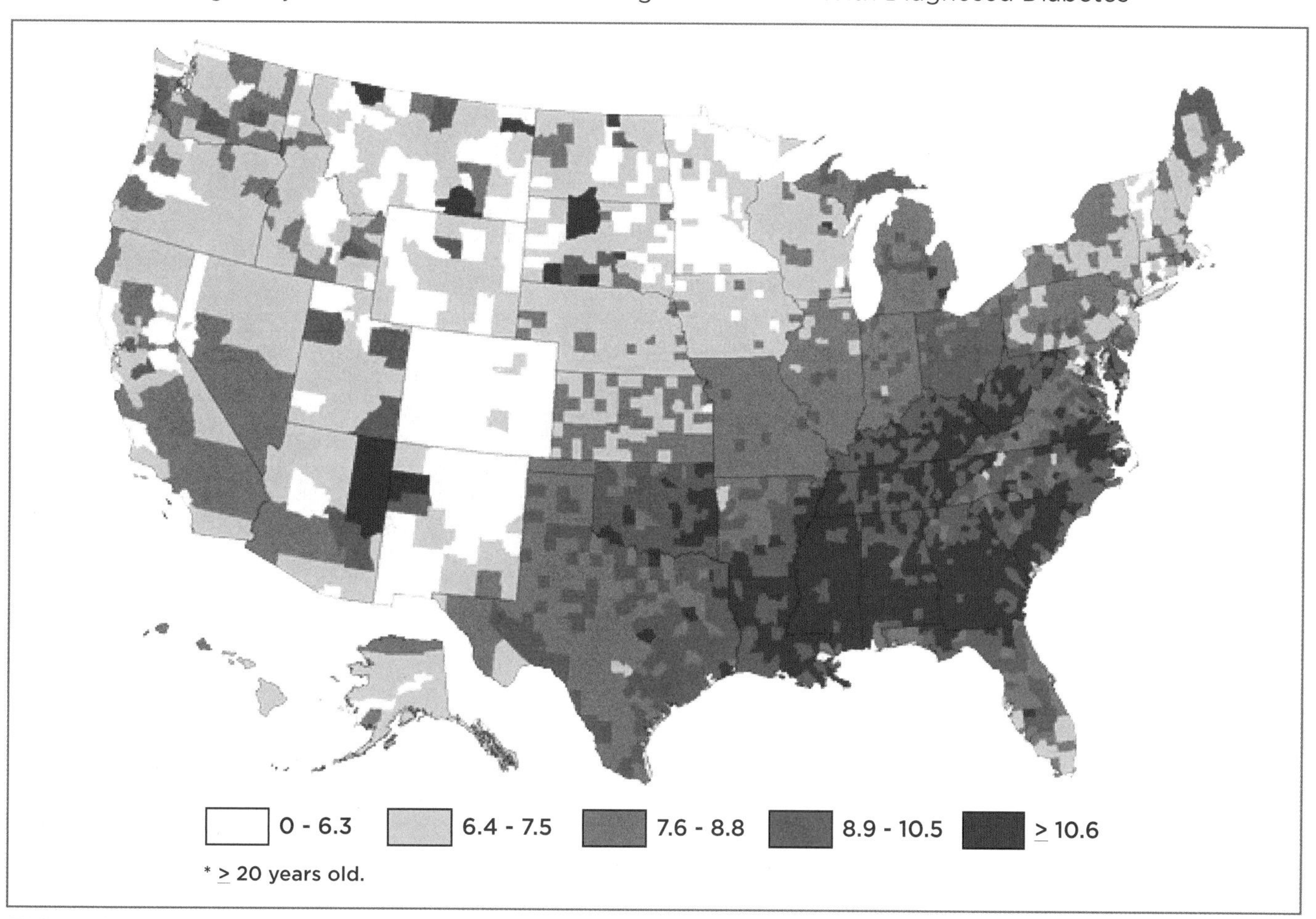

ERS Food Availability (Per Capita) Data System, Report of the DGAC on the Dietary Guidelines for Americans, 2010, D-1, pg. 10. http://www.cnpp.usda.gov/Publications/DietaryGuidelines/2010/DGAC/Report/D-1-EnergyBalance.pdf

Figure 6.16

Plasma Glucose Levels

PLASMA GLUCOSE RESULT (mg/dL)	DIAGNOSIS
99 or below	Normal
100 to 125	Pre-diabetes (impaired fasting glucose)
126 or above	Diabetes*
≥ 200 + symptoms	Diabetes
A1C ≥ 6.5%	Diabetes

** Confirmed by repeating the test on a different day. Source: Centers for Disease Control and Prevention*

GLOSSARY

Type 1 Diabetes Mellitus
When the body's immune system destroys pancreatic beta cells and insulin cannot be made

Type 2 Diabetes Mellitus
Begins as insulin resistance where the cells do not use insulin properly. Gradually the pancreas loses the ability to produce adequate insulin

Type 1 diabetes (T1DM) occurs when a group of cells in the pancreas (beta cells) is unable to make insulin. Clients with Type 1 diabetes depend on insulin injections to control their disease. T1DM is an auto-immune disease—meaning that special cells in the body whose job is to fight disease go awry. They destroy the cells in the pancreas that make insulin. This is determined by genetics or may result from an acute illness. Type 1 diabetes and other auto-immune illnesses tend to run in families. The National Institutes of Health is already testing a vaccine that may prevent this disorder. Only 5 to 10 percent of Americans with diabetes have Type 1. Classic symptoms of Type 1 diabetes appear abruptly and include excessive thirst and urination, hunger, and weight loss.

The most immediately life-threatening aspect of Type 1 diabetes is called ketosis, or the presence of ketones in the blood. Because the cells don't have enough glucose to burn for energy, they start burning fat. In the process of burning fat for energy, they produce ketones. Presence of ketones in the blood is unnatural, and begins to disturb the delicate chemical balance of the bloodstream. If not managed, this condition can lead to coma or even death.

Most cases of diabetes, from 90 to 95 percent, are classified as **Type 2 diabetes (T2DM)**. In this form of the disease, an individual's pancreas does make insulin, but the cells are not as sensitive to it; the body cells don't use the insulin. Type 2 used to be primarily diagnosed in adults over 30 years old. However, with the increasing rates of obesity in youth, there is a trend of Type 2 diabetes being diagnosed in children. As the population gets older and more overweight, the percentage of people with Type 2 diabetes increases. Almost 90 percent of those with Type 2 diabetes are obese. Obesity is a risk factor for Type 2 diabetes, as is advanced age and family history. Symptoms of Type 2 match the symptoms for Type 1, but they are often overlooked because they tend to come on gradually and are less pronounced. Other symptoms that may signal the presence of Type 2 diabetes are tingling or numbness in the lower legs, feet, or hands; skin or genital itching; and gum, skin, or bladder infections that recur and are slow to clear up.

Gestational diabetes is a condition characterized by abnormal glucose tolerance during pregnancy. It begins during the second half of pregnancy and ends after delivery. Most women are tested between the 24th and 28th week of gestation for diabetes with an oral glucose tolerance test. Some individuals with gestational diabetes require medication, including insulin, when meal planning alone is not effective. Previous gestational diabetes increases the risk of a woman being diagnosed with Type 2 diabetes later in life, especially when other risk factors are present.

Prediabetes is a condition when blood glucose levels are higher after fasting but not high enough to be classified as diabetes. People with prediabetes have an increased risk of developing Type 2 diabetes, heart disease, and stroke. About 26 percent of adults over age 20 have prediabetes, and 35 percent of adults over age 60. Studies have shown that this population can prevent or delay diabetes with weight loss and exercise.

Diabetes Management

Diabetes is a chronic disease that can be successfully managed. Treatment is designed to maintain as near-normal blood glucose levels as possible (referred to as glycemic control). Studies show that control of the blood sugar levels slows the progression of the complications of diabetes. People with diabetes may maintain near-normal blood glucose levels through:

- Medications
- Food
- Exercise
- Stress management

The guiding principle is that food (especially carbohydrates) increases blood glucose levels, while medications and exercise help lower them. When these factors are not balanced properly, hyperglycemia can result, and the ongoing risk of complications. Occasionally, these factors become unbalanced in the other direction, causing low blood sugar, or **hypoglycemia**. Characterized by dizziness and weakness, hypoglycemia may occur when medications or exercise are in excess and/or there is not enough food consumed. In other words, factors at play are reducing blood sugar levels too well. Treatment for hypoglycemia is quick administration of foods containing glucose that is absorbed quickly, such as orange juice or glucose tablets.

In healthcare facilities, a diabetes management team provides care for clients. This team usually includes the person with diabetes and his/her family, a registered dietitian nutritionist, a registered nurse, a physician, a pharmacist, and other healthcare professionals. Together, team members perform an assessment, set goals, implement a nutrition intervention, and evaluate and monitor results. Client education for individuals with diabetes is termed diabetes self-management education (DSME). Many clients are taught conventional or intensive management, including the proper use of medications, diet, exercise, stress management, and other aspects of self-care.

GLOSSARY

Gestational Diabetes
Diabetes that is characterized by abnormal glucose tolerance during pregnancy

Prediabetes
Condition where people have higher blood glucose levels after fasting, but not high enough to be diagnosed with diabetes

Hypoglycemia
Low blood sugar

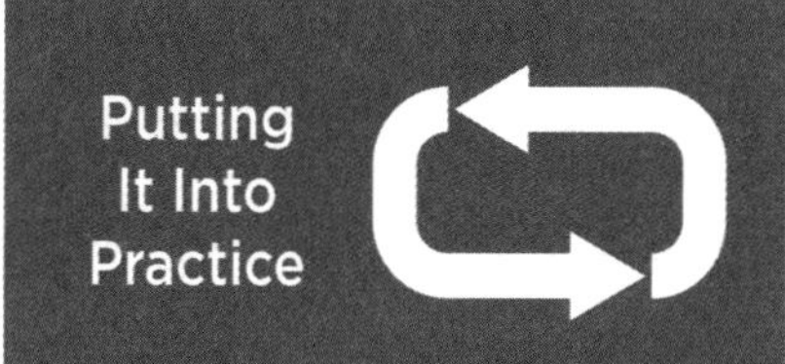

6. Your client mentions that he has "prediabetes," but you notice he has a HgbA1c of 8.7%. What should you do?

Insulin and Oral Hypoglycemic Agents

When the body is not producing enough insulin, a physician may prescribe insulin. Insulin is a hormone, and like many hormones, insulin is a protein. It is normally injected several times each day. It can't be taken by mouth because the digestive enzymes will digest it. People with diabetes normally give themselves insulin by subcutaneous injection (below the skin) at different sites. Insulin may also be administered through an insulin pump, which delivers small doses to the body on a continual basis. Sometimes, insulin preparations are combined in a drug regimen. Preparations of insulin vary by how quickly they act and for how long. Types of insulin include:

- Rapid-acting insulin: starts working in 5-30 minutes and finishes working in 3-5 hours. Examples include Lispro, Aspart, and Glulisine.
- Short-acting insulin: starts working in 30 minutes and finishes working in 5-8 hours. Examples include Regular (R) insulin and Velosulin (for the insulin pump).
- Intermediate-acting insulin: starts working in 1-2 hours and finishes working in 18-24 hours. Examples include NPH (N).
- Basal insulin analogs: start working in 1 hour and finishes working in 24 hours. This type provides even control of blood glucose for 24 hours at a time in most patients (https://www.ncbi.nlm.nih.gov/pmc/articles/PMC4192982/). Examples include glargine, detemir, and degludec.

Oral hypoglycemic agents are drugs taken by mouth to lower blood glucose levels in individuals with Type 2 diabetes. See Figure 6.17 for an overview of oral hypoglycemic medications. Some oral agents stimulate the body to produce more of its own insulin. Oral hypoglycemic agents are generally used for Type 2 diabetes. How these medicines work varies; each is a little bit different. Some need to be taken with meals, while others do not. With some, it is important to avoid alcohol, which may cause stomach upset. Some varieties of oral hypoglycemic medicines come in an extended release form, which provides fairly even control of blood sugar over a long period of time. Typically, these are taken once per day. Other medicines may be prescribed for two or three doses per day, taken at specific times. With insulin, as well as with oral medicines, meals must be planned in conjunction with a medication schedule to optimize control and prevent hypoglycemia. For example, a dose of medicine that has fairly rapid action on blood glucose could lead to hypoglycemia for a client who does not eat a meal shortly afterwards.

Medical Nutrition Therapy

Medical nutrition therapy for diabetes is often complicated because diabetes may be accompanied by other chronic diseases. Those complications might be one or more of the following: heart disease, stroke, high blood pressure, blindness, kidney disease, nervous system disease, amputations, and dental disease. In all of these chronic disease cases, blood glucose control is the foundation of treatment for diabetes.

7. If a client's medical chart shows a fasting blood sugar of 300, what type of diagnosis might you expect to see?

Figure 6.17
Oral Hypoglycemic Agents and Their Action

CLASS OF ORAL HYPOGLYCEMIC AGENT	MEDICATION	PRIMARY ACTION
Biguanides	Metformin	Decrease hepatic production.
Sulfonylureas	2nd Generation • Glyburide/glibenclamide • Glipizide • Glimepiride	Increase insulin secretion.
Meglitinides (glinides)	• Repaglinide • Nateglinide	Increase insulin secretion.
Thiazolidinediones (TZDs)	• Pioglitazone • Rosiglitazone	Increase insulin sensitivity.
Alpha-Glucosidas Inhibitors	• Acarbose • Miglitol	Slow intestinal carbohydrate digestion/absorption.
DDP-4 Inhibitors	• Sitagliptin • Vildagliptin • Saxagliptin • Linagliptin • Alogliptin	Increase insulin secretion (glucose-dependent). Decrease glucagon secretion.
Bile Acid Sequestrants	• Colesevelam	Possibly decrease hepatic glucose production and increase Incretin.
Dopamine-2 Agonists	• Bromocriptine	Modulate hypothalamic regulation of metabolism. Increase insulin sensitivity.
SGL T2 Inhibitors	• Canagliflozin • Dapagliflozin • Empagliflozin	Block glucose reabsorption by the kidney, increasing glucosuria.
GLP-1 Receptor Agonists	• Exenatide • Exenatide (extended release) • Liraglutide • Albiglutide • Lixisenatide • Dulaglutide	E: Increase glucose secretion (glucose-dependent). E-Extended: Decrease glucagon secretion (glucose-dependent). Lir: Slow gastric emptying. A, Lix, D: increase satiety.
Amylin Mimetics	• Pramlinitide	Decrease glucagon secretion. Slows gastric emptying. Increase satiety.

Source: Adapted from the American Diabetes Association. Approaches to Glycemic Treatment, Section 7. In Standards of Medical Care in Diabetes—2015. Diabetes Care 2015; 38 (Supplement 1): 541-548.

The goals of medical nutrition therapy are as follows:

- Maintain as near-normal blood glucose levels as possible.
- Achieve optimal blood lipid levels.
- Provide enough calories to maintain or attain reasonable weight.
- Prevent and treat short-term and long-term complications of diabetes.
- Improve overall health through proper nutrition.

The MNT needs to be custom-tailored to the individual based on type of diabetes, medication(s), nutritional status and needs, weight management objectives, medical treatment goals, food preferences, culture, age, ability to understand the diet, and lifestyle. Meal planning approaches include Carbohydrate Counting, MyPlate, and Exchange Lists for Meal Planning.

Recommendations for macronutrients (CHO, PRO, and FAT) should be based on current eating patterns, food preferences, and metabolic goals. This recommendation and meal pattern determination is done by the Registered Dietitian Nutritionist and the client.

Carbohydrate Counting

Carbohydrate Counting is commonly used in diabetes management. The total amount of carbohydrate is more important than where it comes from. The key is keeping the total carbohydrate content of the meal consistent each day.

Carbohydrate grams can be counted by reading nutrition labels using tables of nutrient content of foods or using the exchange lists. In the exchange lists, one exchange of starch, fruit, or milk each has about 15 grams of carbohydrate. One exchange of each of these foods is called one carbohydrate choice. A meal plan can then be worked out that sets a specific number of carbohydrate choices at each meal or snack for the day.

For example, an individual who needs 1,800 calories requires 225-270 grams of carbohydrate to meet the 50-60 percent of daily caloric intake from carbohydrate. This means 15-18 carbohydrate choices per day would be divided for the meals and snacks needed. The total number of meals and snacks, as well as the timing, is based on the individual's nutritional needs, lifestyle, and type of medication. Anyone counting carbohydrates needs to recognize that this is only part of a healthful eating plan. By focusing on carbohydrate alone, some clients may forget about limiting fat, or consuming adequate vitamins, minerals, and fiber. The MyPlate, Dietary Guidelines for Americans, or similar guidance helps address overall wisdom in developing a healthy diet.

MyPlate and Diabetes

MyPlate can provide an excellent resource for meal planning for those with diabetes. In addition to following MyPlate guidelines, individuals with diabetes should:

- Eat meals and snacks at regular times every day.
- Eat about the same amount of food each day.
- Try not to skip meals or snacks.
- Check blood sugar about 1.5-2 hours after eating to be sure they are not overdoing carbohydrates. The American Diabetes Association suggests 180 mg/dl as a good upper limit for this.

Exchange System

Due to its flexibility to accommodate patient food preferences, Carbohydrate Counting has gained popularity over the exchange system in meal planning for diabetics. However it is important to understand the exchange system. The exchange system classifies foods into groups according to how much protein, fat, and carbohydrate they contain. Serving sizes are specified too. These groups are called **exchange lists**. The exchange lists create a system in which foods within any given group can be swapped or changed for others in the same group. Any of these trades provide the same amount of protein, fat, and carbohydrate. Of course, with these three macronutrients being equal, calories are about equal too. There are seven exchange lists: starch, fruit, milk, other carbohydrates, vegetables, meat and meat substitutes, and fat. The Registered Dietitian Nutritionist sets up an appropriate meal plan in consultation with the client. A typical plan lists how many exchanges of each food group may be eaten at each meal and snack. An exchange plan requires education for the client and others involved in meals. It requires a client to keep careful track of food at every sitting, and to measure food—at least until serving sizes become familiar. As with MyPlate, this system does not require one exchange or serving per meal. For example, an individualized exchange diet may call for two servings from the starch group, one serving from the fruit group, and one-half serving from the milk group at breakfast. Translated into food, this might be:

- 1 whole English muffin (2 bread exchanges)
- 1/2 cup of orange juice (1 fruit exchange)
- 1/2 cup of skim milk (1/2 milk exchange)

One challenge of using the exchange system is that many people do not eat single foods. Instead, they mix and combine foods into stews, casseroles, fajitas, pizza, and much more. Learning to count combination dishes requires education and sometimes nutritional analysis. The American Diabetes Association provides references for counting combination foods in an exchange system. In an exchange system, some basic advice still holds true: It's important to choose a variety of foods to provide needed nutrients.

GLOSSARY

Exchange Lists
A way to classify foods according to nutrients and serving sizes. Foods in each category can be "exchanged" for another food. Used primarily in health care

Exercise

A physician needs to approve an exercise program before a person with diabetes starts the program. This is because when an individual with uncontrolled diabetes (indicated by blood glucose levels of 240 to 300 mg/dl) exercises, the liver releases additional glucose and the hyperglycemia worsens. On the other hand, individuals with good blood glucose control (under 150 and up to 180 mg/dl) can benefit in many ways from exercising. Exercise lowers blood glucose levels because muscle cells use more glucose. Regular exercise results in greater sensitivity of the body to insulin and increases glucose tolerance. Exercise is especially helpful in decreasing cardiovascular risk factors and promoting weight loss. Some individuals with Type 2 diabetes gradually achieve better blood glucose control through weight loss. Individuals using conventional management are usually advised to eat a snack with 10-15 grams of carbohydrate before moderate exercise of an hour or less.

Monitoring

In order to keep an eye on how well the client is maintaining glycemic control, caregivers monitor the following variables:

- **Blood sugar levels:** People with diabetes routinely do self-monitoring of blood glucose (SMBG) by pricking the skin and then applying a drop of blood to a test strip. A glucose meter will read the sugar in the blood and test the blood glucose level. How often a person with diabetes does SMBG depends on the type of diabetes, the degree of glycemic control, and the treatment regimen (medication, diet, exercise).
- **Blood lipid levels** to include total cholesterol, LDL, HDL, and triglycerides.
- **Glycosylated hemoglobin or Hemoglobin A1c (HbA1c):** Hemoglobin is the part of the red blood cell that carries oxygen. During the life span of a red blood cell, glucose in the blood binds to hemoglobin A, the major form of hemoglobin in the red blood cell. When glucose binds to hemoglobin A, the hemoglobin is said to be glycosylated. Glycosylated hemoglobin (HbA1c) values reflect average blood glucose levels during the past six to twelve weeks, and they are a useful indicator of how well a client is controlling his/her blood glucose level. Normal values for the laboratory used by your facility should be consulted.
- **Body weight:** Frequent monitoring of body weight should be a part of the nutrition assessment and monitoring for diabetes management. If a person with diabetes is overweight/obese, it is recommended to lose weight to improve glycemic control. A reduction of 5-10 percent of body weight can result in improvement of glycemic, lipid, and blood pressure control. Follow-up is needed at least every 6-12 months for adults and every 3-6 months for children to assure good control of blood sugar, to evaluate any changes or complications, and to reinforce education.

SECTION D MEDICAL NUTRITION THERAPY AND THE TREATMENT OF CANCER AND HIV/AIDS

Cancer

Cancer is the second leading cause of death in the United States. Over 14 million people in the U.S. have cancer of some type. **Cancer** is a disease characterized by unrestricted and excessive multiplication of body cells. **Tumors** are growths of cancerous cells and may be either **malignant** (meaning cancerous growth is continuing and may be life-threatening) or **benign** (meaning not cancerous). Cancerous cells can also leave their original site of growth and travel through the blood and lymph to spread throughout the body, referred to as **metastasis**.

Sometimes the first signs of cancer are weight loss and anorexia (loss of appetite), and diet is an important part of cancer treatment. Cancer cells require calories and nutrients to grow, and basal energy use is increased in cancer clients. This helps explain part of the weight loss. Cancer clients may need 35 to 50 calories per kilogram of body weight simply to maintain their current weight. To complicate matters more, cancer clients often have little interest in eating. They may experience nausea and vomiting, feel full quickly, and do not taste many foods normally. These symptoms might be caused by the cancer or by the treatment, which may include radiation, chemotherapy, and surgery. Good nutritional status is important to withstand the effects of treatment.

GLOSSARY

Cancer
Disease characterized by unrestricted and excessive multiplication of body cells

Tumor
Growth of cancerous cells that form a mass

Malignant
Meaning cancerous growth is continuing and may be life-threatening

Benign
Growth that is not cancerous

Metastasis
When cancerous cells leave their original site and grow and travel through the blood and/or lymph system to spread throughout the body

The traditional cancer therapies, radiation therapy and chemotherapy, interfere with nutritional status. In radiation therapy, high-energy rays are used to destroy cancerous tissues and stop the growth of cancer cells. Chemotherapy is the treatment of cancer with drugs. Some effects of radiation therapy and chemotherapy include nausea, vomiting, taste alterations, diarrhea, malabsorption, and reduced salivary secretions in the case of radiation treatment of the head and neck. The result can be **cancer cachexia** (malnutrition).

GLOSSARY

Cancer Cachexia
Malnutrition caused by cancer and the treatment of cancer

Surgery is another major approach to treating cancer. Surgery removes cancerous tissue. In these situations, providing proper nutrition will require dietary modifications such as small, frequent meals for clients. About half of cancer clients experience an extreme state of malnutrition and wasting of the body called cancer cachexia. Symptoms include significant weight loss, loss of appetite, feeling full early, abnormal taste and smell abilities, anemia, and other nutritional deficiencies.

Following are approaches to overcome some of the nutritional problems that present in cancer clients.

Loss of Appetite

Causes of anorexia and weight loss include emotional stress and depression, chemotherapy, radiation treatment, and the cancer itself, especially if it is in the gastrointestinal tract. These strategies may help stimulate appetite:

- Ask the physician and nursing staff about effective medications to control nausea and pain. Give these one hour before meals to promote better intake.
- Large amounts of food tend to overwhelm a reluctant eater. Try smaller portions of nutrient-dense food every one to two hours.
- Update food preferences and dislikes often, since these may change during the course of the illness.
- Cater to special requests, even if this means purchasing food not normally stocked.
- Offer high-calorie, high-protein foods.
- Avoid foods with strong odors: use boiling bag and outdoor grill or fans.
- Avoid having favorite foods either right before or right after treatment, as this may put a negative association with previously preferred foods.

Even though many high-calorie foods are high in fat, and in some cases also saturated fat, keep in mind that there are situations where taking in adequate calories is more important than worrying about fat content.

Early Satiety

Feeling full midway through the meal is a common occurrence. These tips may be useful:

- Encourage five or six mini-meals throughout the day.
- Serve a well-balanced, nutrient-dense breakfast since many clients feel better in the morning.
- Instruct the client to save high-fat foods until the end of the meal because these promote satiety.
- Have high-calorie snacks available at the bedside.

Nausea and Vomiting

In addition to medications, the following tactics may help control nausea and vomiting:

- Allow the client to eat when less nauseated; be flexible with mealtimes.
- Eat before cancer treatments.
- Encourage nutrient-dense fluids between meals to prevent dehydration. Use fruit juice, milkshakes, and liquid medical nutritional products.
- Avoid food with strong odors and flavors if these are offensive.
- Offer cold meals rather than hot foods, as this minimizes aromas.
- Bland or dry food (like toast or crackers) may be well tolerated.

Dry or Sore Mouth

Changes in saliva make the client more prone to dental problems. Encourage good oral hygiene and frequent saline (saltwater) rinses. These nutrition tips will help bring relief during meals:

- Drink plenty of liquids at meals; use straws.
- Eat foods that are easy to chew—like cottage cheese, soft fruits, custards, and milkshakes.
- Use sugarless gum to stimulate salivation.
- Analgesics may relieve pain while eating.
- Avoid crisp and raw food, which may scratch the mouth and throat, causing discomfort. Also, acidic and salty food may irritate these areas.
- Soft foods are better tolerated; a pureed texture may be needed temporarily.
- Add liquid, gravy, and sauces to moisten food.
- Drink fruit nectar instead of juice.

Swallowing Difficulties

Swallowing problems occur when the esophagus is exposed to radiation, usually two to three weeks after treatment begins.

- Soft and pureed consistencies are better tolerated.
- Serve food at room temperature or very cold.
- Liquids may be easier to manage; consider liquid medical nutritional products.
- Request an evaluation from the speech pathologist.

Changes in Taste and Smell

Sensations may be decreased or may just be different from normal. Check with the client often to inquire about food aversions, and then make appropriate substitutions for the offending foods.

- Highly seasoned food may be appreciated.
- Meat may be better accepted cold or with something sweet like jelly or applesauce.
- Try soybean-based tofu and dairy products as protein alternatives if meats are refused.
- Plastic disposable utensils may reduce complaints of altered/metallic taste.
- Pay particular attention to the presentation of food on the plate and to mealtime ambiance.
- Rinse mouth before eating.
- Use sugar-free mints, gum, or lemon drops.

Diarrhea

A temporary lactose intolerance may develop, causing diarrhea. Eliminate milk and milk products to determine whether the diarrhea is from lactose intolerance.

- Try low-lactose or lactose-free milk, or a lactose-free medical nutritional product.
- Encourage potassium-rich food to replace potassium losses. Good sources are bananas, apricots, raisins, citrus fruits, and potatoes.
- Avoid high-fat food, which may aggravate the situation.
- Serve soups, broth, sports drinks, and canned fruits to help replace sodium and potassium, which are important electrolytes.

HIV/AIDS

Acquired Immunodeficiency Syndrome (AIDS) is a serious illness that affects the body's ability to fight infection. The human immunodeficiency virus (HIV) causes AIDS. HIV is spread primarily through sexual intercourse with an HIV-infected person, contaminated needles or blood, or from mother to infant during pregnancy or lactation. When first infected with HIV, a client generally has no symptoms. As time progresses, symptoms appear and often include exhaustion, fever, diarrhea, weight loss, muscle pain, and mouth infections. AIDS actually refers to the final stage of HIV infection, when health problems such as recurrent pneumonia, cancers, severe diarrhea, and malabsorption are the most serious.

The wasting and malnutrition just discussed with regard to cancer cachexia are commonly seen in HIV-infected clients. There are many possible reasons for this, such as anorexia, inadequate diet, increased metabolic rate, GI tract infections, drugs, reduced gastric acid secretion, diarrhea, and malabsorption.Early nutrition support is important to build up nutrient stores and body weight. As long as possible, an oral diet is generally preferable, using high-protein, high-calorie foods and supplements as necessary. A concern for HIV-infected and AIDS clients is making sure food is safe to eat. The body ordinarily is well-equipped to deal with bacteria that cause foodborne illness, but these clients are at far greater risk of serious illness. Because of weakened immune systems, these individuals are more susceptible to contracting a foodborne illness. Once contracted, these infections, with their severe vomiting and diarrhea, can be difficult to treat and they can come back again and again. This can further weaken the immune system and hasten the progression of HIV infection, and be fatal for persons with AIDS.

Individuals with AIDS may have inadequate nutrient intakes for reasons similar to those of people with cancer—altered taste perceptions, drug therapy, dry mouth, lack of energy to eat, depression, nausea/vomiting, etc. Accelerated nutrient losses may occur because of diarrhea, drug therapy, infections, or malabsorption. Sound nutritional status may improve a person's response to drug therapy, reduce duration of hospital stays, and promote physical independence. For dietary considerations, follow the same nutritional approaches as cancer patients.

Chapter References

RESOURCES	
Academy of Nutrition and Dietetics*	https://www.eatright.org
Academy of Nutrition and Dietetics. Heart Failure. Academy of Nutrition and Dietetics Evidence Analysis Library.* Published 2017.	https://www.andeal.org/topic.cfm?menu=5289
Academy of Nutrition and Dietetics. Nutrition Care Manual.*	https://www.nutritioncaremanual.org
American Academy of Pediatrics*	https://www.aap.org
American Cancer Society*	http://www.cancer.org
American Diabetes Association*	https://www.diabetes.org
American Diabetes Association. Statistics About Diabetes.* Updated March 22, 2019.	https://www.diabetes.org/resources/statistics/statistics-about-diabetes
American Heart Association*	https://www.heart.org
American Society for Metabolic and Bariatric Surgery. Childhood and Adolescent Obesity.*	https://asmbs.org/patients/adolescent-obesity
Centers for Disease Control and Prevention. Cholesterol.* Updated January 18, 2019.	https://www.cdc.gov/cholesterol/
Centers for Disease Control and Prevention. Diabetes.* Updated July 25, 2019.	https://www.cdc.gov/diabetes/index.html
Centers for Disease Control and Prevention. National Center for Health Statistics.* Updated September 17, 2019.	https://www.cdc.gov/nchs/index.htm
Centers for Disease Control and Prevention. National Diabetes Statistics Report—2017.* Published 2017.	https://www.cdc.gov/diabetes/pdfs/data/statistics/national-diabetes-statistics-report.pdf
Centers for Disease Control and Prevention. National Vital Statistics System. National Center for Health Statistics* Updated September 5, 2019.	https://www.cdc.gov/nchs/nvss/index.htm
Centers for Disease Control and Prevention. Smoking and COPD. Tips from Former Smokers®.* Updated April 1, 2019.	https://www.cdc.gov/tobacco/campaign/tips/diseases/copd.html
Danaei G, Ding EL, Mozaffarian D, et al. The preventable causes of death in the United States: comparative risk assessment of dietary, lifestyle, and metabolic risk factors. PLoS Med. 2011;6(4): e1000058. doi:10.1371/journal.pmed.1000058.	
Dunlay SM, Roger VL. Understanding the Epidemic of Heart Failure: Past, Present, and Future. *Curr Heart Fail Rep.* 2014; 11(4): 404-415.	
Riddle MC, et al. American Diabetes Association Standards of Medical Care in Diabetes—2019. *Diabetes Care.* 2019; 42 (Supplement 1): S01-S193.	
Types of Insulin for Diabetes Treatment. WebMD.*	https://www.webmd.com/diabetes/diabetes-types-insulin#1

** Accessed September 18, 2019*

Continued...

Chapter References *(Continued)*

RESOURCES	
U.S. Department of Agriculture. Scientific Report of the 2015 Dietary Guidelines Advisory Committee. Published February 2015. Accessed September 16, 2020.	https://health.gov/sites/default/files/2019-09/Scientific-Report-of-the-2015-Dietary-Guidelines-Advisory-Committee.pdf
U.S. Department of Health and Human Services and U.S. Department of Agriculture. 2015-2020 Dietary Guidelines for Americans, 8th Edition. Office of Disease Prevention and Health Promotion.* Updated September 18, 2019.	https://health.gov/dietaryguidelines/2015/
U.S. Department of Health and Human Services and U.S. Department of Agriculture. Dietary Guidelines for Americans, 2010. 7th Edition. Office of Disease Prevention and Health Promotion.* Published December 2010.	https://health.gov/dietaryguidelines/dga2010/DietaryGuidelines2010.pdf
U.S. Department of Health and Human Services and U.S. Department of Agriculture. Dietary Guidelines for Americans, 2015. 8th Edition. Office of Disease Prevention and Health Promotion. Published December 2015. Accessed June 28, 2020.	https://www.dietaryguidelines.gov/sites/default/files/
U.S. Department of Health and Human Services and U.S. Department of Agriculture. 2010 Dietary Guidelines for Americans, 2010. 8th Edition. Office of Disease Prevention and Health Promotion Published December 2015. Accessed June 28, 2020.	https://www.dietaryguidelines.gov/sites/default/files/2019-05/2015-2020_Dietary_Guidelines.pdf
U.S. Department of Health and Human Services. Annual Report to the Nation 2019: Overall Cancer Statistics. National Cancer Institute Surveillance, Epidemiology, and End Results Program.*	https://seer.cancer.gov/report_to_nation/statistics.html
U.S. Department of Health and Human Services. National Heart, Lung, and Blood Institute.*	https://www.nhlbi.nih.gov
U.S. Food and Drug Administration. Final Determination Regarding Partially Hydrogenated Oils (Removing Trans Fat). Published May 18, 2018. Accessed September 16, 2020.	https://www.fda.gov/food/food-additives-petitions/final-determination-regarding-partially-hydrogenated-oils-removing-trans-fat

** Accessed September 18, 2019*

Obtain Routine Nutrition Screening Data

Overview and Objectives

Nutrition screening helps a Certified Dietary Manager®, Certified Food Protection Professional® (CDM®, CFPP®) identify healthcare clients in need of nutrition intervention from the Registered Dietitian Nutritionist. It is also required for compliance with regulations and standards in the healthcare setting. After completing this chapter, you should be able to:

- Identify the goals of nutrition screening
- Explain the difference between nutrition screening and nutrition assessment
- Use established guidelines to distinguish between routine and at-risk clients
- Identify appropriate data to be gathered
- Explain the term body mass index (BMI)
- Differentiate between ideal body weight (IBW), usual body weight (UBW), current body weight
- Utilize appropriate data-gathering format/approach for specific client types
- Complete client forms efficiently
- Review examples of common food-drug interactions
- Calculate BEE and total energy needs
- Identify federal regulations related to evaluating patient status and care
- Collect client information from medical record
- Gather client data from relevant sources (e.g., medical record, referrals)
- Complete client forms (e.g., MDS)
- Comply with federal regulations related to evaluating client status and care
- Calculate nutrient intake
- Document relevant nutrition-related information (e.g., laboratory values, BMI)

7

For the first half of the 21st century, Americans will see an unprecedented increase in the number of elderly individuals. As baby boomers grow older, people 85 and over are expected to be the fastest-growing group of elderly persons. Combine that with the fact that elderly persons are at increased risk for nutritional problems, and we see an increased need to identify those who are most at risk. During the 1990s, the American Academy of Family Physicians, the Academy of Nutrition and Dietetics, and the National Council on Aging promoted a Nutritional Screening Initiative. The purpose of the initiative was to use a simple screening tool to discover nutrition concerns before serious illnesses occurred. The tool has been useful in educating the public, but not as beneficial at identifying those who needed immediate intervention.

Nutrition Care Process

The **nutrition care process** is intended to provide a standardized process of providing care to clients and standardized Nutrition Care Process Terminology (NCPT) for documentation of medical nutrition therapy. The Academy of Nutrition and Dietetics defines the nutrition care process in four steps: ADIME. This chapter focuses on Step 1.

1. Nutrition *Assessment* includes collecting information to identify nutrition problems, verify the data, and evaluate that information. This step has two components: nutrition screening and nutrition assessment.
2. Nutrition *Diagnosis* involves defining all nutrition-related problems using standardized terminology defined by the Academy of Nutrition and Dietetics.
3. Nutrition *Intervention* are the actions taken to correct a nutrition problem. This step involves both planning and implementing, and begins with a plan of care followed by a team approach to implement the plan. The nutrition intervention should be directly linked with the information collected in the assessment.
4. Nutrition *Monitoring and Evaluation* should be a measurable outcome that involves follow-up to determine how well the interventions are working.

GLOSSARY

Nutrition Care Process
Four steps to provide a standardized care process: Nutrition Assessment, Nutrition Diagnosis, Nutrition Intervention, Nutrition Monitoring and Evaluation

Nutrition Screening
A component of Nutrition Assessment meant to identify potential nutrition problems

Indicators
Pieces of information, such as weight, measurement, that might suggest a concern or risk

Nutrition Screening

Nutrition Screening is the initial step in a more comprehensive Nutrition Assessment. Nutrition Assessment, including **Nutrition Screening**, is the beginning of the Nutrition Care Process. Nutrition screening is a systematic method for identifying individuals at risk for nutrition problems. Nutrition screening is a process applied to an entire group, and attempts to select members of that group who are candidates for further nutrition intervention. Nutrition screening can be done in public healthcare settings, such as health fairs, or outpatient clinics. In a healthcare facility such as a long-term care facility or hospital, every individual who is admitted should undergo a routine nutrition screening. The nutrition screening process allows nutrition professionals (CDM,CFPP; DTR/NDTR; RD/RDN) to identify clients needing medical nutrition therapy.

One of the primary responsibilities of the Certified Dietary Manager, Certified Food Protection Professional working in healthcare facilities is to obtain routine nutrition screening data. Screening is typically a fairly simple process, based on indicators. **Indicators** are pieces of information (many are numbers and/or measurements) that might suggest a concern or risk. These indicators are built upon statistical data that have been determined to be associated with risk. For example, many research studies have shown that individuals found to be less than 90 percent of their ideal body weight have significantly higher rates of complications from surgery. Based on that, an indicator for nutrition screening may be established as less than 90 percent of ideal body weight. Through research, experts have been able to identify findings and figures that can help to predict the level of nutrition risk. Other indicators might be based on diagnosis, usual food intake, or laboratory data.

If it is determined that some of the indicators are present, what happens next? There are several approaches to determining the level of risk based on indicators. One method is simply to count the risk factors. A screening policy may specify: *If three or more indicators of nutrition risk are present, this patient will be flagged for a complete/comprehensive nutrition assessment. Some screening tools also assess urgency of the follow-up visit or intervention.*

In another scheme, each risk factor receives a point value. Factors judged to increase nutrition risk receive more points. In a nutrition risk scoring system, each risk indicator has a point value, and the total point value identifies the level of nutrition risk. Some systems even define risk levels based on the score. One system may have two levels of risk, such as moderate risk and high risk. Another may have three levels, or even five.

Figure 7.1, A Portion of the Mini-Nutritional Assessment MNA®, provides a nutrition screening tool from Nestle Clinical Nutrition. Note that this example uses a scoring system. In some tools, more points equal greater risk. In the Nestle example, fewer points mean greater risk. Whether to use high scores or low scores for expressing a risk is not important. However, it is important to understand that any tool used in the facility must be interpreted accurately. This is just the nutrition screening portion of the Mini-Nutritional Assessment. To find the complete tool and for more information visit www.mna-elderly.com

Even a nutrition risk scoring system may incorporate certain overrides or automatic flags. Let's say a system specifies 20 points or higher as indicating risk. The system might also say that any individual who has been diagnosed with a pressure ulcer/injury is automatically classified as being at nutrition risk. Even a resident who scores only 16 on the nutrition risk score would be "flagged" for nutrition assessment based on the presence of a pressure ulcer/injury. Overrides or automatic flags can be helpful to be certain that individuals who might benefit from medical nutrition therapy receive appropriate assessment and interventions.

Also, note that the example in Figure 7.1 combines screening and assessment into one document. This can be a simple method of keeping important information together. A nutrition screening result usually becomes part of a permanent medical record. Screening information is thus available to other caregivers. For example, a CDM, CFPP may complete a nutrition screening and place it into the medical record. In follow-up, a Registered Dietitian Nutritionist may gather and evaluate more information to develop a nutrition assessment.

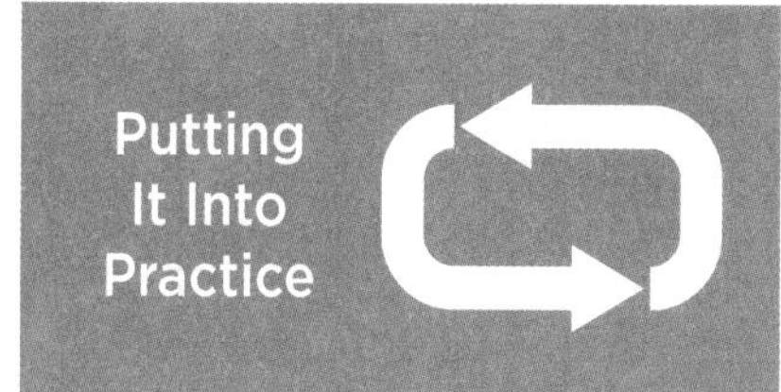

1. If a resident has a weight within the normal range, what other factors could still put her at nutritional risk?

Figure 7.1

A Portion of the Mini Nutritional Assessment MNA®

Mini Nutritional Assessment MNA®

Nestlé NutritionInstitute

Last name: First name:

Sex: Age: Weight, kg: Height, cm: Date:

Complete the screen by filling in the boxes with the appropriate numbers. Total the numbers for the final screening score.

Screening

A Has food intake declined over the past 3 months due to loss of appetite, digestive problems, chewing or swallowing difficulties?

0 = severe decrease in food intake
1 = moderate decrease in food intake
2 = no decrease in food intake ☐

B Weight loss during the last 3 months

0 = weight loss greater than 3 kg (6.6 lbs)
1 = does not know
2 = weight loss between 1 and 3 kg (2.2 and 6.6 lbs)
3 = no weight loss ☐

C Mobility

0 = bed or chair bound
1 = able to get out of bed / chair but does not go out
2 = goes out ☐

D Has suffered psychological stress or acute disease in the past 3 months?

0 = yes 2 = no ☐

E Neuropsychological problems

0 = severe dementia or depression
1 = mild dementia
2 = no psychological problems ☐

F1 Body Mass Index (BMI) (weight in kg) / (height in m)^2

0 = BMI less than 19
1 = BMI 19 to less than 21
2 = BMI 21 to less than 23
3 = BMI 23 or greater ☐

IF BMI IS NOT AVAILABLE, REPLACE QUESTION F1 WITH QUESTION F2.
DO NOT ANSWER QUESTION F2 IF QUESTION F1 IS ALREADY COMPLETED.

F2 Calf circumference (CC) in cm

0 = CC less than 31
3 = CC 31 or greater ☐

Screening score (max. 14 points)

12 - 14 points: Normal nutritional status
8 - 11 points: At risk of malnutrition
0 - 7 points: Malnourished ☐☐

References

1. Vellas B, Villars H, Abellan G, *et al.* Overview of the MNA® - Its History and Challenges. *J Nutr Health Aging.* 2006;**10**:456-465.
2. Rubenstein LZ, Harker JO, Salva A, Guigoz Y, Vellas B. Screening for Undernutrition in Geriatric Practice: Developing the Short-Form Mini Nutritional Assessment (MNA-SF). *J. Geront.* 2001; **56A**: M366-377
3. Guigoz Y. The Mini-Nutritional Assessment (MNA®) Review of the Literature - What does it tell us? *J Nutr Health Aging.* 2006; **10**:466-487.
4. Kaiser MJ, Bauer JM, Ramsch C, et al. Validation of the Mini Nutritional Assessment Short-Form (MNA®-SF): A practical tool for identification of nutritional status. *J Nutr Health Aging.* 2009; **13**:782-788.

For more information: **www.mna-elderly.com**

Nutrition Screening Indicators

Many factors may suggest nutrition risk. By no means is it necessary to use all possible criteria to identify risk. Criteria used in screening are usually representative of a cluster of related findings. In other words, a key indicator used for nutrition screening may represent the tip of an iceberg. If a risk factor exists, it is likely that other risk factors exist along with it. Indicators used in screening (and in nutrition assessment) fall into four basic categories. It may be helpful if you remember it as **A-B-C-D**.

- **A**nthropometric measurements
- **B**iochemical tests
- **C**linical information
- **D**ietary history and information

Anthropometric Measurements. Anthropometric measurements are measurements of the human body. It is typically where nutrition screening begins. The most common examples are height and weight. These two figures are actually very useful, provided that accurate measurements are made. Adults should be weighed on a beam balance scale that is calibrated regularly to ensure accuracy. The best time to weigh a client is in the morning before breakfast and after the bladder has been emptied. For consistency, clients should always be weighed at the same time of day, and on the same scale, wearing the same amount of clothing. This makes comparisons of weight from one date to another most meaningful. There are specialized scales available for clients who are unable to stand. Even when weights are taken correctly, factors such as fluid retention, adaptive equipment on wheelchairs, and wedges or pillows may adversely affect a weight reading. It is important to obtain a weight upon admission and regularly thereafter. Do not simply rely on a weight recorded at a different facility.

An accurate measurement of height is also important. Relying upon the client's self-reported height or a visual estimate is not adequate. Whenever possible, height should be measured with the client standing straight against a measuring tape or stick on a vertical wall or instrument. If this is not possible, using a tape measure to check height from feet to head is an option. For other methods to estimate the height using an individual's knee height, forearm, or demispan, refer to http://www.rxkinetics.com/height_estimate.html.

There are many guidelines and standards that may be used for evaluating body weight. Standards are generally based on height such as Body Mass Index (BMI). In general, a good standard also accounts for differences between males and females, as well as differences in body frame size. For example, a person with a small frame (small bones) should ideally weigh less than a person of the same height who has a larger frame size. Weight alone doesn't tell all, however. Other considerations include body composition of lean and fat mass. A person who exercises regularly and, in particular, someone who does strength training, may accumulate a great deal of muscle mass. This may translate into a high body weight for height, but it may be a healthy condition. Some experts use various methods to evaluate percent body fat.

Using weight and height, we can determine ideal body weight. **Ideal body weight (IBW)** is an estimate of what would be a healthy weight for an individual. It is based on height, gender, and frame size. Check reference tables to determine ideal body weight, or use the simple formula found in Figure 7.2 to calculate IBW. A common

GLOSSARY

Ideal Body Weight (IBW)
An estimate of what would be a healthy weight for an individual according to a standard

Figure 7.2
Hamwi Forumla to Calculate Ideal Body Weight (IBW)

WOMEN	MEN
IBW = 100 lbs for first 5 feet in height + 5 lbs for each inch over 5 feet.	IBW = 106 lbs for first 5 feet + 6 lbs for each inch over 5 feet.

Frame Adjustments (Men and Women)

For a small frame, subtract 10 percent of the total
For a large frame, add 10 percent to the total
For heights less than 60", subtract 5 lbs. for each inch below 60".

formula used today was created by Dr. GJ Hamwi. Here is an example for a 5-foot, 11-inch male with a large frame:

- 106 pounds + (11 x 6) = 172 pounds
- 172 pounds x 0.10 = 17 pounds
- 172 pounds + 17 pounds = 189 pounds IBW

GLOSSARY

Frame Size
Calculated from the ratio of height to wrist circumference

Percent of Ideal Body Weight (% IBW)
A proportion of current body weight as compared to ideal body weight

Actual Weight
What a person weighs now

Usual Body Weight
The weight a person usually is

Notice in the Hamwi formula for ideal body weight an adjustment for frame size. **Frame size** refers to the thickness of bones, or underlying body build and height. To determine frame size, there is a quick and simple measurement. Wrap your hand around your dominant wrist (if you are right handed, wrap your left hand around your right wrist), closing your middle finger and thumb together around the smallest part of the wrist. Then use this gauge:

- If the thumb and finger overlap, it is a small frame size.
- If the thumb and finger meet, it is a medium frame size.
- If the thumb and finger do not meet, it is a large frame size.

There are more exact measurements of frame size that can be done with a tape measure as seen in Figure 7.3. It is important to adjust for a person's frame size when determining ideal body weight.

Once a person's ideal body weight is determined, it can be compared to actual weight. **Actual weight** is what a person weighs right now. When we compare the two figures, we determine **Percent of Ideal Body Weight (% IBW)**. Percent of IBW describes how closely a person's actual weight resembles the ideal.

To calculate a Percent of IBW: (Actual Weight ÷ IBW) x 100

To calculate a Percent of Weight Change:
[(Usual weight - Actual weight) ÷ usual weight] x 100

In addition, it might be valuable to know usual body weight. **Usual body weight** is the weight the client "usually" weighs.

Here are two examples of calculating percent of IBW:

1. Marla weighs 156 pounds. Her IBW is 115 pounds. Percent of IBW = (156 pounds ÷ 115 pounds) x 100

   = 1.36 x 100

   = 136%

   Marla is at 136 percent of her IBW.

Figure 7.3

Frame Size from Height-Wrist Circumference Ratios (r)[a]

FRAME SIZE	MALE r VALUES	FEMALE r VALUES
Small	>10.4	>11.0
Medium	9.6-10.4	10.1-11.0
Large	<9.6	<10.1

[a] $r = \frac{\text{height (cm)}}{\text{wrist circumference (cm)}}$

The wrist is measured where it bends (distal to the styloid process) on the right arm (see illustration).

Place tape here

Styloid process ("wristbone")

Source: Metropolitan Life Insurance Company

2. Jacob weighs 137 pounds. His IBW is 148 pounds. Percent of IBW = (137 pounds ÷ 148 pounds) x 100

   = 0.93 x 100

   = 93%

   Jacob is at 93 percent of his IBW.

Note that in these examples, it is alright to round calculations to the nearest whole number. IBW and related calculations are only estimates, so it is not necessary to extend decimal places. Roughly speaking, percent of ideal body weight gives an indication of whether a person is potentially undernourished or overweight. For example, one rule of thumb says that a person at or below 90 percent of IBW may be a nutritional risk.

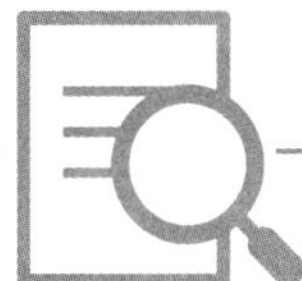

View the Supplemental Material for the Focus on Formulas video to calculate ideal body weight (IBW) and to calculate % of ideal body weight (IBS).

However, this measurement alone does not tell all. Imagine Jacob from the example above. Currently, he is below his IBW. To better understand his nutritional state, what is missing is what the recent trend has been. Jacob weighs 137 pounds right now. Has he always been a thin man? If so, maybe there is not a concern here. On the other hand, what if Jacob weighed 159 pounds just six months ago and is now down to this weight? This should be of great concern because it indicates a severe downward trend in his weight. If this is the case, it would be assumed that his weight will continue to fall without intervention. This rapid weight loss may be due to health conditions such as cancer, dysphagia, or depression. Furthermore, if he is losing weight at a rapid clip, he may be losing some of his lean body mass. **Lean body mass** describes the weight of all parts of the body that are NOT fat, e.g. muscle, bones, and organs. If Jacob is losing lean body mass, his body systems may not be functioning at their best. He is likely at risk.

A final way to measure body mass is to examine the percentage of body weight that is fat. Obviously, as body fat percentage increases, so does the health risk. Figure 7.5 shows BMI classifications and desirable body fat percentage.

If needed, this calculation can be done by hand or using a calculator.
Method 1: BMI = 703 x weight in pounds ÷ height in inches ÷ height in inches.
Method 2: Height in inches x height in inches = height in inches squared. BMI = Weight ÷ Height in inches squared x 703.

Can it be determined what is really going on here? The answer is by calculating percent weight change. **Percent weight change** indicates by what proportion the body weight has changed over a certain period of time.

GLOSSARY

Lean Body Mass
The weight of all parts of the body not including the fat (e.g., the weight of muscle, bones, and organs)

Percent Weight Change
Indicates by what portion the body weight has changed over a certain period of time

Let's use Jacob again as an example:

Jacob weighs 137 lbs. now. He weighed 159 lbs. six months ago.

Percent weight change = [(159 lbs - 137 lbs) ÷ usual weight] x 100

= [22 ÷ usual weight] x 100

= [22 ÷ 159] x 100

= 0.14 x 100

= 14 percent

Jacob has experienced a 14 percent weight change over six months. Another way to say this is: He has lost 14 percent of his body weight over the past six months.

To calculate percent weight change, it's important to find the most reliable weight information possible for past data. Sources may include a medical record, the report from the client, or a report from a family member. Unfortunately, it is not always possible to obtain highly reliable information about past weights. Also, there is no specific time frame for a percent weight loss calculation. The following percent weight changes indicate nutrition risk:

- A weight loss of 5 percent over the past one month,
- A weight loss of 7.5 percent over the past 90 days, or
- A weight loss of 10 percent over the past six months.

Another method for comparing weight with height to gauge overweight or underweight is the body mass index (BMI). BMI is often used today as a measure of overweight and obesity, which is related to the risk of development of chronic diseases. It is calculated from a person's height and weight. The National Heart, Lung, and Blood Institute describes BMI as an estimate of body fat. The higher the BMI, the higher the risk for certain diseases such as heart disease, high blood pressure, Type 2 diabetes, gallstones, breathing problems, and certain cancers. Although BMI can be used for most men and women, it does have some limits:

- It may overestimate body fat in athletes and others who have a high muscular mass.
- It may underestimate body fat in older persons and others who have lost muscle.

Figure 7.4 shows a reference table for determining BMI. Please note that current research suggests significantly decreased morbidity and mortality for a target BMI of 25-29 for individuals age 65 years or older. A final way to measure body mass is to examine the percentage of body weight that is fat. Obviously, as body fat percentage increases, so does the health risk. Figure 7.5 shows BMI classifications and desirable body fat percentage.

Body fat is most often measured using special calipers to measure the skinfold thickness of the fat fold under the skin and other parts of the body. Skinfold thickness is a measurement of the fleshy part of the body at a specified location. Because half of all body fat is under the skin, this method is quite accurate if it is performed by a

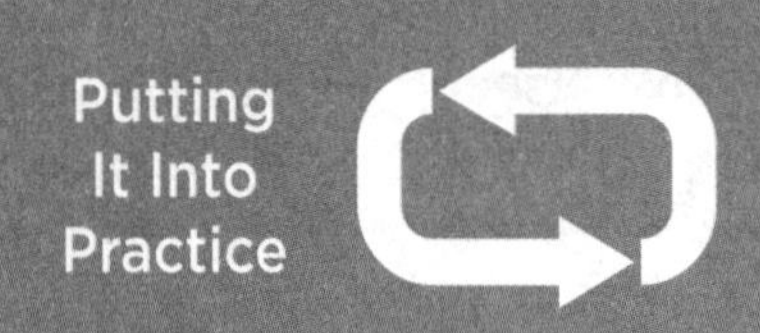

2. Your male client is 6'3" tall and has a medium frame. He weighs 150 lbs. What is his IBW and percent of IBW?

Figure 7.4

Body Mass Index Table

To use the table, find the appropriate height in the left-hand column labeled Height. Move across to a given weight (in pounds). The number at the top of the column is the BMI at that height and weight.

	BODY MASS INDEX																					
HEIGHT	19	20	21	22	23	24	25	26	27	28	29	30	31	32	33	34	35	36	37	38	39	40
58"	91	96	100	105	110	115	119	124	129	134	138	143	148	153	158	162	167	172	177	181	186	191
59"	94	99	104	109	114	119	124	128	133	138	143	148	153	158	163	168	173	178	183	188	193	198
60"	97	102	107	112	118	123	128	133	138	143	148	153	158	163	168	174	179	184	189	194	199	204
61"	100	106	111	116	122	127	132	137	143	148	153	158	164	169	174	180	185	190	195	201	206	211
62"	104	109	115	120	126	131	136	142	147	153	158	164	169	175	180	186	191	196	202	207	213	218
63"	107	113	118	124	130	135	141	146	152	158	163	169	175	180	186	191	197	203	208	214	220	225
64"	110	116	122	128	134	140	145	151	157	163	169	174	180	186	192	197	204	209	215	221	227	232
65"	114	120	126	132	138	144	150	156	162	168	174	180	186	192	198	204	210	216	222	228	234	240
66"	118	124	130	136	142	148	155	161	167	173	179	186	192	198	204	210	216	223	229	235	241	247
67"	121	127	134	140	146	153	159	166	172	178	185	191	198	204	211	217	223	230	236	242	249	255
68"	125	131	138	144	151	158	164	171	177	184	190	197	203	210	216	223	230	236	243	249	256	262
69"	128	135	142	149	155	162	169	176	182	189	196	203	209	216	223	230	236	243	250	257	263	270
70"	132	139	146	153	160	167	174	181	188	195	202	209	216	222	229	236	243	250	257	264	271	278
71"	136	143	150	157	165	172	179	186	193	200	208	215	222	229	236	243	250	257	265	272	279	286
72"	140	147	154	162	169	177	184	191	199	206	213	221	228	235	242	250	258	265	272	279	287	294
73"	144	151	159	166	174	182	189	197	204	212	219	227	235	242	250	257	265	272	280	288	295	302
74"	148	155	163	171	179	186	194	202	210	218	225	233	241	249	256	264	272	280	287	295	303	311
75"	152	160	168	176	184	192	200	208	216	224	232	240	248	256	264	272	279	287	295	303	311	319
76"	156	164	172	180	189	197	205	213	221	230	238	246	254	263	271	279	287	295	304	312	320	328

Source: National Institutes of Health

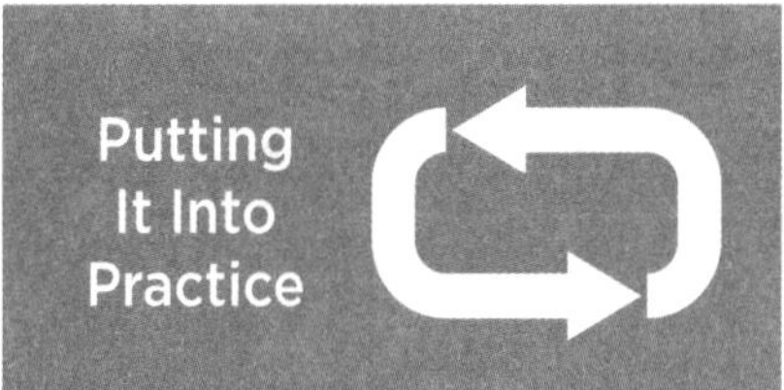

3. How would you classify a BMI of 27 for an 82 year-old client?

Figure 7.5
BMI Classifications and Desirable Body Fat Percentage

BMI CLASSIFICATION		DESIRABLE BODY FAT PERCENTAGE	
Risk Category	BMI Measurement	Men	Women
Underweight	BMI <18 Kg/m^2	13-25%	17-29%
Healthy Weight	BMI 20-25		
Overweight	BMI 25-29.9		
Obese	BMI $\geq$ 30		

Source: Centers for Disease Control and Prevention

person who has a lot of experience. Standards exist for comparing the measurements and using them to gauge not only percent body fat, but also overall nutritional status (protein and calorie nutrition). Other anthropometric measurements to assess muscle mass include mid-arm circumference and mid-arm muscle circumference.

Biochemical Tests. Biochemical tests, or laboratory tests, can be very helpful in assessing a client's nutritional status. Some typical standards for interpreting these test values appear in Figure 7.6. The normal values for each of these tests are determined by the facility. Various laboratories will have their own "normal ranges" for lab values. Some values may also be interpreted or adjusted for elderly clients based on health status and treatment goals. Figure 7.6 shows some of the laboratory tests with nutritional significance.

Serum Albumin. More than half of all the protein in the blood is albumin. Serum albumin is not a direct indicator of nutritional status, particularly protein status, but it takes time to change and there are several factors that can affect the albumin levels. Therefore, a client with a low serum albumin may have been in poor nutritional status for some time or the albumin could be low as a result of systemic inflammation. Serum albumin decreases in systemic inflammation (chronic and acute), trauma, edema, severe infection, or protein-calorie malnutrition. Serum albumin can also be affected by hydration. However, since it takes a long time to change, or may not be nutrition-related at all, it is not the best indicator of nutritional status.

Serum Prealbumin. This is a protein made by the liver and is considered one of the most sensitive and reliable indicators of protein status. Unlike serum albumin, it is not affected by hydration. It is a good measure for effectiveness of nutrition support, because it will begin to change within approximately four days. Even though it is produced by the liver, prealbumin is not affected by most forms of liver disease.

Serum Transferrin. Like albumin, transferrin is a protein found in the blood. Transferrin carries iron to where red blood cells are made. Serum transferrin levels

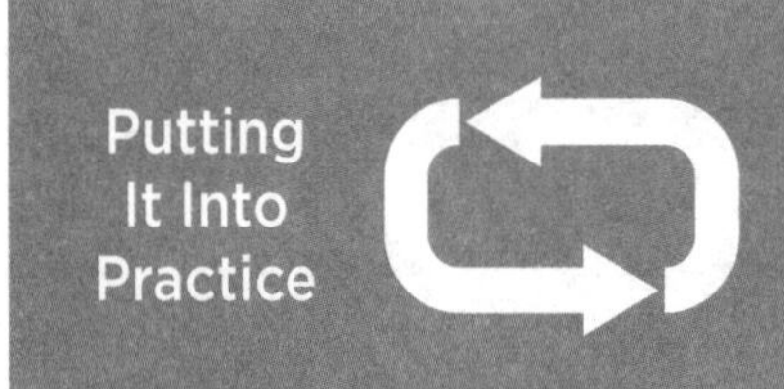

4. Steven weighs 240 lbs. and measures 6'2". What would be his risk category based on his BMI? He weighed 201 lbs. when he was admitted. What is his percent weight change?

Figure 7.6
Selected Laboratory Tests with Nutrition Significance

Serum Albumin
Normal Range*: 3.5-5.0 gm/dl (Centers for Medicare & Medicaid Services uses 3.4–4.8 gm/dl for individuals over 60 years of age)

Significance: Can measure protein status; but is also altered by edema and chronic or acute inflammation. Should not be used as a direct nutritional status indicator. May appear high due to dehydration, which concentrates the blood. Takes about 2-3 weeks to change in response to protein status.

Serum Prealbumin (PAB)
Normal Range*: 16-35 mg/dl

Significance: Can measure protein status; 11-15 mg/dl may indicate mild protein depletion; <10 mg/dl suggests significant protein depletion. PAB takes only a few days to change in response to protein status. With adequate nutrition support of a malnourished client, this value should rise approx. 2 mg/dl each day.

Serum Transferrin
Normal Range*: 180-380 gm/dl

Significance: Can measure protein status; takes about 10 days to change in response to protein status; may be elevated with iron-deficiency anemia.

Total Lymphocyte Count
Normal Range*: 3,000-5,000 cells/mm

Significance: This is a count of lymphocyte cells in the immune system; can measure protein status; 1,500-1,800 may indicate mild protein depletion; 900-1,500 suggests moderate depletion. TLC may be high in infection.

Fasting Blood Sugar/Glucose (FBS or FBG)
Normal Range*: 70-99 mg/dl

Significance: Elevated FBS suggests diabetes or poor control of blood sugar for a person with diabetes. Slight elevations may occur with age. Note that random blood sugar (e.g. after a meal) may be higher (up to about 140 mg/dl). BS of approx. 300 mg/dl is dangerously high, leading to severe confusion and possible coma. Very low BS (< 60 mg/dl) is hypoglycemia and requires immediate treatment.

Glycosylated Hemoglobin (HbA1c)
Normal Range*: < 5%

Significance: This value indicates control of blood glucose/sugar over a recent period of two to three months. It is valuable in evaluating ongoing blood sugar control for a person with diabetes. A low figure indicates good control. A high figure (e.g. > 7%) suggests blood sugar may have been consistently or frequently high. Current recommendations for this lab value are related to individualization and liberalizing within established parameters for elderly in the LTC setting.

Hemoglobin (Hgb or Hb)
Normal Range*: 12-15 g/dl (adult woman); 14-17 g/dl (adult man)

Significance: Low Hgb with low HCT together often indicate anemia due to inadequate iron, folate, vitamin B6, vitamin B12, or other nutrients in the body. It is also low following blood loss, e.g. from internal bleeding, trauma, or surgery, and during cancer. Slightly low levels may occur with aging.

Hematocrit (HCT)
Normal Range*: 36-46% (adult female); 41-53% (adult male)

Significance: Measures number and size of red blood cells; low Hgb with low HCT together often indicate iron-deficiency anemia; may be high (or appear normal) in dehydration.

Serum Cholesterol
Normal Range*: < 200 mg/dl

Significance: High levels represent risk of cardiovascular disease.

High Density Lipoprotein (HDL) Cholesterol
Normal Range*: 40–60 mg/dl

Significance: "Good" cholesterol; < 40 mg/dl represents risk of cardiovascular disease; high levels are desirable (see Chapter 6).

Low Density Lipoprotein (LDL) Cholesterol
Normal Range*: < 100 mg/dl optimal; 100–129 mg/dl near optimal

Significance: "Bad" cholesterol; elevated levels represent risk of cardiovascular disease (see Chapter 6).

Serum Triglyceride
Normal Range*: < 150 mg/dl

Significance: High levels may mildly increase risk for cardiovascular disease; very high levels may suggest a blood lipid disorder; can lead to fatty deposits in the body (e.g. in liver); can also suggest uncontrolled diabetes.

Serum Potassium
Normal Range*: 3.5–5.0 mEq/L

Significance: Becomes elevated during renal failure and other conditions; may become low with medications (e.g. potassium-wasting diuretics) or diarrhea; elevated or very low levels can become life-threatening; important to monitor for a client placed on either a high or low potassium diet or those receiving dialysis.

Blood Urea Nitrogen (BUN)
Normal Range*: 8-20 mg/dl

Significance: An important measure of renal function; high levels may indicate renal failure, dehydration, or other medical conditions.

** Note: Standards for normal ranges are set by the institution and may vary. Many clinical factors, such as fluid retention, dehydration, medication regimens, diseases of major organs, and many others can affect laboratory value readings. It is important to review the entire clinical picture, and consult with other members of the healthcare team in interpreting laboratory values.*

Sources: National Institutes of Health, Centers for Medicare & Medicaid Services (CMS), American Academy of Family Physicians

are considered a more sensitive indicator of protein deficiency than albumin because transferrin levels change more quickly in response to changes in nutritional status.

Total Lymphocyte Count (TLC). Lymphocytes are white blood cells involved in fighting infection. In the case of protein deficiency, the total number of lymphocytes decreases. Certain drugs also decrease total lymphocyte count.

Hematocrit and Hemoglobin. Hematocrit is the percent of packed red blood cells in blood. Hemoglobin is the oxygen-carrying pigment of the red blood cells. A low hemoglobin level may indicate iron-deficiency anemia.

Clinical Information. Some of the clinical information that can have a bearing on nutrition screening and assessment is available in the medical record. Certain diagnoses or conditions, for example, may indicate a need for nutritional evaluation. For example, pressure ulcers are one of the conditions that require medical nutrition therapy for treatment. Additionally, a client whose symptoms include ongoing diarrhea and/or fever would be another. A client on a tube feeding would be yet another example. Figure 7.7 lists medical and social factors that may affect nutritional status.

Yet another type of clinical information that is important in understanding the nutritional picture for any client is medications. The effects foods and drugs have on each other can determine whether medications do their jobs and whether the body gets the nutrients it needs. Medications can interfere with the way the body digests, absorbs, or uses a nutrient. A medication that causes taste changes or gastrointestinal discomfort may reduce a person's food intake over time. This may cause weight loss and/or loss of nutritional well-being. Conversely, dietary factors can affect how medicines function in the body. This interchange can be mild or life-threatening. It depends on the medication and many other factors. Figure 7.8 provides sample food/drug interactions. Figure 7.9 lists some commonly-used drugs that may have nutrition-related effects.

Figure 7.7
Nutrition-Related Clinical Information

MEDICAL FACTORS		SOCIAL FACTORS
• Cancer • Diabetes • Heart and circulatory disease • High blood pressure • Kidney disease • History of alcohol use and/or abuse • GERD • History of depression • Liver disease • Lung disease • Illness with increased metabolic needs: burns, infection, trauma, protracted fever	• Malabsorption syndromes • Surgery of gastrointestinal tract • Overweight • Underweight • Recent unplanned weight loss • Certain medications • Chemotherapy/radiation therapy • Pressure ulcers • Chewing/swallowing problems • Inadequate fluid intake • Declining cognition	• Living and eating alone • Not enough money for food • Inadequate facilities for storing and preparing food • Problems shopping for food • Declining mobility • Alcohol use

Figure 7.9

Medications with Possible Nutrition-Related Effects

DRUG	POSSIBLE EFFECTS
Analgesic (Pain Killer)	
Aspirin	Gastric pain or bleeding, nausea and vomiting
Acetaminophen	Gastrointestinal disturbance, liver toxicity
Antibiotic	
Amoxicillin	Diarrhea, nausea and vomiting
Ampicillin	Diarrhea, glossitis (inflammation of the tongue), stomatitis (mouth ulcers), nausea and vomiting
Cephalexin	Abdominal pain, diarrhea, nausea and vomiting
Erythromycin	Abdominal cramping, diarrhea, nausea and vomiting
Penicillin	Diarrhea, glossitis, stomatitis, nausea and vomiting
Tetracycline	Anorexia, diarrhea, dysphagia, glossitis, nausea and vomiting, decreases vitamin K synthesis
Antipsychotics/Antidepressants	
Nearly all affect appetite and/or weight change	
High Blood Pressure	
Atenolol	Diarrhea, nausea
Propranolol	Abdominal cramping, constipation, diarrhea, nausea and vomiting, decreased carbohydrate tolerance
Bronchodilator	
Theophylline	Anorexia, gastric irritation, nausea, vomiting
Diuretic	
Chlorthalidone	Anorexia, constipation, cramping, diarrhea, gastric irritation, electrolyte imbalance
Furosemide	Abdominal cramping, anorexia; constipation; diarrhea; dry mouth; thirst; fluid and electrolyte imbalance; nausea and vomiting; decreased blood potassium, magnesium, sodium; increased urinary potassium, magnesium, sodium
Hydrochlorothiazide	Anorexia, constipation, diarrhea, gastrointestinal irritation and ulceration, nausea and vomiting
Estrogen Replacement Therapy	
Estrogens	Abdominal cramping, bloating, edema, nausea and vomiting, carbohydrate intolerance
Non-Steroidal Anti-Inflammatory	
Ibuprofen	Abdominal cramping, constipation, diarrhea, edema, flatulence, gastrointestinal bleeding and ulceration, heartburn, nausea and vomiting
Naproxen	Abdominal pain, constipation, diarrhea, gastrointestinal bleeding and ulceration, heartburn, nausea and vomiting, stomatitis
Steroidal Anti-Inflammatory	
Prednisone	Abdominal distention, fluid and electrolyte imbalance, fluid and sodium retention, indigestion, nausea and vomiting, negative nitrogen balance, peptic ulcer, decreased carbohydrate tolerance, less vitamin D activity, increased appetite, increased weight

Source: US Public Health Service

Diet History and Information. Diet history is the final part of nutrition screening. A diet history and information may include one or more tools designed to develop a snapshot of a client's eating habits.

A Registered Dietitian Nutritionist may request a **food record**, which is a diary of food and beverages consumed. A common food record is kept for any number of days. A meaningful food record must include all condiments and additions to foods— such as mayonnaise used on a sandwich, or margarine and jelly spread on toast. Also, measurements of foods consumed are important. If a client has to tell how many ounces of roast beef he consumed, for example, this can be challenging. Sometimes, it helps to go over measurements and reporting with a client before the record begins. Food models (pieces of plastic molded to look like real foods) are useful for explaining portion sizes. The food record is then reviewed with the client to be sure all foods are listed and all portion sizes and preparation methods are accurate. Figure 7.10 shows a sample food record form.

This same form could be used as another tool often referred to as a **24-hour recall**. With a 24-hour recall, the interviewer guides the client through the last 24 hours and has him/her recall what was eaten. Again, it is important to use food models to help clients determine amounts eaten, condiments used and other items that may not be included as part of a "meal or snack" (e.g. a handful of nuts from the bowl on the table), how food is prepared (grilled, fried, served with sauce, etc.). One limitation to using a 24-hour recall is that all of the foods are not recalled or recorded. If a client has memory loss, this might not be the most appropriate tool to use. As with other nutrition tools, this could also be completed with a family member to increase reliability.

Another tool is a **food frequency questionnaire**. This is a checklist that identifies how often a client eats each of a variety of foods. This provides information about eating habits and preferences that may not show up on a brief food record. Today there are many programs on the Internet to enter food frequency information, such as MyPlate Super Tracker at www.choosemyplate.gov.

In addition to diet histories, the Registered Dietitian Nutritionist, CDM, CFPP, or nursing staff can record what the client eats and drinks for three days and then do a nutrient analysis to quantify intake of calories, protein, and/or other nutrients. This is called a **calorie count**, with a *nutrient intake analysis*. Observing and/or recording actual intake as in a food record is extremely important for understanding a client's nutritional needs. Industry research shows that about 75 percent of nursing home residents eat less than three-quarters of their food, which can have a tremendous impact on health.

Now, remember that water is a nutrient and that dehydration is a major risk among older Americans. Thus, monitoring fluid intake is important, too. Nursing staff and other team members may monitor fluid intake for certain patients. From a clinical perspective, they may also want to know more about how kidneys or other body organs are functioning. Thus, a typical review of fluid becomes an In and Out (I/O) record. An **I/O record** is a document of all fluids consumed and excreted over a 24-hour time period.

In a healthcare setting, nursing, foodservice, and other caregivers also review a resident's ability to eat and feed himself. **Meal observation** is a key assessment tool that helps to identify individuals who are having problems with appetite, chewing,

GLOSSARY

Food Record
A diary of food and beverages consumed, usually for a given number of days

24-Hour Recall
What was eaten in the past 24-hours as determined by personal interview and recall, or that of a family member regarding the client's intake the day before

Food Frequency Questionnaire
A checklist or questionnaire that tracks how often a client eats each of a variety of foods

Calorie Count
Documented results from direct observation at meal and snack times (usually in a hospital or nursing home) which are then tallied to reveal calories consumed in a day

In and Out (I/O) Record
A document of all the fluids consumed and excreted over a 24-hour period

Meal Observation
A key assessment tool that helps to identify individuals who are having problems with appetite, chewing, swallowing, alertness, self-feeding, or many other factors

View Supplemental Material to see Figure 7.8, Sample Food-Drug Interactions.

swallowing, alertness, self-feeding, or many other factors that may influence nutritional well-being. Based on observations, members of the team may begin to form strategies for helping a client eat well and enjoy meals.

Finally, a nutrition assessment includes a broader background on lifestyle and social factors that may influence nutrition. Many of the factors described in Chapter 8—such as cultural influences, religious beliefs, attitudes, and more—may be relevant in a diet history. For example, a person's ability to shop for and prepare food at home is very important.

Awareness of support systems and knowing who is responsible for meals sets groundwork for nutrition education that may be needed later in the nutrition care process. Developing a solid diet history usually involves gathering information directly from the medical record, from other caregivers in a healthcare facility, from the client, and sometimes from family or significant others. The ability to gather accurate information depends on interpersonal rapport and solid communication skills. Talking with others to gather information requires interviewing skills. Upon completion of a nutrition assessment, a caregiver lists all nutrition problems identified, and then recommends a plan for addressing each problem.

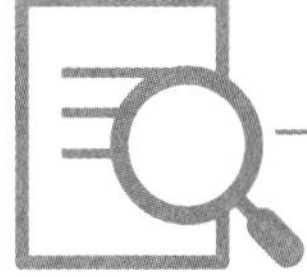

View Supplemental Material to see Figure 7.10, Sample Food Record Form.

Nutrition Assessment

Once the nutrition screening is completed, the next step is dependent upon the results of the screening. If the nutrition screening suggests a concern such as overweight, high blood sugar, cancer, etc., then an in-depth evaluation of a client's nutritional well-being will need to be done by the Registered Dietitian Nutritionist (RDN). This is called a **nutrition assessment**. The Registered Dietitian Nutritionist uses a comprehensive approach to determine nutritional status and will need the screening information you provide. The RDN uses interviews, laboratory data, clinical information, body measurements, information gathered from healthcare team members, and other tools to develop an assessment. The CDM, CFPP and the RDN work as a team, and the determination of specific duties should be made as a team and stated in the facility policy and procedure manual. Figure 7.11 shows the Scope of Practice for Nutrition Screening as defined by the Association of Nutrition & Foodservice Professionals. In some facilities, other members of the healthcare team may help to gather information for the nutrition assessment. It is typically the responsibility of the RDN to make a final evaluation utilizing all information. The nutrition assessment forms a basis for determining a nutrition diagnosis and developing a personalized nutrition care plan. Further chapters will address nutrition care planning and explain some of the follow-up required to assure effectiveness of a nutrition care plan.

BEE and Nutrient Needs

Another aspect of nutritional assessment is an estimation of nutrient needs. Some assessments involve comparing these estimations with actual intake, in order to evaluate whether a client is able to nourish himself adequately. Estimating nutrient needs also forms a foundation for planning individual menus and meals, as well as for planning tube feedings and parenteral nutrition regimens. Most often, the estimation of nutrient needs will be the responsibility of a Registered Dietitian Nutritionist. However, here is some background that helps to demystify these seemingly magic numbers.

GLOSSARY

Nutrition Assessment
A comprehensive approach by a Registered Dietitian Nutritionist using multiple data sources to determine nutrition status

Basal Metabolism
A term that describes how much energy the body needs when it is completely at rest

Basal Energy Expenditure (BEE)
The energy (in the form of calories) needed to maintain basic bodily functions such as breathing, brain function, and keeping the heart beating

Figure 7.11
Nutrition Screening

CDM, CFPP

NUTRITION SCREENING*

If Low-Risk
(per facility standard)

- Completes Minimum Data Set (MDS) Section K
- Completes Resident Assessment Protocols (RAP)
- Develops Care Plan

OR

If Risk Warrants
(per facility standard)

- Implements Established Protocols**
- Completes MDS Section K
- Completes RAP
- Develops an Initial Care Plan (refer to RDN)

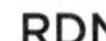

RDN

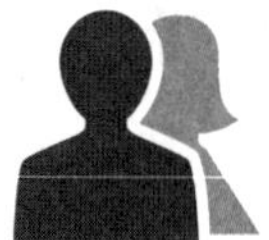

NUTRITION CARE PROCESS

- Initiates Nutrition Care Process (including in-depth assessment, nutrition diagnosis, nutrition intervention, nutrition monitoring and evaluation)
- Reviews MDS
- May Update RAP
- Updates Care Plan; May Revise Goal

** Per systematic, documented policies and procedures developed/approved by RDN and Standards of Professional Practice developed by ANFP*

*** These protocols would be facility-specific*

Basal or Resting metabolism is a term that describes how much energy the body needs when it is completely at rest. **Basal energy expenditure (BEE)** is the energy (calories) needed to maintain functions such as breathing, brain function, and keeping the heart beating or body functions at rest. It is usually expressed as calories per day. There are many formulas for calculating BEE, which differs between men and women and varies according to age. Figure 7.12 shows a sample set of formulas for adults. BEE calculations may also be automated through use of computer software. These calculations are based on weight in kilograms (kg) and height in centimeters (cm). To convert pounds to kilograms, divide by 2.2 lb./kg and to convert inches to cm, multiply inches by 2.54 cm/inch. BEE accounts for only about two-thirds of calories in an average person's daily needs. Above and beyond the total resting state, the body needs more calories for digesting food, for moving and exercising, for growing or healing, and more. When a fever is present, the body uses a tremendous amount of energy to produce the fever. A fever is heat, and heat is energy. A caloric needs estimate is an estimate that accounts for the total amount of calories needed, e.g., for one day. It is built on the BEE, but includes additional factors to account for other energy needs. As with BEE, there are many models and formulas for calculating this. Figures 7.12 and 7.13 identify some guidelines. Note that these guidelines are for adults only and are quite general. Furthermore, an estimate is only an estimate. In practice, any nutritional plan must be monitored. Follow-up assessment always includes weight monitoring, and adjustments to an initial plan are common.

View the Supplemental Material for the Focus on Formulas video Calculating Daily Protein Needs.

Figure 7.12
Formulas for Calculating BEE for Clients Over 18 Years Old

MEN	WOMEN
Harris-Benedict Equation: BEE = 66 + (13.7 x weight in kg) + (5 x height in cm) - (6.8 x age in years) Alternate Formula: BEE = 1.0 x (weight in kg) x 24	**Harris-Benedict Equation:** BEE = 655 + (9.6 x weight in kg) + (1.8 x height in cm) - (4.7 x age in years) Alternate Formula: BEE = 0.9 x (weight in kg) x 24
Mifflin-St. Jeor Equation: BEE = (10 x weight) + (6.25 x height) - (5 x Age) + 5	**Mifflin-St. Jeor Equation:** BEE = (10 x weight) + (6.25 x height) - (5 x Age) - 161

Notes: *To convert pounds to kilograms, divide by 2.2 (2.2 lb. = 1 kg). To convert inches to centimeters, multiply by 2.54 (1 in = 2.54 cm). There are height-weight percentile tables for clients under age 18.*

Figure 7.13
Nutrition-Related Clinical Information

ACTIVITY FACTORS (Add these to the BEE)	INJURY FACTORS (Add these to the BEE)
• 0.2 x BEE for a patient who is in bed most of the time • 0.3 x BEE for an individual who is ambulatory and/or moderately active • 0.5 x BEE for an individual who is very active	• 0.2 x BEE following surgery • 0.35 x BEE following skeletal trauma (bone fractures) • 0.1 - 0.4 x BEE following other trauma • 0.1 x BEE for each degree (F) of fever • 2.1 x BEE for severe burn

For protein-calorie malnutrition: *Add an amount for weight gain/growth. This might be 500-1,000 calories per day.*
To achieve weight loss (for an overweight individual): *Subtract 500-1,000 calories per day to promote a loss of 1-2 lbs./week.*

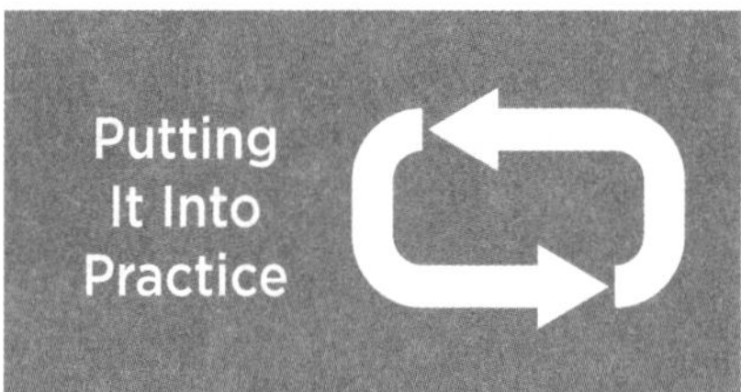

5. Why would knowing what medications someone is taking be relevant to screening for nutritional risk?

Other common clinical nutrition calculations include an estimation of protein needs (Figure 7.14) and an estimation of fluid needs (Figure 7.15) For additional nutrient needs estimates, search the Internet for the RDIs. Many medical conditions can alter the needs for calories, protein, fluids and other nutrients. For fluids it is particularly important to be aware of a physician's order. Fluid restrictions are common among healthcare clients.

Figure 7.14
Estimating Daily Protein Needs

- For a healthy adult: 0.8 grams x body weight in kg
- For a malnourished client: 1.2-1.5 grams x body weight in kg
- Following surgery: 1.0-2.0 grams x body weight in kg
- Following trauma, severe burn, or multiple fractures: 2.0 grams x body weight in kg

Source: Adapted from Nutrition 411

Sources for Nutrition Screening Tools

As Chapter 7 draws to a close, it has been determined that many sources and standards exist for nutrition screening. Tools vary from one facility to another. As a staff member of a healthcare facility, determine if there is a nutrition screening tool in place. Then, become familiar with the tool and apply it. Often, a Registered Dietitian Nutritionist or Clinical Nutrition Manager will help to locate and/or develop a screening tool. Some facilities develop nutrition screening tools in-house, drawing on the expertise of the Registered Dietitian Nutritionist and healthcare team members. On the other hand, a screening tool may come from professional organizations, such as the Academy of Nutrition and Dietetics or other dietetics group. It may come from researchers or educational institutions. It may come from a provider of products to support medical nutrition therapy. Nutrition screening standards and forms are sometimes components of diet manuals. Finally, nutrition screening may be built into a clinical nutrition management software package. Software-based systems may have default screening criteria and scoring values built-in. Typically, however, a Registered Dietitian Nutritionist can select indicators and thresholds in the software in order to customize scoring to institutional policies and procedures. Another advantage of using software support in the screening process is that most programs can then generate a report or list for follow-up assessment. If a priority system is used (e.g. Level 1 Risk, Level 2 Risk, etc.), software may sort the list by priority level. Software also automates the calculations involved in nutrition screening.

Regardless of the choice of tools, an effective nutrition screening process:

- Uses meaningful screening criteria, as identified by a qualified individual (e.g. Registered Dietitian Nutritionist)
- Sets meaningful thresholds that correspond to known risks

6. How much protein per kg would a 76 year-old patient with a low percent of IBW need?

- Is applied to every client
- Is implemented quickly upon admission
- Is implemented uniformly and consistently

The screening process is implemented uniformly and consistently through the use of standardized forms, such as the example in Figure 7.1. Using a form ensures consistency in screening, review of the same key indicators among all clients, without overlooking any piece of the screening standard. It's like a shopping list; it ensures that nothing will be forgotten. A software program accomplishes the same objective, but through an electronic process. By following a methodical process for nutrition screening, you can be reasonably confident that you are finding the clients whose personal health may benefit from medical nutrition therapy. When following protocol with nutrition screening, this ensures that each of these clients receives a nutrition screening and, if warranted, a nutrition assessment.

View the Supplemental Material to see Scope of Practice and Practice Standard.

Furthermore, nutrition screening is generally dictated by relevant healthcare regulations, both federal and state. Guidelines from The Joint Commission also apply to most healthcare facilities. Standards may require that nutrition screening be conducted within a given timeframe after admission and again at prescribed intervals. Based on regulations, the role of a CDM, CFPP in screening may vary from one facility to another. Likewise, the method of documenting screening activities may also vary. Thus, it is imperative to become familiar with all relevant regulations and standards at any place of employment, and to follow them. Each healthcare facility needs to develop a policy and procedure for nutrition screening that achieves the objective of identifying clients at risk, and stipulates a mechanism for assuring regulatory compliance and documentation.

The Nutrition Screening and Nutrition Assessment information needs to be documented in the medical record. Please review the ANFP Practice Standards: Documenting in the Medical Record, as well as the Scope of Practice for the Certified Dietary Manager, Certified Food Protection Professional found in the Nutrition Supplemental Materials.

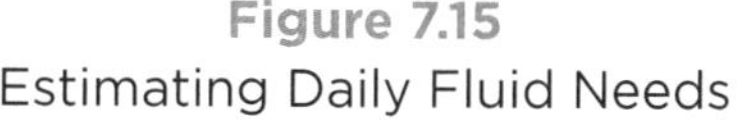

Figure 7.15
Estimating Daily Fluid Needs

FORMULA	DISEASE FACTORS that Increase Fluid Requirements	DISEASE FACTORS that Decrease Fluid Allowed
For Average Adults: 30 mL/kg **For Adults with Infection or Draining Wounds:** 35 mL/kg **For Adults with CHF or Renal Disease:** 25 mL/kg	Fever Draining wounds Diarrhea Vomiting Hyperventilation Respirator Excessive perspiration Pressure ulcer/injury (stages II, III, IV)	Congestive heart failure (CHF) Cardiac disease Renal disease Edema or ascites

Indicators of Dehydration

- Client has clinical signs of dehydration
- Client loses more fluids through vomiting, fever, diarrhea than he/she consumes

Source: Adapted from Nutrition 411

Chapter References

RESOURCES	
Academy of Nutrition and Dietetics*	https://www.eatright.org
Association of Nutrition & Foodservice Professionals	www.ANFPonline.org
Centers for Medicare & Medicaid Services**	https://www.cms.gov
Certifying Board for Dietary Managers	www.CBDMonline.org
Hermann J. Drug-nutrient interactions. Oklahoma State University Extension.** Published October 2019.	https://extension.okstate.edu/fact-sheets/drug-nutrient-interactions.html.
Mueller C, Compher C, Ellen DM. A.S.P.E.N. clinical guidelines: nutrition screening, assessment, and intervention in adults. JPEN J Parenter Enteral Nutr. 2011;35(1):16-24.	
Nestlé Nutrition Institute. MNA® Mini Nutritional Assessment.**	https://www.mna-elderly.com
Nutrition 411—Daily Protein Needs and Daily Fluid Needs	https://www.consultant360.com/nutrition411
Posner BM, Jette AM, Smith KW, Miller DR. Nutrition and health risks in the elderly: the nutrition screening initiative. *Am J Public Health*. 1993;83(7):972-978.	
Stang J, Story M. Nutrition Screening, Assessment, and Intervention. In: Stang J, Story M. *Guidelines for Adolescent Nutrition Services*. University of Minnesota: Center for Leadership, Education and Training in Maternal and Child Nutrition; 2005: 35-54.**	https://pdfs.semanticscholar.org/8fc2/97a0c9f9120247785d421ab139fbb89673e7.pdf
U.S. Department of Agriculture. Food and Human Nutrition. National Agricultural Library.*	https://www.nal.usda.gov/food-and-human-nutrition
U.S. Department of Health and Human Services**	https://usphs.gov
Weerts S. Aging and Nutrition. Diet.com.**	https://www.diet.com/g/aging-and-nutrition

** Accessed September 18, 2019; **Accessed March 21, 2020*

Interview Clients for Nutrition-Related Information

Overview and Objectives

After gathering nutritional data, the next step is to interview clients. You determine who your clients are and will use at least one technique to gather information about client needs . You will use this information to examine how clients' needs influence the foodservice operation. In addition, in order to provide nutrition care, the Certified Dietary Manager®, Certified Food Protection Professional® (CDM®, CFPP®) needs to understand what motivates people to eat and how foods are chosen. Culture, religion, and regional influences may have a direct impact on what is consumed. After completing this chapter, you should be able to:

- Identify different types of clients
- Plan and ask appropriate questions of clients
- Gather information from the client and/or family member(s)
- Identify significant information and problems
- Recognize nonverbal responses and communication cues
- Record information gathered
- Utilize ethical and confidentiality principles and practices
- Gather client information from relevant sources (multi-disciplinary team members)
- Address food customs and nutritional needs/preferences of various racial, cultural, and religious groups
- Use ethical and confidentiality principles and practices

8

If asked to describe your customers/clients, what would you say? Everyone who is provided meal service would be considered a client. This might be hospital patients or nursing home residents. They are a very important part of the clientele. Another part of the clientele is the staff that works and eats at the facility. If the facility prepares meals for members of the community, such as "Meals on Wheels," they are also considered customers/clients. Are meals prepared for family members on special occasions? Are there other groups served that aren't mentioned here? Each of these groups has different needs and different expectations. A successful foodservice department knows who their clients are and routinely surveys each group. This chapter will discuss interviewing patients/clients/caregivers for nutrition-related information.

Interviewing Clients Begins With Good Communication Techniques

GLOSSARY

Communication
The exchange of information by writing, speaking, or gestures

In this discussion about interviewing clients, let's start with some basics about good communication. Communicating clearly is the key to success when working with clients. **Communication** is a two-way process. There are six basic steps in communication that are important in interviewing clients:

1. Prepare for the communication
   - Plan what you intend to ask before you interview the client.
   - Anticipate how your client might be feeling.
2. Conduct the interview
   - Explain why you are interviewing the client.
   - Speak slowly, clearly, and confidently.
   - Explain clearly what you expect/need.
   - Ask the client to relate back to you the purpose of your visit.
3. Review the message
   - Don't judge what they are telling you or judge the person.
   - Look for the key points or specific answers to your questions.
   - Give feedback to acknowledge your understanding.
   - Listen carefully to what the client has to say.
   - Have non-judgmental collaborative conversation.
   - Engage to build and strengthen motivation to share thoughts and ideas.
   - Build relationship that conveys a partnership, acceptance, compassion, and a belief in the client's own potential for positive interactions.
4. Evaluate the effectiveness of your communication
   - Periodically ask for questions or clarify with client any questions.
   - Ask questions to evaluate client understanding.
   - Ask client to repeat important information to evaluate learning.
5. Communication can break down due to these common communication barriers:
   - **Message quality:** Have you used words the client understands? Were the instructions clear? Did you ask enough questions to get all of the information you need?
   - **Noise:** Did the client have a television/radio/other multimedia on while you were trying to communicate? Were other people in the room talking? Is there equipment running in the room?

- **Time:** Were you in a hurry? Was the client in a hurry? Is the interview tool too long for one session? Is the client overwhelmed or fatigued?
- **Conflict:** Is the client angry? Are you having a bad day; is something bothering you?

6. Overcome the communication barriers
   - **Message quality:** If using technical terms, make sure to explain them (even the phrase "diet history" might seem foreign or they may not understand the word "fat" in food). Continue to seek feedback and encourage shared dialog in the interview by asking questions such as, "Would you like to go through that again?" or "What are some things we've discussed that make the most sense to you?" Focus clearly on what is needed and why it is needed.
   - **Noise:** Ask if appropriate, that they minimize their multimedia equipment in order to conduct the interview. If other people or equipment in the room contribute to distracting noise, ask to go somewhere else to conduct the interview.
   - **Time:** Before beginning the interview, make sure that there is enough time to complete the questions/interview.
   - **Conflict:** Don't take it personally and remain patient and professional.

There are three types of communication: **written, verbal,** and **nonverbal**. The steps above can be used with both verbal and written communication. Non-verbal communication is the communication that occurs without language such as gestures, facial expressions or the way voices are used—speaking softly or loudly. Nonverbal communication is just as important as verbal and written communication because it gives clues as to how well you are communicating. What if a client won't look at you

GLOSSARY

Written Communication
Expressing thoughts, messages, or information by writing

Verbal Communication
Expressing thoughts, messages, or information by speaking

Nonverbal Communication
The form of communication without speaking or writing that include gestures, facial expressions, and body language

Figure 8.1
Basic Communication

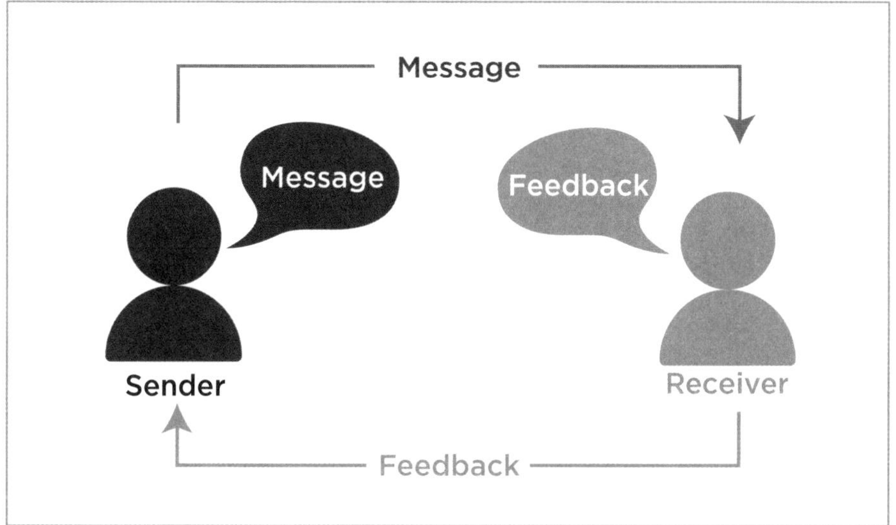

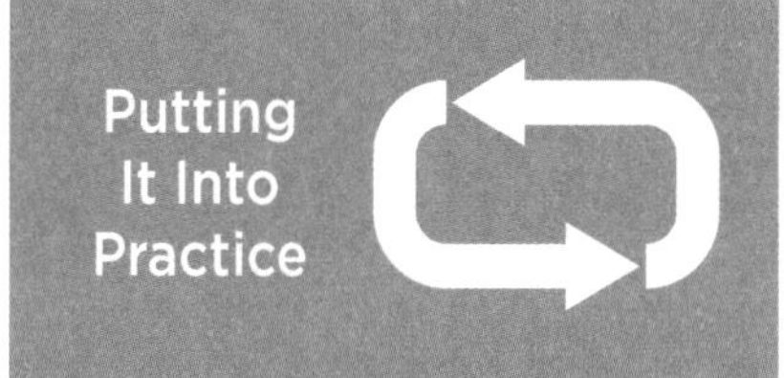

1. You are interviewing a client in their room. What type of communication is this? You notice their arms are crossed during one of the questions. What type of non-verbal communication is this?

during an interview? What does this mean? Are they interested in the information? Could it be a part of their cultural beliefs? Let's review the common types of nonverbal communication:

- **Facial expressions:** smiling, frowning, sneering, rolling the eyes, raising the eyebrows all convey how one is receiving the message. As the sender, watch for changes in facial expression to make sure you are communicating clearly.
- **Eye contact:** Are your clients looking you directly in the eye? That can mean they are interested and being attentive to what is being said. It is important to know that in some cultures (e.g. Asian, Latin American, African, and Native American), direct eye contact can only be used between certain people; with some cultures, direct eye contact could be considered rude and inappropriate.
- **Gestures:** If you are interviewing people of different cultures, be aware that they may have a different meaning for some gestures. Become aware of how you gesture when you talk so you will use appropriate hand gestures.
- **Physical contact:** Shaking hands is a typical American greeting. Touching, holding, embracing, patting on the back all convey messages, and those messages may be different in different cultures. Be careful about how you use physical contact with clients.
- **Distance:** How close you stand to a client while interviewing is another form of nonverbal communication. If you stand too close, it may violate the client's 'personal space.'
- **Posture:** If your client is sitting up and looking at you, you can conclude they are interested. If they are slouching or leaning away from you, if their arms are crossed and they are looking away, you might conclude that they are not interested.

As you begin your career as a CDM, CFPP, consider developing a checklist that will be a reminder of the basics needed for good communication. This can be part of any interview or survey instrument you use. See Figure 8.2 for an example.

Interviews for Nutrition Information

Each facility will have its own process for when the CDM, CFPP and/or Registered Dietitian Nutritionist first visits a person as a new admission. Some facilities have an immediate visit to gather food preferences. Some facilities visit after the first week to gather diet information and assess the quality of their foodservice (see Figure 8.3 for an example). Long-term care facilities conduct a diet history within the first 14 days as part of nutrition screening.

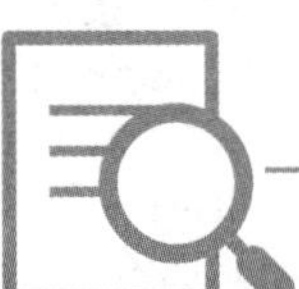

View the Supplemental Material to see Figure 8.3, Sample Page From an Electronic Diet History Questionnaire.

Figure 8.2
Checklist for Good Communication Skills

- I care about how clients respond to my messages.
- I don't use jargon in my messages.
- I don't judge people.
- I watch for nonverbal communication cues.
- I try to make each person feel important by listening to his or her messages.
- I am sensitive to feedback.
- My message is simple, direct, and clear.

Diet History. A diet history is a unique assessment of the client's food intake patterns. A diet history has two features: it describes actual intake, and it gives information about why the client makes certain food choices. It also includes a review of many factors that may have an impact on nutrition, such as lifestyle, social factors, medical conditions, and more.

A diet history usually begins with a series of questions. A Registered Dietitian Nutritionist or CDM, CFPP may ask:

- Where do you usually eat?
- How often do you usually eat?
- When do you usually eat?
- Do you eat by yourself or with others?
- Who does the food shopping in your household?
- Who does the cooking?
- How is your appetite?
- Have you had any appetite changes in the last month? 6 months?
- Do you have hunger or cravings during the day?
- Are you having any problems or concerns with eating?
- Are you having any problems chewing?
- Are you having any problems swallowing?
- Are you experiencing any digestive concerns, such as nausea, vomiting, constipation, or acid indigestion/heartburn?
- Have you experienced any weight changes within the past month or past 6 months?
- Do you have any food allergies or intolerances?
- Do you currently follow a special diet?
- Do you currently take any nutritional supplements?
- Are there any foods you avoid? If so, why?
- What foods do you consider a comfort and are part of your daily routine?
- What are your favorite foods and beverages?

Questions such as these and many others begin to build a picture of a person's overall dietary intake. A diet history may include one or more tools designed to develop a snapshot of a client's eating habits. Additional methods of collecting food records were covered in Chapter 7 (Obtain Routine Nutrition Screening Data). When conducting the interview, remember to focus on the checklist for guidance and on the client in order to maintain good communication. The diet history may be your first opportunity to make a great impression.

Some facilities have adopted electronic means of collecting diet history information. See Figure 8.3 for a sample from an electronic diet history questionnaire. The Diet Calc Diet History Questionnaire II and Analysis software are available free of charge from the National Institutes of Health: http://appliedresearch.cancer.gov/dhq2/dietcalc

- Electronically compute calorie information
- Document more detailed information
- Expedite analysis of the data for problems

What happens if the client is unable to communicate because they cannot speak or are not cognitive? If they are unable to speak, use pictures or food models and ask them to respond in writing to the questions, if they can. If they are not cognitive, ask close family members to assist you in completing the diet history. If there are no family members available, observe them during several meal times to collect diet information and review transfer information in the medical record.

Some clients may not speak English but can understand what is said. Sometimes speaking slower and very clearly, in addition to using gestures, facial expressions, etc., can be useful. Use pictures or draw it. Food models may also be helpful. Be patient. In some areas or cases where clients do not speak English, an interpreter may be necessary. Also, refer back to the discussion about cultural sensitivity.

Conducting Effective Interviews

In addition to the checklist for good communication, there are other tips for conducting effective interviews that will lead to success (see Figure 8.4—Tips for Conducting Effective Interviews). A function of a diet history is to gather information about why a client eats what they do.

During the interview, it is important to address food customs that are cultural, racial, or religious in origin. If you work in an area with a diverse population, the interview should have specific questions relating to their culture. Investigate the factors that affect the food intake of your clients. Let's take a closer look at some of the factors that influence what foods are chosen, and how feelings relate to dietary choices. These factors include: cultural heritage, regional trends, religious practices, social and emotional meanings.

Cultural Heritage

First, consider food as part of every culture. To understand this aspect of food, try asking some questions. You could have the client begin by closing his or her eyes, think of a time when the family all ate together. Describe that ... the smells, what it looked like, the sounds. Now think about a wedding celebration. What food will always be served? Most people will answer: a wedding cake. Or, in China, the answer may be: roasted pig. Maybe ask about how birthdays are celebrated in their families, and ask if there are any special foods served then. From these examples, many regard food choices

Figure 8.4
Tips for Conducting Effective Interviews

- Plan questions in advance and use a form to keep track.
- Introduce yourself by name and title.
- Avoid yes-or-no questions. Instead, use open-ended questions, such as: "Tell me more about..."
- Ask for more information or clarification when needed. This can be done by paraphrasing (summarizing and rephrasing what has been said).
- Allow the client time to give an answer. Silence can be helpful.
- Use nonverbal language to show the client you are listening. For example, maintain good eye contact and lean slightly toward the client to demonstrate your attention.
- Avoid leading questions that give the client the answer you expect. For example, do not ask, "You don't eat pizza often, do you?"
- When closing the interview, express appreciation to the client and review the next steps, if appropriate.

as cultural symbols. The meaning of these foods is much deeper than a sum of protein, carbohydrate, fat, vitamins, and minerals—the sheer nutritional values.

Many food choices arise from what is learned through cultural experiences. Holidays, festivals, and important events each have associated foods. In addition, daily food choices vary by culture: Traditional German cuisine, for example, might include sausage, schnitzel, spaetzel, beer, and other specialties. Japanese cuisine typically includes sushi, tempura, and rice. Swedish cuisine might include pancakes, even at meals other than breakfast. Mexican cuisine includes staples such as tortillas, rice, and refried beans. Creole cuisine, popular in New Orleans, represents a synthesis of French cooking with locally available foods, and the influences of Caribbean and Spanish cultures.

Cultural contributions to cuisine include the choices of ingredients, the style of preparation, the equipment used to cook food, the seasonings, and styles for displaying and serving. Dining itself is also cultural. Washing hands at the table with a warm, moist cloth is a common practice in some cultures. Choices for dining room décor, table settings, eating utensils, ambiance, music, lighting, accepted dress, and even the timing of meals, or the degree to which conversation is encouraged or discouraged all reflect cultural patterns.

As a land of immigrants, the United States enjoys multi-faceted cultural diversity. Our food choices are as rich and complex as our population itself. See Figure 8.5 for cultural food influences. Here are more examples of cultural and ethnic food influences.

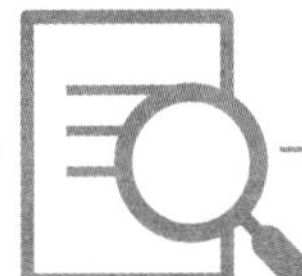

View the Supplemental Material to see Figure 8.6, Questions to Ask a Hispanic Client.

Hispanics/Latinos. The United States Census Bureau defines Hispanics as those who indicate their origin to be Mexican, Puerto Rican, Cuban, Central or South American (e.g., Dominican, Nicaraguan, Colombian), or other Hispanic origin. The largest of these is the Mexican-American population, which represents at least two-thirds of all Hispanics/Latinos. Hispanics often consume more rice and less pasta and ready-to eat cereals than non-Hispanics. They also are likely to eat less processed meats and more likely to eat beef. They often include more vegetables in their diet, especially tomatoes, and drink more whole milk than low-fat or skim milk, compared to their non-Hispanic white counterparts. Legumes and corn in combination are a good source of protein, and cheese is a frequent ingredient. When working in an area with a large minority population, the interview questions should reflect the cultural practices. Figure 8.6 provides an example of questions that could be asked to a Hispanic client.

East Indians. Staples of the Indian diet include rice, beans, lentils, and bread. Rice is usually served steamed and mixed with flavorings. Indian breads include chapatis, round flatbread made of whole wheat flour; and naan, a bread that uses yeast. India's religious beliefs have also influenced the diet of Indians (e.g. Hindus believe that cows are sacred so they do not eat beef). Chicken or lamb, in moderation, is augmented with vegetables, dried beans, lentils, and split peas. Curry powder, a mixture of spices, is often used to flavor Indian foods. The heart of Indian cooking is the combination of spices that gives each dish its unique flavor. Indian cuisine has become increasingly popular during the first decade of the 21st Century with over 1,200 Indian food products now available in the United States.

Chinese. Vegetables, rice and noodles, fruits, and foods made from soybeans (such as tofu and soy milk) are very important foods in the Chinese-American diet. Plain rice is served at all meals. Sometimes fried rice is served. Pork, poultry, and fish are popular and used in small amounts to flavor the rice. Foods are often seasoned with soy sauce,

Figure 8.5

Examples of Cultural Influences on Food Intake in the United States

GROUP	GRAINS	VEGETABLES	FRUITS	MEAT	DAIRY
Hispanic/Latino	Tortillas (may be made with lard), rice	Cactus, cassava, chayote, jicama, peppers, pinto beans, tomatoes (salsa)	Avocado, bananas, guava, mango, papaya, plantain, citrus fruits	Chorizo (sausage and other processed meat), goat meat, tongue, pork	Goat cheese, goat milk, whole milk
Asian (China, Japan, Korea, Southeast Asia)	Rice noodles	Garlic, ginger, mung beans, sprouts, bamboo shoots, bok choy, cabbage, carrots	Mango, banana, citrus fruit, coconut, pineapple	Small amounts of meat, especially fish; eggs, tofu	Soy milk
Middle Eastern	Couscous, tahini, pita bread, filo dough	Tomatoes, olives, lentils, hummus, grape leaves, eggplant	Dates, figs, citrus fruits	Small amounts of lamb, fish, chicken	Yogurt, feta cheese
East Indian	Rice, whole wheat flat bread (naan)	Red lentils, pigeon peas, legumes, curries	Coconut, watermelon, mango	Many East Indian people are vegetarian, some mutton chicken, fish	Milk, butter, yogurt

Please note that this is not meant to be an exact or comprehensive list of foods. All of these cultures have diets that vary from one region/country to another. Modification of table, Foodservice Management By Design, Chapter 2.

which is high in sodium. (Low-sodium versions can be purchased.) Corn oil, sesame oil, and peanut oil are used. Tea is the main beverage and it is always enjoyed black—without sugar, cream, or milk. Cow's milk and dairy products are not used often. Fruits are important and few sweets are eaten.

Japanese. Some people are surprised to learn that Japanese food is quite different in appearance and taste from Chinese food. While Chinese food is often stir-fried, Japanese food is often simmered, boiled, steamed, or broiled. Also, Japanese foods are not as highly seasoned as Chinese dishes. Sushi, a rice wrapped in seaweed, has become a popular food choice in the Unites States in the past decade. Rice is the staple of many Japanese-American diets, along with a variety of noodles. As in Chinese cooking, soybean products, such as soy sauce, are important. Seafood is generally more popular than meat and poultry. Vegetables, such as watercress and carrots, are an important part of most meals. Tea is the most popular beverage, especially green tea, an excellent source of antioxidants.

Middle Eastern. Foods of choice in a traditional Middle Eastern diet include yogurt, cheeses (such as feta and goat cheese), lamb, poultry, chickpeas, lentils, lemons, eggplant, pine nuts, olives, and olive oil. A Greek specialty is baklava, a baked dessert made with nuts, honey, and filo dough. Common cooking styles are grilling, frying, and stewing.

Culture Change Movement

How many times do Americans get together socially without food? A culture change movement is spreading across the United States that involves many of these cultural contributions. This culture change movement is transforming nursing home care from an institutional setting to a home setting. With the increase in the 'senior' population, nursing care facilities will have to focus on the opportunities to make choices and allow customers to express preferences. As we have seen in this chapter, these choices are fundamental to our basic quality of life.

Regional Trends

Within the United States' unique cultural heritage is the development of regional culinary trends which are often a mix of foods local to that area and ethnic traditions passed down through the generations. For example, the Northeast is known for lobster and maple syrup; in the Southwest, Mexican-style food is popular.

Religious Practices

Religious beliefs, customs, and rituals can have a strong influence on eating habits. Fasting is one practice that many religions observe and the of time one fasts varies with his/her religion and can range from one day to a month. One example is Muslims who observe Ramadan. Ramadan lasts for one month and fasting occurs from sun up to sun down. Think about how this practice might affect Muslim clients in a long-term care facility. The following information explains several religious beliefs and food laws.

Jewish Dietary Laws

The Jewish dietary laws are called kashrut or keeping **kosher**. Some Jews follow all the Jewish dietary laws all the time; others follow the laws not at all or to varying degrees, perhaps only on special holidays. The word kosher means clean or pure, proper, or in agreement with religious dietary laws. Basic concepts include the following:

- Pig and pork products are not kosher so they are not eaten. Also, birds of prey are not kosher (this includes wild chickens and turkey). Domestic chicken, turkey, goose, pheasant, and duck are fine.
- According to Jewish dietary laws, only fish that have fins and scales are considered kosher. All finfish are acceptable, but shellfish, crustaceans, and fish-like mammals are not allowed. This includes shrimp, lobster, oysters, clams, scallops, crab, catfish, shark, and frog. Fish do not have to be koshered like meats and poultry.
- Meat and meat products may not be cooked or served with any dairy products. For example, chicken a la king and creamed chipped beef are forbidden unless made with nondairy products. Pots and pans in which meat is cooked and dishes on which meat is served may not be used for dairy products. Separate sets of utensils and dishes are necessary. Dairy products may be eaten from one to six hours after meat is eaten (the amount of time depends upon an individual's traditions).

GLOSSARY

Kosher
Fit, proper, or in agreement with Jewish dietary law

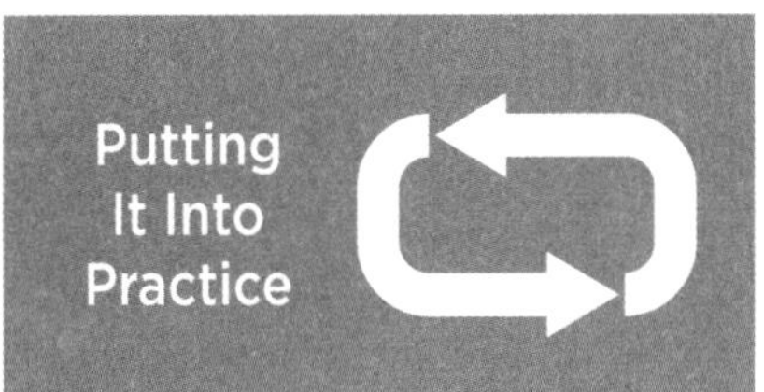

2. List some ways you can provide an inclusive menu to recognize cultural differences in your facility.

- All fruits, vegetables, and starches are considered kosher as well as pareve (meaning neutral), so they can be served with meat or dairy meals. A foodservice operation offering kosher food must be sure that all aspects of the operation are in accordance with kosher dietary laws.

Figure 8.7 is a summary of different Religious Dietary Practices.

Muslim/Islamic Dietary Laws

Five Pillars of Islam

There are five main pillars of the Islamic faith. The first is faith, which is the belief that the purpose of life is to serve God, and that there is only one God: Allah, and Muhammed is His messenger. The second pillar is prayer. Salah are the prayers that are said five times each day: dawn, noon, mid-afternoon, sunset, and nightfall. They are recited facing Mecca, and can be said almost anywhere. Friday is a day of public prayer; Muslims pray in the mosque, a building that is used for public worship. There are no priests in Islam and prayer is usually led by a knowledgeable person chosen by the congregation. The third pillar is zakat, or the giving of alms, which are offerings to the poor, an act of piety. In some Islamic cultures, Muslims are expected to give a substantial amount of their net worth to the poor. Sharing of wealth is an important part of being Muslim. The fourth pillar is fasting or sawm. Fasting is done to fulfill a religious obligation, to earn the pleasure of Allah, to wipe out previous sin, and to appreciate the hunger of the poor and their needs. The fifth pillar is a pilgrimage to Mecca or hajj. This is a requirement of those who are physically and financially able. Pilgrims to Mecca wear seamless white garments, go without head coverings or shoes, abstain from shaving or having their hair cut, and avoid harming any living thing—animal or vegetable.

Dietary Laws

In Islam, eating is considered to be a manner of worship. Self-indulgence is not permitted, eating for survival and good health is. The customary rule is to eat to about two-thirds of capacity, and share the rest of the food with others. Food is never wasted or thrown away. The hands and mouth are always washed before and after meals. If utensils are not used for eating, a person would only use their right hand because the left hand is considered unclean.

In the Islamic culture, permitted foods are called **halal**, or lawful. Meat must be slaughtered in a specific manner for it to be considered halal. This involves slitting the throat and allowing the blood to drain completely from the animal. The person that kills the animal must recite this phrase, "In the name of God, God is great." Unlawful or prohibited foods are called **haram**. Foods considered haram include swine, four-footed animals that catch their prey with their mouths, and birds of prey. Also, improperly slaughtered animals are haram.

GLOSSARY

Halal
Foods permitted in the Islamic culture

Haram
Unlawful or prohibited foods in the Islamic culture

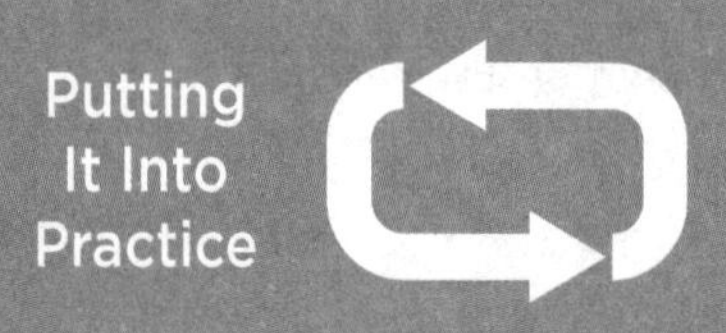

3. What are some adjustments to your menu that should be made to accommodate a person who practices the Seventh Day Adventist faith?

Figure 8.7
Religious Dietary Practices

RELIGION	DIETARY PRACTICE OR LAWS	UNDERLYING PRINCIPLE
Buddhism	Avoid animal products, sometimes even fish; many Buddhists are vegetarians; fasting practiced by monks.	Like many other religions, plant foods or foods of the earth are considered most wholesome.
Eastern Orthodox Christianity	Restrictions on meat and fish during fasting, which for the strict Orthodox Christian can be over half of each year.	Fasting, especially on holy days, is part of their faith.
Hinduism	Beef is not eaten. Other meat and fish are restricted or avoided including pork, poultry, and shellfish. Many are strict vegetarians or vegans. They also practice fasting.	The cow is considered a sacred animal so eating beef is forbidden. Dairy products are allowed.
Islam/Muslim	Pork or birds of prey are excluded. Alcohol, coffee, tea, and other stimulants are avoided. Eating for health is important. Fasting is considered to have a cleansing effect.	Following prescribed dietary laws is an important part of their faith.
Judaism U PARVE	Pork and shellfish are excluded. Meat and dairy are not allowed to be served at the same meal. Leavened bread such as yeast bread is also restricted. Fasting promotes spiritual growth.	Following prescribed dietary laws is an important part of their faith.
Mormonism	Strict Mormons avoid alcohol and caffeinated beverages including coffee, tea, and chocolate. Fasting is practiced and plant-based foods are highly encouraged.	Addictive behaviors are believed to cause poor physical and emotional health. Fasting promotes spiritual growth.
Rastafarianism	Foods may only be slightly cooked so meats and canned foods are excluded. Most seafood is restricted.	Foods that are permitted are Biblical based or I-tal, which means slightly cooked.
Roman Catholicism	Red meat is restricted on certain days such as Fridays during Lent. Fasting is practiced by some.	Fasting and food restrictions are observed according to the church calendar.
Seventh-Day Adventist	Pork and most meat and fish are excluded; eating a plant-based diet is prescribed. Low-fat dairy products and eggs are allowed.	Eating and drinking are done to 'honor God' and preserve one's health.

Source: Adapted from www.faqs.org/nutrition/pre-sma/religion-and-dietary-practices.html.

Alcohol and drugs are prohibited, including food prepared with alcohol, such as vanilla extract, unless medically necessary. Muslims are encouraged to refrain from stimulants such as coffee, tea, or other beverages containing caffeine.

Feast and Fast Days

Ramadan is a holy month of fasting, occurring in the ninth month of the Islamic calendar. It is a time of worship to recognize when the Qur'an was first revealed to Muhammad. During Ramadan, Muslims abstain from food, drink, smoking, and sexual activity from dawn until sunset. Food can only be eaten before the sun comes up or after it sets. All Muslims who have reached puberty are required to fast. Exceptions are allowed for pregnant women, nursing mothers, and travelers. Muslims are also encouraged to fast six days during the month following Ramadan.

Feasts are not common because Muslims do not believe in overconsumption. The end of Ramadan is celebrated by a feast called the Festival of Sacrifice. A sheep, cow, or goat is slaughtered and the meat is shared with neighbors and the poor.

Social and Emotional Meanings

Eating has many social and emotional meanings to us. In the heritage of every human culture, a meal is enjoyed with family and friends and is often an event unto itself. Even the food preparation can be a social event complete with rituals and traditions. With today's fast-paced lifestyles, however, more people eat while doing something else—such as while working, driving, or walking. Companionship, though, makes a meal more satisfying. Its importance can be seen when thinking about food and social events. Food is always part of a celebration. Food is part of courtship and dating. People go to restaurants to have fun together. When a visitor comes to your home or place of work, the custom is to offer food or drink. Food is fundamental to hospitality.

GLOSSARY

Comfort Food
Food that imparts a unique sense of emotional well-being, such as chicken soup

Emotionally, foods can represent comfort. Many adults associate particular foods with happy childhood memories, or talk about the favorites that "mom (or dad or another family member) used to make." Food that imparts a unique sense of emotional well-being, like chicken soup, is called a **comfort food**. Which foods provide comfort vary from one person to the next, but some foods have built a reputation for comfort. For some people, mashed potatoes and fried chicken are comfort foods. Other comfort foods may include things like chocolate cake, or grilled cheese sandwiches and cream of tomato soup. Whatever a person associates with good feelings and family routines can become a comfort food.

When someone is not feeling well, physically or emotionally, the value of comfort foods increases. Often, a food that is well tolerated has emotional meaning, too. Chicken noodle soup, for example, not only has some medicinal value for someone suffering from a cold, it may also feel emotionally soothing. Sometimes, food as comfort plays a strong role in an individual's nutrition. Food has such powerful emotional overtones that it can take on its own meaning. Some people eat when they feel lonely, nervous, or stressed.

Social and emotional meanings of food can exert strong influence on the foods each of us choose to eat. Meanings such as these play an important role in dietary care. We all need a comfortable social environment, companionship, and a certain amount of familiar fare to feel satisfied from a meal. In fact, research shows that in a long-term care environment, residents eat better when they are with others and in a relaxed environment.

All of us have biases when working with a diverse client base. If one follows the checklist for good communication skills in Figure 8.2, he/she will be open and engaged with the client. If a client is hostile regarding his diet, you can deflate that hostility by acknowledging their feelings.

Supplementing the Diet History

Once the diet history is complete, gather additional client information from other interdisciplinary team members. Who are the members of the **Interdisciplinary Team (IDT)**? Generally, it is the Director of Nursing; Registered Dietitian Nutritionist and/ or Certified Dietary Manager, Certified Food Protection Professional; Certified Nursing Assistant (CNA); Physical Therapist; Occupational and/or Speech Therapist; Social Worker; client; and/or family members. Information gathered from the client and/or family members is just the beginning. Contact the Physician or primary care clinic of the client if you need information on usual body weight, unless the client is being admitted from home, then the client or family may be a better source. The Occupational or Speech Therapist may know if the client has a swallowing disorder or needs adaptive equipment. The Social Worker can provide information on how the client is adjusting to his or her new environment. Nursing staff may provide information about the amount of food consumed at meals/snacks and information on medicines. It is also important to work with the Pharmacist and the Registered Dietitian Nutritionist regarding food-drug interactions.

GLOSSARY

Interdisciplinary Team (IDT)
Team members that may include the Director of Nursing; Registered Dietitian Nutritionist and/or Certified Dietary Manager, Certified Food Protection Professional;Certified Nursing Assistant; Physical Therapist; Occupational and/ or Speech Therapist; Social Worker; client; and/or family members

Talking with others is one method of gathering additional diet history information and also requires good communication skills. Solid working relationships built on mutual respect are essential. In the course of a work day, a Certified Dietary Manager, Certified Food Protection Professional interacts with many members of the team. This provides an opportunity to ask questions and relate observations. Information communication can play a strong role in client care. However, these interactions must be managed professionally. Team members need to exert care to protect client confidentiality at all times. They need to avoid discussing client needs in public areas.

Each facility has its own policies regarding sharing client information. In addition, it will be critical to know and follow HIPAA guidelines (Health Insurance Portability and Accountability Act). This act requires the provision for security and privacy of client data.

Another way team members share information is through a client's medical record. To gather information from a medical record, first become acquainted with how records are organized in the facility. Most facilities maintain records electronically on a computer system. A typical medical record includes the following components:

- An admission sheet listing patient information, admission date, reason for admission, and names and contact details for family members
- A section for physicians' orders, including diet, medications, tests, and treatments
- A page listing problems
- A section for test results
- A section for progress notes from all disciplines

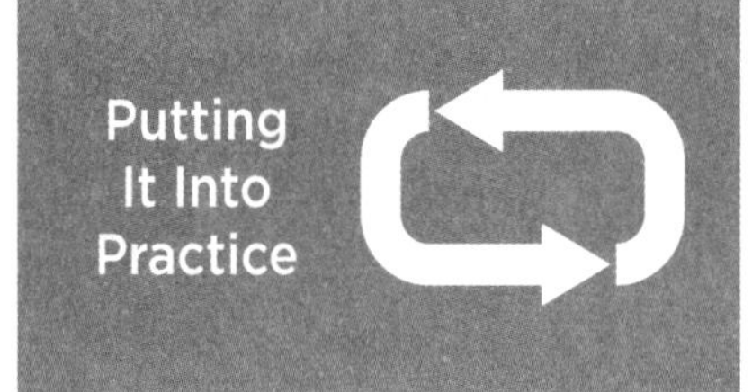

4. Which interdisciplinary team members could you involve if a new client seems to have some memory issues, but also mentions some difficulty swallowing?

Documenting Interview Information

Every time an interview is conducted, it is important to record the information systematically and carefully. Create a note in the medical record per the facility's process. Create paper or electronic food preference information to assist the foodservice staff when preparing trays. Interviewing the client and/or family members is the first step in obtaining nutrition information for the Nutrition Screening and Assessment. Further data collection will be discussed in the next chapter.

Chapter References

RESOURCES	
Centers for Disease Control. Cultural and Diversity Considerations.*	https://www.cdc.gov/tb/education/skillscourse/participant/slidehandouts/day2/Day2_Cultural_and_Diversity_Considerations.pdf
FEMA. IS-242.b: Effective Communication.	https://training.fema.gov/emiweb/is/is242b/visuals/visuals_01.pdf
How to Set & Achieve Your Goals. Smart Goals Guide.*	https://www.smart-goals-guide.com
National Cancer Institute. Diet History Questionnaire II (DHQ II) for U.S. & Canada. National Cancer Institute Division of Cancer Control & Population Science. Updated January 13, 2020.	https://epi.grants.cancer.gov/dhq2/
National Cancer Institute. Diet History Questionnaire II (DHQ II): Diet*Calc Software. National Cancer Institute Division of Cancer Control & Population Science. Updated July 24, 2020.	https://epi.grants.cancer.gov/dhq2/dietcalc/
The Ohio State University Extension*	https://extension.osu.edu/home
Waibel RA. Religion and Dietary Practices. Faqs.org.	http://www.faqs.org/nutrition/Pre-Sma/Religion-and-Dietary-Practices.html

**Accessed March 21, 2020*

Document Nutrition Information in Medical Record

Overview and Objectives

Documenting of nutritional data and using standardized language are critical practices for medical management as well as regulatory compliance. The Certified Dietary Manager®, Certified Foodservice Protection Professional® (CDM®, CFPP®) needs to under- stand the process of gathering and documenting nutrition information in the electronic health record. After completing this chapter, you should be able to:

- Explain the uses of common documents including a diet manual, health record, and an MDS form
- Chart in medical records using appropriate forms and formats
- Translate commonly used abbreviations into medical terms
- Enter and retrieve data using a computer
- Describe the impact of HIPAA regulations on medical documentation
- Use nutrition information
- Complete client forms (eg. nutrition screening, Minimum Data Set [MDS])
- Document relevant nutrition-related information (e.g., laboratory values, BMI, etc.)

In a healthcare environment, it is not enough to provide excellent care. It is also crucial to document all medical care, including nutrition-related care. Documentation serves a number of purposes:

- It provides a standardized reference that caregivers can use on an ongoing basis for providing care. It helps focus details in implementing a plan of care. It also helps compare information over time and track changes in nutrition status.
- It is a primary communication tool with other members of the healthcare team. This is important because effective teamwork is required to achieve high-quality care for any individual.
- Documentation within healthcare facilities is mandated by government funding agencies who require key information about the client, the facility, types of provider, and reason for assessment of the client.
- It lays groundwork for a healthcare facility to receive reimbursement for the services it provides (e.g. from insurance companies and Medicare).
- It is a legal record.
- It is part of quality standards for healthcare facilities.
- It is also a resource for monitoring quality of services.

Documentation has multi-faceted rationale. The need to document care applies not only to CDM, CFPPs, but to all members of the healthcare team. In fact, most care documents are shared by members of the team. It is also apparent that when a CDM, CFPP writes down what is done, it is not only for him/her and other members of the nutrition care team. Much of the documentation will be read and used by other interdisciplinary team members. Thus, following the guidelines that are universally used and understood in the healthcare professions is imperative. Medical documentation is guided by policies and procedures in the facility. While the principles are universal, details about how, where, and what to document vary. Wherever a CDM, CFPP may work, it is an excellent idea to become familiar with all policies and procedures regarding documentation and to follow them closely.

What types of nutrition service records does a CDM, CFPP use and maintain? Among the most common are a diet manual, a health record, a dietary reference card or tray card, and an MDS form (used in long-term care).

Diet Manuals

A **diet manual** specifies therapeutic diets and their application. Usually, a diet manual is used like a reference book. Today, diet manuals such as the Academy of Nutrition and Dietetics Nutrition Care Manual, are available for purchase online. The manual standardizes names for diets. A **diet order** is the diet prescribed by the physician (or other authorized healthcare professional) for an individual client. The diet order is usually documented in the health record and notification sent to the nutrition services team. When a physician orders a diet, standard terminology allows communication among the physician, the nutrition care team, and the entire healthcare team. For example, a physician orders a "diabetic diet." How would this diet order be implemented? There are many dietary interventions for diabetes, so the term "diabetic diet" is not specific enough. But perhaps the facility develops a diet for diabetes centered on MyPlate. Perhaps the diet manual will describe a diet such as "Diabetes MyPlate Diet." The diet manual will outline in detail how each food group is used in developing menus and serving meals. For some diets, the manual may specify foods to be used and foods to omit. In some ways, a diet manual may resemble an expanded

GLOSSARY

Diet Manual
Standardized document that specifies therapeutic diets and their application; each facility will specify the diet manual they intend to use

Diet Order
Diet prescribed by the physician (or other authorized healthcare professional) for an individual client

version of the last chapters in this textbook, minus the background on medical conditions. The diet manual will also give more information about how to dictate an order. A carbohydrate counting diet, for instance, must include a level of carbohydrate or daily goal. It may read: "Carbohydrate Counting—210 grams of carbohydrates per day." This form of control is helpful so that a physician's intent and the actual result coincide.

Most healthcare facilities adopt or adapt a diet manual from an outside source. The Academy of Nutrition and Dietetics, as well as many state and local chapters of dietetic associations, develop diet manuals and offer them in the professional marketplace. Usually, very large healthcare facilities develop their own manuals however, this is a massive undertaking. Whatever the source, as a CDM, CFPP in health care, you will need to identify this standard for diet planning. Deciding on a diet manual and nutrition care specifications is done in communication with physicians, RDNs, and other members of the healthcare team. In a large facility, a formal approval process may be required. In a small facility, the medical director alone may approve the diet manual. A diet manual should be readily available for reference by all caregivers, and should form the basis for the facility's menu planning and meal service. The diet manual also serves as a reference for what information might be used in nutrition education sessions for a client following a specific diet order.

Health Record

A **health record** is a formal, legal account of a client's health and disease, intended to promote continuity of care among healthcare providers. It contains information to:

- Identify the client
- Support the assessment and diagnosis (findings)
- Justify the treatment (test results)
- Document the diagnosis and treatment

A health record may also be called a medical record, medical chart, or a chart. Each facility has its own procedures and guidelines for recording in the health record. As of 2014, long-term care facilities receiving Medicare/Medicaid funds began using an electronic health record.

The CDM, CFPP may still encounter paper medical records in some facilities (private pay nursing homes, assisted living senior centers, adult daycare, etc.). Another reason to maintain paper copies may be to provide nutrition/medical care in case the electronic health record (EHR) system were to "go down."

There are a variety of formats for recording information in the health record. Many facilities use the **problem-oriented medical record (POMR)**. The POMR is a system of collecting data and planning client care that focuses on the client's problems. The POMR promotes standardization and organization of the client record and gives a clear view of the care provider's line of reasoning. Much of the information in a POMR is organized according to problems. The POMR includes:

- Collection of data
  - Information from an interview with client, family, and caregiver
  - Health assessment or physical exam information of the client
  - Results from various laboratory and radiologic tests

GLOSSARY

Health Record
The formal, legal account of a client's health and disease

Problem-Oriented Medical Record (POMR)
A medical record that utilizes a system of collecting data and planning client care focused on a client's problems

- A problem list
  - > Chronologic list of problems that the healthcare team will need to treat
  - > Date of each problem's onset
  - > The action taken
  - > The treatment outcome or resolution
  - > Date of the treatment
- Plans for addressing each problem/progress notes (Nutrition Care Process)
- Evaluation summary including plans for follow-up or referral

GLOSSARY

Progress Note
A notation in the medical record by a health professional

Nutrition Care Process
Method of documenting nutrition data with five steps: Nutrition Assessment, Nutrition Diagnosis, Nutrition Intervention, Monitoring, and Evaluation

The problem list is continually updated. Physicians and professionals from various disciplines (nursing, nutrition, physical therapy, etc.) write progress notes in the chart. A **progress note** summarizes a client's progress related to a specific problem. For example, imagine a client has a problem identified as poor nutrition status (protein and calories). A progress note will review this problem, evaluate the effectiveness of the plan for improving the nutrition status, and state how the condition has changed. Progress notes are written at key intervals during the course of a client's stay or anytime a client's condition changes.

The Academy of Nutrition and Dietetics has implemented the **Nutrition Care Process (NCP)** that impacts documenting nutrition data. The purpose of this process is to standardize the provision of care and standardize the language so that communication among team members is more uniform. This is very advantageous with electronic health records. The Nutrition Care Process has five steps known as ADIME:

1. Nutrition *Assessment*—this step includes nutrition screening
2. Nutrition *Diagnosis*
3. Nutrition *Intervention*
4. *Monitoring*
5. *Evaluation*

The first step, nutrition assessment, consists of five areas:

1. Food/Nutrition-Related History
2. Anthropometric Measurements
3. Biochemical Data, Medical Tests, and Procedures
4. Nutrition-Focused Physical Findings
5. Client History

Nutrition assessment begins after nutrition screening data indicates that the client may benefit from nutrition care. These five areas include information that CDM, CFPPs can collect and document.

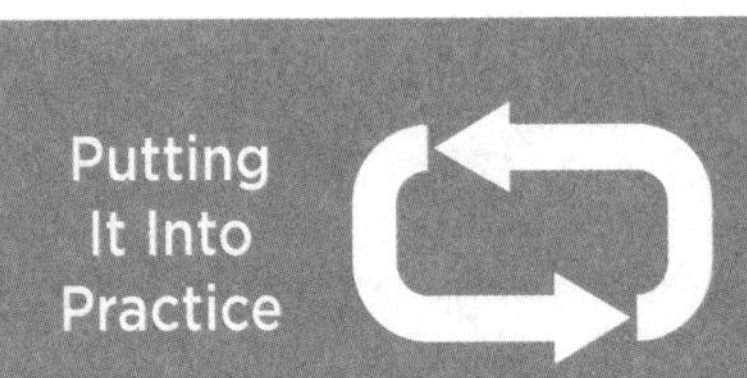

1. In the medical record you notice the patient's blood sugar is high. What type of data is this?

Historically, using the POMR method, notes in the client's chart were structured according to the SOAP format. **SOAP** is an acronym for information types. It stands for: Subjective, Objective, Assessment, and Plan.

- **Subjective:** Data from the client's point of view or as told by the client or family members
- **Objective:** Data that is acquired by inspection, examination, from the laboratory, and radiologic tests
- **Assessment:** Analysis based on the subjective and objective data
- **Plan:** Recommended actions of the caregivers to further information, therapy, education, or counseling

This method, while considered outdated, is still useful as a way to organize nutrition screening data for Step 1 of the Nutrition Care Process. Figure 9.1 gives examples of each type of information in SOAP format.

With the implementation of the electronic health record, most of the documentation is done electronically. It is very important to work with the interdisciplinary team (IDT) at the facility to determine who is going to enter what data in the electronic health record; consistency is essential. Each department may have data to enter under separate tabs. Discuss with the Registered Dietitian Nutritionist what information should be collected and entered into the health record, in accordance with facility policy.

Using the nutrition screening information, the first determination is whether the client is at nutrition risk. Depending upon the process in the facility, a referral may come from nursing. The Registered Dietitian Nutritionist, using the screening information that has been entered, will complete the NCP Assessment Step 1 (Nutrition Assessment). From there, the Registered Dietitian Nutritionist determines the nutrition diagnosis. With the NCP, there are many diagnoses (identified by NCP code number) from which to choose.

The diagnosis should be a specific nutrition-related problem that can be addressed through nutrition intervention. An example of a nutrition diagnosis is N1-5-3. Inadequate Protein Intake. This is not the medical diagnosis, but it is a problem that can be addressed through nutrition intervention. The Registered Dietitian Nutritionist will also write what is called a PES (Problem, Etiology, Signs and Symptoms) statement. The PES is written to describe the nutrition-related "problem," then to identify the probable "related" root cause, and followed with the statement "as evidenced by," which specifies signs and/or symptoms that connect the assessment data to support the diagnosis. For instance, a PES statement for a client in a nursing home who has difficulty feeding himself might read:

- **PES Statement:** Self-feeding difficulty (Problem), related to decreased dexterity (Etiology or cause), as evidenced by inability to feed himself with regular dishes and utensils (Signs and/or Symptoms).

  This type of clear PES statement would lead to how to proceed (our "intervention") and how to follow any progress (Monitoring and Evaluation).
- **Interventions:** Scoop plate, large-handled utensils, spill-proof drinking cups
- **Monitoring & Evaluation:** Meal intake 95 percent

A client may have several PES statements if he/she has several nutritional problems. However, these would generally be prioritized to help determine which problem should be addressed first.

GLOSSARY

SOAP
A structured way of collecting data—stands for subjective, objective, assessment, and plan

Figure 9.1

Nutrition-Related Components of SOAP Data

SUBJECTIVE INFO.	OBJECTIVE INFO.	ASSESSMENT	PLAN
• Eating habits and patterns • Food preferences • Appetite • Reaction/adherence to diet • Problems chewing or swallowing • Food allergies • Usual weight • Changes in eating habits • Changes in weight • Previous diets and instructions • Habits—activity, sleep, bowel • Use of vitamin/ mineral supplements • Use of medications **Examples:** • *Client reports feeling nauseated and wants less food.* • *Client reports feeling better and is requesting more food.* • *Client reports difficulty swallowing due to sore mouth. Has requested liquids or soft foods only.*	• Height • Actual weight • Ideal body weight • Percent weight change • BMI • Diet order • Pertinent laboratory values • Nutritional needs (calories and protein) • Calorie count or food intake information • Medications (as they pertain to nutrition) • Observed feeding or eating ability • Diet history taken • Diet instruction given **Examples:** • *Client is blind.* • *Diet order: 2 gram low sodium.* • *Client given diet instruction on low-fat diet.*	• Evaluation of weight as it compares to standards and usual past weight • Evaluation of appropriateness of prescribed diet • Evaluation of nutrient and drug interactions • Evaluation of laboratory values • Evaluation of diet history • Evaluation of eating/ feeding ability • Evaluation of client's compliance with diet • Evaluation of any other problems that are nutrition-related **Examples:** • *Client is able to make menu selections consistent with 4 gram sodium diet.* • *Diet history shows client's daily intake of sodium is over 10 grams due to frequent consumption of high sodium foods.* • *Client's low albumin indicates significant malnutrition.*	• Goal weight • Initiate/recommend supplemental feedings • Initiate/recommend vitamin/mineral supplements • Initiate/recommend diet instruction prior to discharge • Initiate/recommend calorie counts (intake records) • Request more laboratory tests • Request daily weights • Referral to other health team members **Examples:** • *Provide liquid, complete nutrition supplement between meals.* • *Design a low fat, low cholesterol diet with client.* • *Start calorie count tomorrow (insert date) A.M.*

Another charting format is the narrative format, in which the caregiver simply writes a narration or description of all relevant data, findings, and care in a logical format. A narrative note should be brief and concise. The narrative format may be what the CDM, CFPP uses in preparation for the Nutrition Care Process. Figure 9.2 shows an electronic narrative chart note that includes a narrative note from both the Certified Dietary Manager and the Registered Dietitian Nutritionist.

No matter which charting format a facility uses, the total content of the chart notes should be very similar; it is helpful if the charting language is standardized. In long-term care facilities, care plans are written separately. The care plan form is used by all disciplines, such as nursing and physical therapy. Writing in the progress notes and the care plan is often the responsibility of the Registered Dietitian Nutritionist. State regulations vary as to who is responsible for writing progress notes and care plans. In some states, the Certified Dietary Manager, CDM, CFPP may update care plans and chart in the medical record. State regulations also vary as to how often the progress notes and care plans must be updated. It may be 30 days, 90 days, or another interval of time. This process may vary with corporate or facility policy. For example, state regulations may say that the CDM, CFPP may complete the Minimum Data Set (MDS) or care plan, but per facility/ corporate policy the CDM, CFPP may not be allowed to do this. It may be that facility policy only allows the RDN or MDS-RN to complete the progress note or care plan.

Charting Standards

There are some standard rules to use in charting, along with specific guidelines for the type of progress notes you should use in your facility. Always sign your entries in the health record and include your credentials. Keep in mind that if you do not document something, it has—for legal and regulatory purposes—not occurred. Figure 9.3 lists some standard rules for keeping good nutrition-related records.

Document to show what information has been reviewed and researched. For example, a note might indicate that you are attempting to obtain the usual weight for a client, but are not being able to do so. Another example might include that the client's medications have been reviewed to see if any of these might be affecting the client's nutrition status. These notations are important to demonstrate that you did not simply forget or overlook important aspects of nutrition care. As a shortcut, healthcare professionals use many abbreviations for medical and clinical terms in medical records. Figure 9.5 lists some common abbreviations. In any facility, accepted standards for abbreviations may vary slightly; it's important to be consistent with what your facility uses. It is also important to remember that the medical record is a legal document that will be read by many people. Maintain professionalism; do not criticize the facility, the client, or others or appear to be assuming a role that the CDM, CFPP is not qualified for in a progress note. For example:

- Client did not receive her lunch tray because nurse forgot to pass it.
- Think this client has diabetes—please check.
- Client is a jerk!

All of these examples are inappropriate and unprofessional to use in progress note charting.

Figure 9.2

Electronic Chart Note in Narrative Format Using Nutrition Care Process Standardized Language

DATE	NARRATIVE
01/19/2021	New Resident Admission
Recorded by the CDM, CFPP	Question was asked of resident: "What did you eat on a typical day prior to admission?" Resident was having a hard time remembering question I was asking him from the past. As to foods he had at home, he stated whatever was around to eat he ate. Updated meal card choices with the resident: Comments from resident regarding facility: Stated he enjoys the food. Also stated he enjoys the activities he has been attending. Explained the guest tray policy to him, happy hours, and monthly birthday parties. Resident has been coming to the dining room for meals. He likes to use clothing protector with meals. Talked about his carbohydrate counting diet. Additional food/nutrition-related information from resident: • Do you have trouble swallowing? *No* • Do you have trouble chewing? *No* • Do you like to drink liquids? *Yes, like juices and milk; states he's not been drinking coffee.* • How would you rate your appetite? *Good* • Do you use/need any assistive devices to help with eating? *Yes, has been using Kennedy cups, large handled utensils, and a scoop plate.* • Did you drink nutritional supplement at home prior to admission? *No*
01/23/2021 Recorded by the IDT	**Dietary Progress Note:** Other purpose: care conference **Family/Resident Visit:** Met with resident, discussed: meals, no trouble eating per resident, food is good and he gets enough to eat. **Assessment:** Same as previous note dated 11/18/20 was 155.5# so weight is stable. Intakes are good. Medications: Lantus Insulin was decreased to 12 units at HS from 20 units D-stix; since insulin change = 70-76 mg/dl in the a.m., 183-261 at noon, 96-320 mg/dl in the afternoon, and 219-279 at HS. Skin condition: B=18 **POC Recommendations:** See Care Plan and CAAs
01/24/2021 Recorded by the RDN	**Dietary Progress Note:** PPS: 14 day: Assessment dates: 11/19/20 - 11/24/20 **Assessment:** Diet Order: carbohydrate counting diet; Supplement: none. Dietary Bowel Aides: None; Chewing/ Swallowing Difficulty: none; Adaptive Eating Devices: Special Utensils: large-handled utensils, Scoop Plate, Other: Kennedy cups; Weights: 11/19/20: 155.6#—no wt change; Usual Body Weight: current wt; Height: 73"; BMI: 20.5—normal; Dining Area: Willow dining room; Medications: include: simvastatin, Dyazide, Lantus, Humalog; Labs: none; D-stix: (11/18-24/20) AM range: 60-92 mg/dl—improved after change in Lantus to 12 units at hs on 11/19/20; noon range: 146-302 mg/dl; supper range: 96-320 mg/dl; hs range: 130-315 mg/dl. Receives Humalog sliding scale at meals and separate Humalog sliding scale at HS. Meal Intake: 95%—18 meals; Self Feeding Ability 7: set up; Fluid: 1080 ml/3 meals; Dehydration Risk: 0, Skin Condition: intact; Braden: 18 Stable nutritionally as evidenced by good meal intake, feeds self with adaptive devices, wt is stable for resident, and skin is intact. Continue to work with blood sugars and insulin orders.
01/24/2021 Recorded by the RDN	**Estimated Needs:** Kcalorie: 1440 x 1.3 = 1873; Protein: 84 grams per day; Fluids: 2100 ml/24 hours. **Goal:** Maintain wt at 155 +/- 5# x three months. Achieve and maintain A1c< or = 7% x three months. **Progress to Goals:** Met goal re: wt; unable to assess A1c— no new orders at this time. Detail Goal Changes: Goal will be retained. **PES Statement:** Problem altered nutrition labs—glucose/A1C Related to: Diabetes, recent CVA Manifested by: elected blood sugar and A1C. **Interventions:** Carb counting diet, insulin as ordered, collaboration with MD re: suggested insulin changes. **Monitoring and Evaluation:** labs/blood sugar—improving.

Thank you to Joan Bahr, MS, RDN, Source: Epione Pavillion, Cuba City, WI and to Cindy Morrissey, CDM, CFPP for sharing nutrition documentation from their long-term care center electronic records for the narrative notes.

Figure 9.3
Rules for Keeping Good Client Records

- Write legibly, spell words correctly, and use spell checking tools.
- Use the color ink your facility requires (usually, this is black).
- Include direct quotes from clients (marked with quotation marks) as appropriate in the Subjective portion of a SOAP note.
- Aside from documenting subjective information obtained from a client, place only objective or factual information (actual numbers, such as height, weight, BMI, etc.) in the medical record. Do not speculate.
- Complete all blocks and spaces on forms.
- Use facility-approved abbreviations; do not invent your own.
- Date all entries accurately.
- Refer to days of the week as dates.
- Do not erase anything. If you need to make a correction, just cross through it with a single line and write "error" with your initials above it.
- Document missed appointments or any other acts of poor compliance.
- Be complimentary in remarks about the client or client's family.
- Record only information that pertains to the client, particularly nutrition-related.
- Use the medical records in a professional manner to help guide your nutrition-related recommendations.
- Be complete and accurate.
- Be as brief as possible. Remember that others have to read your notes, and everyone is busy. Complete sentences are not necessary.
- Make only nutrition-related diagnoses; remember that diagnoses of medical conditions is the physician's role.
- Always sign your entries with your name and your credentials.
- Document all relevant information. If something is not documented, it is presumed it did not occur.

Nutrition Services Records

Nutrition Services Records are maintained by the Nutrition Care Team. These records include any or all of the following: 1) a diet order, 2) a filing system, or 3) diet office software and the tray cards. In a healthcare facility, a designated nutrition services team member receives and reviews the diet order. A diet order is the diet prescribed by the physician for an individual client. This is usually a written order in the medical record. Often, it is the responsibility of a nurse or someone on the nursing staff to notify the nutrition services department of a diet order. Diet orders are most often transmitted via electronic record, perhaps in an internal document called a diet sheet or diet notification, and are sometimes transmitted by phone in what is called a verbal order. Verbal orders from the nursing units should be discouraged, because they do not provide solid documentation. Both nursing and nutrition services need to develop and jointly approve a policy and procedure for communicating and documenting diet order transmission. If policies and procedures permit verbal orders, the name of the person transmitting and receiving the diet order and the time it is received should be documented. Verbal orders should be verified in writing prior to the next meal to confirm accuracy.

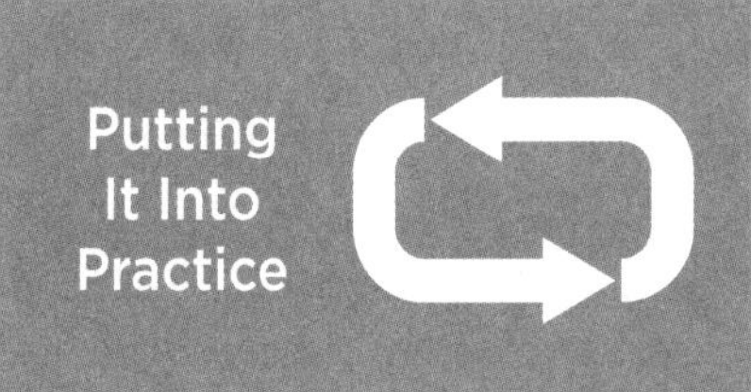

2. A nursing assistant verbally asks you to send lunch to Mr. Brown, a new resident who was admitted that morning. His diet notification was not sent by the nurse yet. In your facility, it is policy that a diet notification be sent to Food Service with all new diet orders. What should you do?

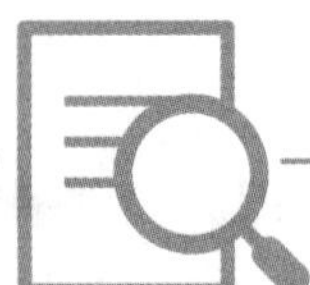

View the Supplemental Material to see Figure 9.4, Sample Dietary Kardex Card.

GLOSSARY

Kardex System
Small portable file system for nutrition information: diet order, food preferences, allergens/intolerances, and other meal information

Tray Cards/Meal Cards
Cards used in tray assembly that indicate preferences and diet-related guidelines for individual client meals

Resident Assessment Instrument (RAI)
Consists of three components and is utilized to assess each client's functional capacity and needs

Minimum Data Set (MDS)
The starting point of the RAI and is a standardized tool for collecting information that is the core of the RAI

Care Area Assessment (CAA)
The second component of the RAI and is used to make decisions about areas suggested by the MDS

RAI Utilization Guidelines
Guidance for when and how to use the RAI, including instructions for completing the RAI and structured frameworks for synthesizing MDS and other clinical information

In almost all healthcare facilities, diet orders are written by the physician, although sometimes the Registered Dietitian Nutritionist can change an order. As explained earlier in this chapter, a physician should order only diets listed in the facility's approved diet manual. In a typical healthcare facility, the diet manual is reviewed and/or updated on a regular basis and approved by the Registered Dietitian Nutritionist and the medical director of the facility.

Now that the diet order has been sent to dietary services, it must be recorded in nutrition services records. The facility may use a computer-based meal management system. Within nutrition services, the staff maintain an internal record of the meal-related information. In many facilities this will be computer-based and automated. A sample of an electronic card appears in Figure 9.4. A **kardex system** (a small, portable file system) may still be used. It may be part of a diet office software, maintained on a computer system. Typically, a computerized format of the Kardex Card lists food preferences, allergies or intolerances, and meal planning patterns used in meal service. It also lists the diet order as copied from the physician's order in the health record. It may also contain other information about the plan of care and relevant clinical data used in monitoring nutrition status. Alternately, some long-term care operations maintain **tray cards** or **meal cards** indicating preferences and diet-related guidelines for individual client meals. Tray cards and menus may be color-coded to indicate a specific diet. The color-coding helps foodservice workers assemble trays quickly, as they can glance ahead at the color and anticipate which foods are needed. Documents such as these exist primarily as a convenience for carrying out meal service. Maintaining a kardex card or tray card does not substitute for formal, legal documentation as required of the entire healthcare team.

Federal Regulations Concerning Nutrition and Documentation in Nursing Facilities

Nursing homes and non-critical access hospital swing beds participating in the Medicare and Medicaid programs must follow federal regulations developed by the Centers for Medicare & Medicaid Services (CMS). Regulations address quality of care. CMS requires certain documentation in a standardized format. Both institutional licensure and reimbursement for services depend on proper documentation. Individual states enforce the regulations, and sometimes adapt them. States also enforce regulations controlling licensure for the facilities. Thus, in any state where you work, you need to become familiar with the standards.

A centerpiece of the CMS regulations is the **Resident Assessment Instrument (RAI)**. This is a specialized form of medical documentation required of every healthcare facility that is receiving funding from Medicare and/or Medicaid. The RAI helps healthcare team members assess and plan high-quality care, and is required above and beyond the medical record that is already being maintained. The RAI includes three basic components: the **Minimum Data Set (MDS)** and **Care Area Assessment (CAA)** process and **RAI Utilization Guidelines**.

Minimum Data Set (MDS)

The MDS is a standardized reporting form used by members of the healthcare team to do an assessment of each resident. MDS 3.0 has been used since 2010 and was intended to "improve reliability, accuracy, and usefulness of the MDS." MDS 3.0 actively engages the client in interviews and conversations. Members of the healthcare team work together to complete the form, which may be maintained on paper or in a computerized system. Regulations require a facility to transmit MDS forms to CMS

Figure 9.5
Common Abbreviations for Medical Records

ABC	Ambulatory/Bed/Chair	**FBS**	Fasting Blood Sugar	**PT**	Physical Therapy
A/C	Alert/Confused	**fl**	Fluid	**pt**	Patient
ac	Before food or meals	**g/c**	Geriatric Chair	**qAM**	Every morning
ADL	Activities of Daily Living	**gd**	Good	**qh**	Every hour
ADR	Adverse Drug Reaction	**GI**	Gastrointestinal	**qid**	Four times a day
ad lib	As desired	**gm**	Gram	**resp**	Respiration
AHD or ASHD	Arteriosclerotic Heart Disease	**GTT**	Glucose Tolerance Test	**Rx**	Treatment
alb	Albumin	**hb/ Hg/ Hgb**	Hemoglobin	$\bar{s}$	without
bid	Two times daily	**HCT**	Hematocrit	**sob**	Shortness of breath
BM	Bowel Movement	**hs***	Bedtime	**stat**	Immediately
BP	Blood Pressure	**V**	Intravenous	**supp**	Suppository
BUN	Blood Urea Nitrogen	**K**	Potassium	**tab**	Tablet
$\bar{c}$	with	**liq**	Liquid	**tid**	Three times a day
CBC	Complete Blood Count	**mg**	Milligram	**Tx**	Treatment
CHF	Congestive Heart Failure	**ml**	Milliliter	**URI**	Upper Respiratory Infection
co, c/o	Complains of	**Na**	Sodium	**UTI**	Urinary Tract Infection
CRF	Chronic Renal Failure	**noc**	At night	**via**	By way of
CV	Cardiovascular	**NPO**	Nothing by Mouth	**WBC**	White Blood Count
Dx	Diagnosis	**OOB**	Out of Bed	**WNL**	Within Normal Limits
ECG, EKG	Electrocardiogram	**OT**	Occupational Therapy	**wt**	Weight
eg	For example	**po**	By Mouth		
et	and	**prn**	As necessary		

on a regular basis. By current regulations, this transmission is an electronic (not paper) process.

The Minimum Data Set (MDS) form outlines a minimum amount of data that caregivers must collect and use. It is designed for use by a number of healthcare professionals as an interdisciplinary care tool. The MDS includes a fact sheet and a full assessment form that is used upon admission and once a year, or more often if there is a significant change in the client's condition. A shortened version of the MDS, called the MDS Quarterly Assessment Form, is filled out every three months. The MDS form collects basic information such as:

- Disease diagnoses
- Health conditions
- Physical and mental functional status
- Sensory and physical impairments
- Nutritional status and requirements

- Special treatments or procedures
- Mental and psychosocial status
- Discharge potential
- Dental condition
- Activities potential
- Drug therapy

The Registered Dietitian Nutritionist or CDM, CFPP may complete Section K, "Oral/Nutritional Status," on the MDS 3.0, and become involved in helping with nutrition-related components in other sections of the MDS form as well. According to regulations, the CDM, CFPP may complete the Minimum Data Set (MDS). Confirm with your facility or corporation who is designated to complete the MDS as some facilities have policies which only allow the RDN or MDS-RN to complete it. A sample page from the MDS form appears in Figure 9.6.

Section K asks for information on the following:

1. Swallowing disorder/Nutritional status
2. Height and weight
3. Weight loss/Weight gain
4. Nutritional approaches
5. Percent intake by artificial route

The client's assessment must be coordinated by a Registered Nurse. Every facility should assign MDS items or portions to a specific health professional such as the Registered Dietitian Nutritionist or CDM, CFPP for Section K.

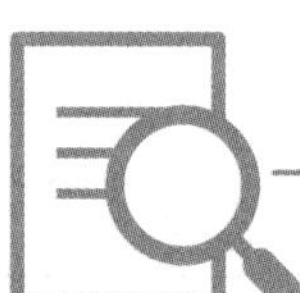

View the Supplemental Material to see Figure 9.10, CMS Guidelines for Completing the MDS—Section K.

Role of the CDM, CFPP in Completing Section K

- To ensure accurately assessed and calculated information
- To communicate with Registered Dietitian Nutritionist and healthcare team
- To facilitate and follow up on recommendations by team (Registered Dietitian Nutritionist and speech, OT, physician, medical director, nursing)
- To participate in the RAI Process, including ongoing evaluation, progress, decline, trends

The intent of this section is to prevent malnutrition and dehydration, and to ensure the appropriate use of feeding tubes. See Supplemental Material for CMS Guidelines for Section K. Note that in CMS forms, "cc" is the standard unit of measure for fluids.

Care Area Assessment (CAA) Process and Care Planning

CAA is the second part of the Resident Assessment Instrument (RAI). The CMS's RAI Version 3.0 Manual, Chapter 4, has a great diagram, shown below in Figure 9.6, that illustrates the RAI process. As can be seen from this figure, the CAA process is the decision-making process. The interdisciplinary team (IDT) reviews the responses to items coded on the MDS, and then interprets and addresses specific care areas to provide additional information that can be used for the care plan. There are 20 areas of care that must be addressed. There are no specific tools or forms for the additional assessment of the triggered areas. Teams are encouraged to use clinical practice guidelines and critical thinking skills. Since the RAI must be completed within 14 days, the CAAs, as part of the RAI, must also be completed and documented within the same 14 days. See Figure 9.9 for the timeline to complete an RAI.

RAI Utilization Guidelines

Utilization Guidelines are instructions concerning when and how to use the RAI. As an example, if the MDS identifies dehydration that is a Care Area Trigger (CAT), further evaluation through the Care Area Assessment (CAA) is warranted. For each CAT, there is "CAT logic" to be used as you review the trigger in the Care Area Assessment process. See Supplemental Material for MDS—Section K for CAT Logic Table. "CAT" logic. Dehydration may have an impact on specific issues, the risk of issues or conditions for the client. As you assess the dehydration, your interdisciplinary team may identify the cause, any risk factors, and the complications associated with dehydration. Once you have completed the Care Area Assessment, you can then decide whether or not to develop a care plan. Not every Care Area Trigger (CAT) needs a care plan, but you must assess every Care Area Trigger.

A significant change is defined as a major change in the client's status that is not self-limiting, has an impact on more than one area of the client's health status, and requires interdisciplinary review or revision of the care plan. Examples include unplanned weight loss of 5 percent or more in 30 days or 10 percent in 180 days; emergence of a pressure ulcer at Stage II or higher (where no ulcers were previously present at Stage II or higher); a need for extensive assistance or total dependence when eating; or a condition in which the resident is judged to be unstable.

Figure 9.6
Overview of the Resident Assessment Instrument (RAI) and Care Area Assessments (CAAs)

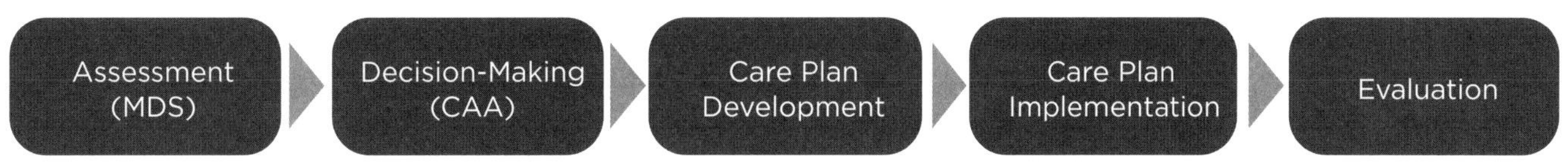
Assessment (MDS)
Decision-Making (CAA)
Care Plan Development
Care Plan Implementation
Evaluation

Source: CMS's RAI Version 3.0 Manual

Figure 9.7
CAA in the Resident Assessment Instrument (RAI)

1. Delirium
2. Cognitive Loss/Dementia
3. Visual Function
4. Communication
5. Activity of Daily Living (ADL) Functional/Rehabilitation Potential
6. Urinary Incontinence and Indwelling Catheter
7. Psychosocial Well-Being
8. Mood State
9. Behavioral Symptoms
10. Activities
11. Falls
12. Nutritional Status
13. Feeding Tubes
14. Dehydration/Fluid Maintenance
15. Dental Care
16. Pressure Ulcer/Injury
17. Psychotropic Drug Use
18. Physical Restraints
19. Pain
20. Return to Community Referral

Source: CMS's RAI Version 3.0 Manual

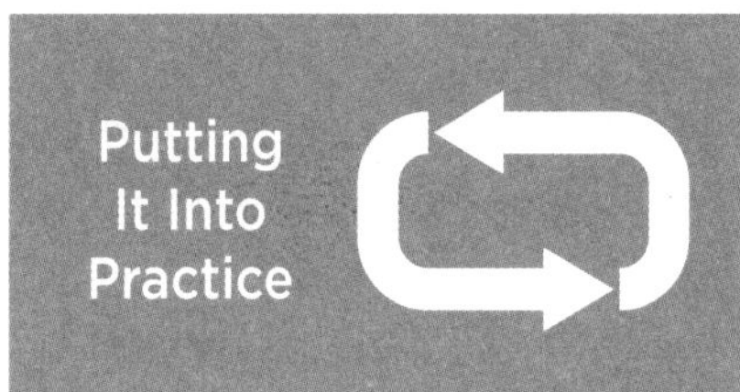

3. A new resident was admitted on a feeding tube with confusion, inability to communicate, and she was unable to walk. The IDT team completes the RAI by the end of the 14 days. By day 20, the resident has made dramatic improvements and she is eating and drinking with good intake, her feeding tube has been removed, and she is alert and oriented. When would you need to complete another RAI?

Figure 9.8
Timeline for Resident Assessment Instrument (RAI)

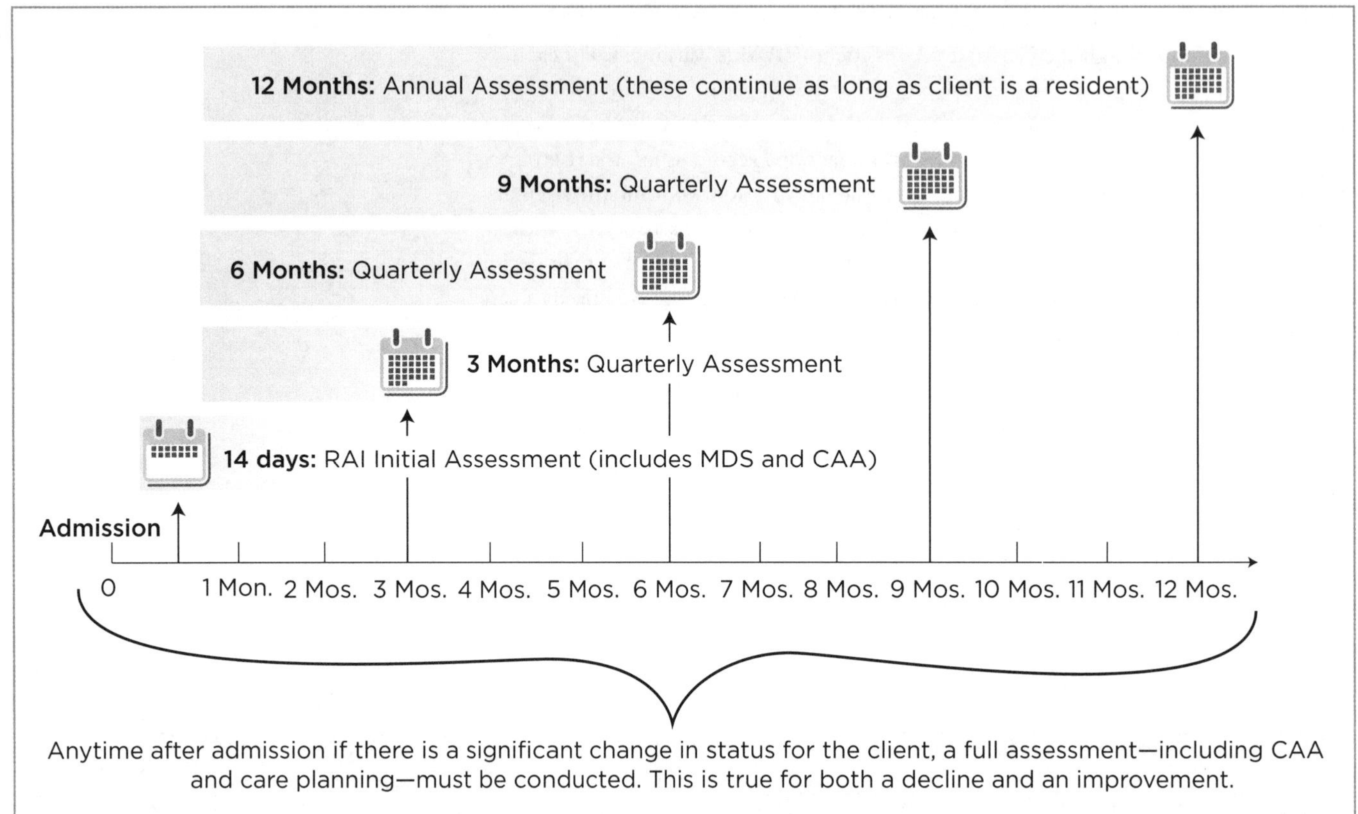

Documentation should support decision-making regarding whether to proceed with a care plan for a triggered CAA and, if so, the type(s) of care plan interventions that are appropriate for a particular client. Documentation may appear anywhere in the clinical record (e.g. progress notes, consults, flowsheets, etc.), as dictated by the charting policies and procedures of your own facility.

For each triggered CAT, indicate whether a new care plan, care plan revision, or continuation of current care plan is necessary to address the problem(s) identified in the assessments. The Care Planning Decision column must be completed within seven days of completing the Resident Assessment Instrument (MDS and CATs).

To summarize, when a CAA is triggered, the Registered Dietitian Nutritionist or CDM, CFPP must participate in an additional assessment using the CAA process. RDN or CDM, CFPP must still document the nature of the condition, risk factors, factors to consider in care planning, referrals, and the reasons to proceed or not proceed with care planning.

Excerpts from the CAA/CATs for Nutritional Status, Feeding Tubes, and Dehydration/Fluid Maintenance appear in Supplemental Material for MDS Section K. This provides key information for healthcare team members.

Several other CATs may require dietary services interventions including the following:

- Cognitive Loss or Dementia. Cognitive loss may put residents at risk for eating problems.
- ADL Function Rehabilitation Potential. A resident may have difficulties feeding himself or herself.

- Mood State. A mood state problem may cause loss of appetite and weight.
- Activities. Offering nutrition supplements can be part of an activity program.
- Dental Care. A client's teeth/dentures affect his or her ability to eat.
- Pressure Ulcer. Pressure ulcers have nutritional implications.
- Psychotropic Drugs. Drugs can decrease appetite or change a client's ability to taste and smell foods.

Assessments on Return Stay/Readmission

If a facility has discharged a client without the expectation that the client would return, then the returning client is considered a new admission (return stay) and would require an initial admission RAI comprehensive assessment within 14 days of admission. This typically occurs when a client bed has not been held while they are out of the facility.

If a client returns to a facility following a temporary absence for hospitalization or therapeutic leave, it is considered a readmission. Facilities are not required to assess a client who is readmitted, unless a significant change in the client's condition has occurred. However, in most situations the event that triggers a hospital stay is a significant change for the client. In most cases, a new assessment is warranted/needed. In these situations, follow the procedures for significant change assessments.

HIPAA

HIPAA stands for **Health Insurance Portability and Accountability Act**, a bill signed into law in 1996, and designed to protect health insurance coverage for workers and their families when they change or lose their jobs.

A new security regulation was added to HIPAA, which took effect in April 2003. This was intended to protect the privacy of healthcare clients, while also standardizing exchange of healthcare information. When working in a healthcare facility, the manner in which medical records and related documents are handled is guided, in part, by HIPAA.

HIPAA dictates that client information and health-related data will be kept secure. "Secure" as defined in the law refers to the key ideas of:

- Patient privacy and the right to keep personal and medical information confidential
- Safeguard information, such as computer files, from physical and technical hazards
- Maintain a computer system that holds clients' nutrition care records, with security features to be sure that access is limited and protected, and be sure the system itself is safely maintained. Here are some examples of how this might be accomplished:
  - Control access to computers by requiring a login with user names and passwords. Do not keep a written record of these (or keep one in a highly secured location).
  - Control availability of user names and passwords, and delete access if, for example, someone leaves employment.

GLOSSARY

Health Insurance Portability and Accountability Act (HIPAA)
Standardizes the exchange of healthcare information and assures client/patient privacy and the right to keep information confidential

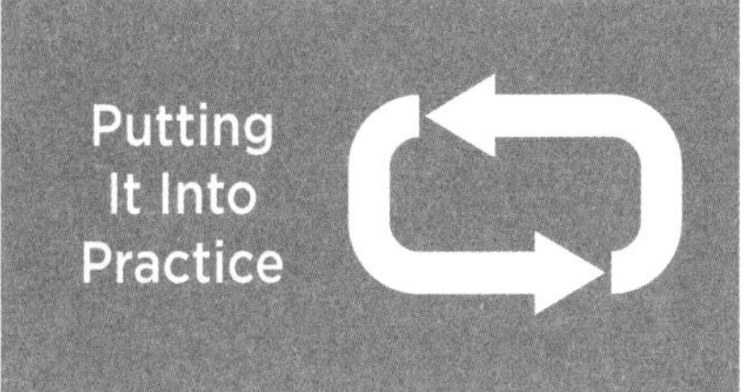

4. You are visiting a newly-admitted resident with dementia. The resident has a visitor who is a close friend of the family. The visitor asks you what type of diet the resident is on because she wants to bring some food in for her. She also wants to know if the resident is going home soon. What do you say?

- If client information is held on laptops, personal digital assistants, phones, or other portable computers, make sure these computers are secured and locked to prevent unauthorized use.
- Maintain routine back-ups of computer data. Use virus and worm protection, as well as other safeguards, to prevent data destruction.
- Check your insurance coverage; some companies will not cover you for a violation.

GLOSSARY

Electronic Health Record (EHR)
One of the methods to adopt the full exchange of healthcare information where all records are updated and maintained electronically

The Centers for Medicare & Medicaid Services (CMS) had a plan to establish a national **Electronic Health Record (EHR)**. Most facilities have already adopted part of the plan by establishing shared electronic health records. The national plan makes patient information from multiple providers readily available to improve client outcomes and safety. Diet office software that integrates with the EHR will become more fully implemented in the effort to fulfill a national EHR.

On a more general level, every employee of a healthcare facility must adhere to an established policy addressing privacy. Refrain from discussing client information in public areas where others could overhear it. If needing to destroy client records, check your facility's policies and procedures. Most records will need to be shredded. Handle all documents in such a way that individual records, care plans, MDS forms, etc., cannot be seen by others (except authorized members of the healthcare team). For example, do not lay a printout with patient names and diagnoses on a chair while chatting with a patient and a family member.

Another fundamental HIPAA concept is called chain of trust. Healthcare facilities and related organizations have to exchange data in order to accomplish many tasks, such as insurance reimbursement. An organization must establish a chain of trust with others, meaning that it transmits data only to other organizations that have committed to following HIPAA regulations.

To develop a plan for complying with HIPAA, first examine where security of information is vulnerable. Then, develop procedures for protecting information at each of these points. HIPAA compliance strategies and policies are evolving rapidly. All employees in a healthcare facility will want to become familiar with HIPAA-related policies and procedures and follow them carefully. You may be called upon to help develop policies and procedures related to records in the foodservice department. Any time there is a change in the way health information is handled, re-evaluation and possible revision of HIPAA policies and procedures may be needed.

Summary

Standardized documentation of nutritional data is a critical practice for medical management as well as regulatory compliance. The information and strategies presented here provide the tools to help the Certified Dietary Manager, Certified Food Protection Professional understand and implement the processes involved.

Chapter References

RESOURCES	
ANFP Practice Standard: Documenting in the Medical Record. Certifying Board for Dietary Managers (CBDM).*	https://www.cbdmonline.org/cdm-resources/practice-standards/competency-area-1-nutrition/documenting-in-the-medical-record
CDM, CFPP Scope of Practice. Certifying Board for Dietary Managers (CBDM)	https://www.cbdmonline.org/cdm-resources/cdm-cfpp-scope-of-practice
HIPAA - United States Department of Health and Human Services. HHS Office of the Secretary,Office for Civil Rights, Ocr. HIPAA for Professionals.* Published June 16, 2017.	https://www.hhs.gov/hipaa/for-professionals/index.html
MDS 3.0 Centers for Medicare & Medicaid Services (CMS) MDS 3.0 RAI Manual. Accessed March 30, 2020.	https://downloads.cms.gov/files/MDS-30-RAI-Manual-v115-October-2017.pdf
MDS 3.0 Centers for Medicare & Medicaid Services (CMS) MDS 3.0 Training.*	https://www.cms.gov/Medicare/Quality-Initiatives-Patient-Assessment-Instruments/NursingHomeQualityInits/NHQIMDS30TrainingMaterials

*Accessed March 27, 2020.

Identify Nutrition Problems and Client Rights

Overview and Objectives

As a prospective Certified Dietary Manager®, Certified Food Protection Professional® (CDM®, CFPP®), you should see a pattern emerging with these chapters. You have interviewed clients, conducted screening, utilized the nutrient intake information, and now you are going to identify clients who might need nutrition interventions and honor client rights in the process. After completing this chapter, you should be able to:

- Explain the role of the CDM, CFPP in identifying nutrition problems and client rights
- Classify the types of information that are relevant to nutrition care
- Verify information to ensure accuracy
- Explain the rationale for reviewing medications
- Compare nutrient intake to nutrient standards
- Review documentation for nutrition care follow-up
- Honor client rights while providing nutrition care
- Identify significant nutrition-related laboratory values

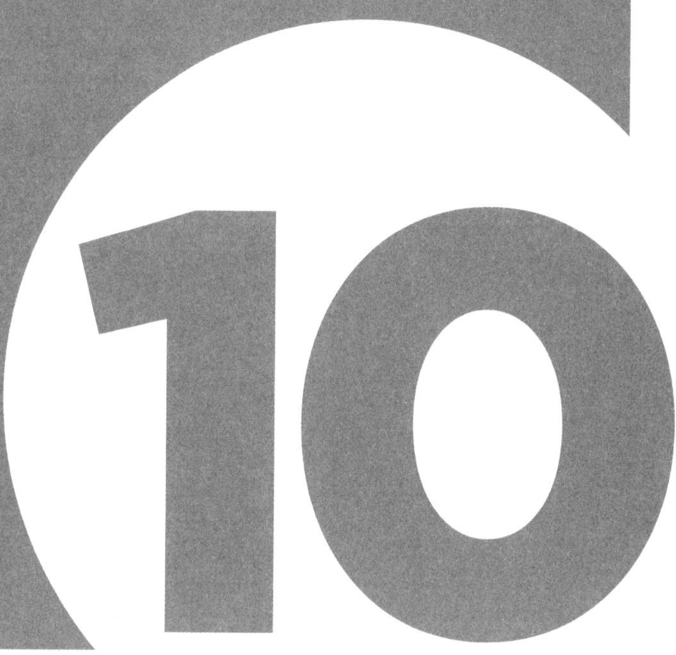

These past few chapters have focused on some of the clinical responsibilities of a CDM, CFPP. Clinical nutrition tasks that may appear in a CDM, CFPP's job description include: obtaining a diet history, performing nutrition screening, reviewing medical records for information relevant to nutrition, calculating nutrient intake, documenting nutrition care, planning individualized menus according to diet orders, counseling clients about basic dietary restrictions, and communicating with the client and the healthcare team. In many long-term care facilities, a CDM, CFPP attends to nutrition-related needs on a daily basis, while a part-time or consulting Registered Dietitian Nutritionist provides intermittent assessment and planning. The CDM, CFPP will be the first to identify nutrition problems and may be responsible for bringing them to the attention of others. Providing clinical nutrition care requires an understanding of what information to look for and using that information to identify potential problems.

Nutrition-Related Information

Nutrition-related information may take the form of anthropometric measurements, biochemical tests, clinical information, and diet histories. Sources for this information include the medical record, direct observations and interviews, nutrition care documents, and communications with the healthcare team. Let's examine the process of gathering information from these sources to identify nutrition problems.

Health Record

The health record contains the formal documentation of all aspects of care for each individual client. Members of the healthcare team, including the CDM, CFPP, record their activities here. It is the communication tool that allows everyone on the healthcare team to provide continuity of care. The record contains all orders written by the physician, including diet orders. The health record is the first document a CDM, CFPP will review in performing nutrition screening. Pertinent data includes a report of laboratory tests and the medical history forms completed by the physician, the nurse and other team members, including the Registered Dietitian Nutritionist. Be alert to overlaps in these records with some of the pertinent questions for a diet history. For example, a nurse may note the client's concerns with eating and previous diet patterns. Height and weight are usually in the medical history and/or the nursing intake notes, and weight must be measured (not just estimated or copied) using standardized procedures. How the record is organized is somewhat unique to each facility. However, the job of the CDM, CFPP is to become familiar with the health record and use it as a resource for gathering information on an ongoing basis. Remember that it is a legal document so record information legibly in black ink. All changes must be visible with a modified message. Do not use liquid white-outs, instead draw a single line across the information to be modified and write above this line with a new message. It must contain enough evidence to justify the progress and care of the client. Also note that electronic medical records are becoming more often used, which will replace the paper record. Figure 10.1 summarizes information to check in the health record.

Direct observation and interviews. The best way to understand and relate to clients, including their nutrition-related needs and their progress, is to visit with them and observe them. It is a good idea to observe and visit with them at meal times, as much as possible. It is important to make contact several times. The first contact should be a simple meal observation. The second contact should be a visit with the client to discuss meals, eating habits, and the client's food preferences. In the third contact, it will be important to include family in the discussion about how the client was doing prior to being admitted to the facility, as well as the family's wishes for the client.

Figure 10.1
Nutrition-Related Information in the Health Record

- Diet order
- Diagnosis
- Medical history
- Social history
- Laboratory tests
- Height and weight
- Laboratory values
- List of medications
- Care plan
- Physician orders
- Progress notes
- Nursing intake notes
- Nursing notes
- MDS form
- Speech therapy, physical therapy, occupational therapy notes

In these contacts, what should the CDM, CFPP be looking for to learn about the client?

- Focus on Food. What is the client eating; how much; what foods are they avoiding, enjoying; is the client chewing and swallowing without any problems?
- Focus on Fluid. How much is the client drinking; any coughing, drooling, or choking occurring? Is the amount of fluid affecting how much the client is eating?
- Focus on Feeding Issues. Is the client able to initiate eating; can the client position him/herself for a meal; can the client open/handle food packages; can the client use utensils? Does the client need adaptive utensils, bowls, etc.?

If a client does not consume 75 percent or more of food for two out of three days, or does not consume all/almost all of the fluids for two out of three days, there is cause for concern. When a visual observation of intake suggests a problem, the next step is often a calorie count, and review with the healthcare team.

A visit with clients at meals or at other times is a perfect opportunity to ask them if they have any questions or concerns regarding the diet. A client may not understand why bacon is not being offered on his low sodium diet, presenting an opportunity to explain why certain foods are omitted. Another important question to ask the nursing staff and family members is if the client may be consuming other food (not provided by the facility). Family members can be a valuable source of information because they may be bringing food for the client. The CDM, CFPP can explore what foods are brought and why they are being provided. The associated reasons may give insight into a diet order.

When visiting with the client and family it is important to include questions about alcohol consumption in the social history portion of the interview. All alcoholics are at nutritional risk. Alcoholism is a common cause of undernutrition in the United States, even among the elderly population. Alcohol affects digestion of food, absorption, metabolism, transport of nutrients, and excretion. The diet history is often the best way to reveal a history of alcohol issues. Involving and asking the family is important, as many clients may deny use or not recall the alcohol consumed.

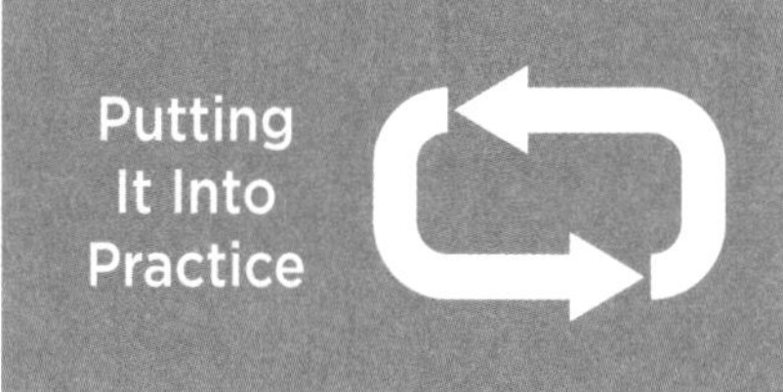

1. A client's diet order would typically be listed in the ____________ section of the medial record.

Nutrition Care Documents

In most facilities, the foodservice department maintains its own detailed documents for managing day-to-day nutrition care. The system varies, but may include a nutrition care plan as part of the electronic health record. Here, the Registered Dietitian Nutritionist; Certified Dietary Manager, Certified Food Protection Professional; Nutrition and Dietetic Technicians, Registered; and other dietary personnel note information that will help with planning and meal management. A diet history may be recorded here. A CDM, CFPP or Registered Dietitian Nutritionist may copy pertinent facts from the medical record to this portion of the medical record. A weight record is important. Each weight should be recorded with a date for ongoing monitoring. If certain laboratory values are being monitored, it would be appropriate to include these in the nutrition care plan. Having a policy and procedure for weight monitoring helps to assure consistency in weight records. See Figure 10.2 for a sample weight monitoring policy.

In addition, weight monitoring may be done using daily, weekly, or monthly weights. Using IBW and %IBW are common ways to track weight change over time.

Meal planning details that appear in a nutrition care document include: the physician's diet order, a list of food likes and dislikes, the diet order (if the client is following a specific diet/menu plan), and any special requests or needs. Foodservice staff use this information when planning individual menus for each meal. In some long-term care facilities, food preferences are recorded on a printed menu for each client or a tray card, which accompanies a tray along a conveyor during tray assembly. In other facilities, nutrition care documents are maintained in a dietary computer system. The menu itself is also a critical nutrition care document. Whether by computer or by hands-on intervention, foodservice staff review menu offerings or nutritionally equivalent alternatives for clients and assure that each meal served meets the diet order and client preferences.

After reviewing weight records and diet histories, the next step is to identify clients who meet the criteria for at-risk weight loss or those who are having obvious problems eating. As was learned from the chapter on nutrition screening, this is the information that the CDM, CFPP would share with the Registered Dietitian Nutritionist, take to the care planning meeting, and/or share with the interdisciplinary team members.

Drug-Nutrient Interactions

A CDM, CFPP needs to devote specific attention to the topic of drug- nutrient interactions. The effects foods and drugs have on each other can determine whether medications do their jobs, and whether the body receives the nutrients it needs. The extent of interaction between foods and drugs depends on many factors: the drug, the dosage, the individual's age, size, and specific medical condition. Adverse interactions occur more likely under the following circumstances:

- Drugs are taken over many years
- Several drugs are taken daily
- Nutrition status is poor

Medications should be taken as prescribed. Some medication should be taken with food, and some should not be taken at mealtime. For example, the presence of food in the stomach and intestines may influence a drug's effectiveness by slowing down or

Figure 10.2
Policy on Weight Monitoring

Policy:
Each resident or patient's weight will be monitored consistently and closely by the interdisciplinary team. All residents with patterned or significant weight change will be assessed by the facility's interdisciplinary team as indicated. Interventions to address nutritional issues will be initiated and incorporated into the resident's care plan and re-evaluated on a timely and periodic basis.

Procedure:

1 Upon admission to the facility, the nursing staff will weigh each resident, establish an accurate weight, and document the weight. The dietetics professional will determine ideal/desired body weight and document in the medical record.

2 Weights are to be taken (by nursing staff) at least monthly, weekly, as ordered by the physician, or as outlined in the nutrition risk protocol. If a patterned or significant weight loss or gain is noted, the resident is to be re-weighed using consistent scale.

3 Scales should be checked routinely for accuracy. Nursing or other designated staff is responsible for reviewing weekly weights, notifying appropriate disciplines of significant changes, initiating corrective actions, and completing documentation.

4 In the event of a patterned or significant unplanned weight loss/gain of at least 5% in 30 days, or 10% in 180 days, the following interventions will be carried out:
   - Notification of attending physician and family member/responsible party by nursing staff.
   - Notification of dietetics professional by nursing staff. The dietetics professional will assess the resident, document the assessment, and make recommendations in the resident's medical record. Orders may be obtained for nutritional supplements or other interventions.
   - Nursing staff will initiate a new MDS if indicated, schedule an interdisciplinary conference, and revise the care plan.
   - The Director of Nursing is responsible for determining the need for initiation or discontinuation of weights other than weekly or ordered by physician.
   - Request lab work if necessary.
   - Nursing will initiate a 3-day calorie count.

5 If the resident's weight significant loss/gain is explainable (i.e., weight reduction program, dialysis, diuretic therapy), then the facility will not be required to complete a new MDS. If the facility does not complete a new MDS, documentation must be entered into the resident's medical record to support this determination, with appropriate revisions made to the resident's care plan.

Source: Nutrition411

speeding up the time it takes the medicine to go through the gastrointestinal tract to the site in the body where it is needed.

Food may also contain substances that can react with certain drugs in ways that make the drugs virtually useless. Alternately, components in foods can enhance the action of certain drugs, sometimes triggering a medical crisis or, in rare instances, even death.

Food-drug interactions can be described in a variety of ways:

- Effects of foods on medications
  > Drug absorption
  > Drug metabolism (breakdown)
  > Drug excretion

- Effects of drugs on nutrients
  - > Nutrient absorption
  - > Nutrient metabolism
  - > Nutrient excretion

Medications can also have side effects that have nutrition complications. Let's take a look at some examples of these drug-nutrient interactions. For a summary of drug-nutrient interactions, see Figure 10.3.

A major way food affects drugs is by impeding absorption of the drug into the bloodstream. A classic interaction is the one between tetracycline (an antibiotic) compounds and dairy products. The calcium in milk, cheese, and yogurt impairs absorption of tetracycline. The solution is to avoid dairy products close to the time of taking tetracycline. Another example is a drug called Fosamax®. It must be taken without food, especially coffee and orange juice. Otherwise, it may not be used by the body.

Excessive consumption of foods high in vitamin K, such as liver and leafy green vegetables, may hinder the effectiveness of anticoagulants. Vitamin K, which promotes clotting of the blood, works in direct opposition to these drugs, which are intended to prevent blood clotting.

Some of the potassium-sparing diuretics (drugs that remove excess water from the body) can interact with large quantities of potassium in the diet. As potassium builds up in the bloodstream, heartbeat can become irregular. Even though high-potassium foods are ordinarily a great idea, a patient taking one of these medications must moderate potassium intake by avoiding excess orange juice, bananas, potatoes, tomatoes, and other high-potassium foods. However, other types of diuretic drugs remove potassium from the body. These are called potassium-wasting diuretics. Clients taking these drugs need to boost potassium intake to help maintain safe blood potassium levels.

Perhaps the most hazardous food-drug interaction is the one between monoamine oxidase inhibitors (MAOI), drugs prescribed for depression and high blood pressure, and tyramine in foods. The reaction can raise blood pressure to dangerous levels, sometimes causing severe headaches, brain hemorrhage and, in extreme cases, death. To prevent a possible reaction, anyone taking MAOI drugs should avoid high tyramine foods. (Note: tyramine is an amino acid found in fermented products like beer, and aged cheese and cured meats like salami, or fish. High tyramine diet is rarely prescribed today.)

Alcohol, which is a drug itself, does not mix well with a wide variety of medications, such as antibiotics; anticoagulants; hypoglycemic drugs, including insulin; antihistamines; high blood pressure drugs; MAOIs; and sedatives. Alcohol combined with antihistamines, tranquilizers, or antidepressants causes excessive drowsiness that can be especially hazardous to someone driving a car, operating machinery, or performing some other task that requires mental alertness. Alcohol can also dissolve coatings on time-released medications. The result is that a medication surges into the bloodstream too quickly.

Just as some foods can affect the way drugs behave in the body, some drugs can affect the way the body uses food. Drugs may act in various ways to impair proper nutrition by hastening excretion of certain nutrients, by hindering absorption of nutrients, or

Figure 10.3
Summary of Drug-Nutrient Interactions

Drugs can alter food intake absorption, metabolism, or excretion by:	**Food** can alter drug absorption, metabolism, or excretion by:
• Changing the acidity of the digestive tract (pH may change to alkaline too) • Changing digestive juices (both quantity [amount] and quality [dilution]) • Altering the movement of the digestive tract • Damaging the lining of the digestive tract • Binding with nutrients • Interfering with the metabolism of vitamins	• Changing the acidity of the digestive tract • Increasing the secretion of digestive juices • Changing the rate of absorption of the drug • Binding with drugs and decrease absorption

SPECIFIC CONCERNS

- Grapefruit with Fosamax®, Statins
- Foods high in vitamin K (leafy greens, cauliflower, broccoli, Brussels sprouts, kale) with Coumadin®
- Folate deficiency with cancer therapy (Methotrexate)
- MAOIs with foods containing tyramine (aged cheese, alcohol, liver, figs, bananas, avocados, soy sauce, fava beans, colas, coffee, chocolate, raisins)
- Alcohol and any medications

WHAT THE CDM, CFPP CAN DO

- Look for long-term drug usage.
- Review drug and diet histories of clients.
- Identify clients who are likely to develop drug-nutrient interactions (e.g. the elderly, those taking multiple medications).
- Reassess nutrition status often for clients who might be at risk.

by interfering with the body's ability to convert nutrients into usable forms. Nutrient depletion of the body occurs gradually, but for those taking drugs over long periods of time, these interactions can lead to deficiencies of certain vitamins and minerals, especially in children, the elderly, those with poor diets, and the chronically ill.

Some drugs inhibit nutrient absorption. Among these are colchicines (drugs prescribed for gout) and mineral oil (an ingredient used in some over-the-counter laxatives). Mineral oil can interfere with absorption of vitamin D, vitamin K, and carotene.

A number of drugs affect specific vitamins and minerals. The antihypertensive drug hydralazine and the antituberculosis drug Isoniazid (INH) can deplete the body's supply of vitamin B6. They can do this by inhibiting production of the enzyme necessary to convert the vitamin into a form the body can use, or by combining with the vitamin to form a compound that is excreted. Similarly, anticonvulsant drugs that are used to control epilepsy can lead to deficiencies of vitamin D and folic acid because they increase the turnover rate of these vitamins in the body.

Quite a few drugs—such as the antibiotic neomycin and oral hypoglycemic agents—can impair absorption of vitamin B12. But because most Americans have good stores of vitamin B12 in their livers, it takes prolonged ingestion of these drugs to cause a deficiency. Anticonvulsant medications, such as dilantin, reduce the body's supplies of vitamin D and folate. To prevent deficiency, clients may need to drink more milk, eat folate-rich foods, and/or take vitamin supplements. Medications and the intake of these foods must be timed appropriately. Drugs readily available without a prescription can also lead to nutrition problems. For example, chronic use of antacids can cause phosphate depletion, a condition that in its milder form produces muscle weakness and in more severe form leads to a vitamin D deficiency. Aspirin can cause vitamin C loss. Modifying the diet to include more foods rich in the vitamins and minerals that may be depleted by certain drugs is preferable to taking vitamin or mineral supplements. In fact, supplements of some vitamins can counter the effectiveness of certain drugs. For a summary, refer back to Figures 7.10 and 7.11 in Chapter 7.

Consult with the Registered Dietitian Nutritionist and the Pharmacist to determine food-drug interactions and the recommendations for nutrition care.

Comparing Nutrient Intake to Standards

Often, a CDM, CFPP needs to use the results of nutrient calculations to identify nutrition problems. The one-day food record for a client has been calculated and analyzed. Does the client's intake meet his/her nutritional needs? The first step in the determination is to select nutrients that need to be reported. Using the same nutrients ordinarily displayed on a Nutrition Facts Label is usually a good start, however it is important to look at a broader range of nutrients and complete a nutritional analysis. A facility often has nutrient analysis software provided. This software can calculate the DRI-RDA for nutrients. For each nutrient, identify the Dietary Reference Intake—Recommended Dietary Allowances (DRI-RDA) for your client's age and gender. Then, calculate total intake as a percentage of the DRI-RDA. To calculate percentage, divide the actual intake of a nutrient by the recommended intake of the nutrient, then remove the decimal point. Following is an example.

Case #1: Mary

Mary consumes 11 mg of iron in one day. Her DRI-RDA is 18 mg of iron. Percentage of DRI-RDA is 11 ÷ 18 = 0.61 or 61 percent. What is her energy intake, estimate energy needs, and then compare intake and energy expenditure.

Is it necessary to have 100 percent of the DRI-RDAs for each nutrient? Not always. Consider Mary again, with the low iron intake for one day. Here are conclusions that cannot be drawn, based on a one-day food record:

- Mary is deficient in iron.
- Mary never eats foods containing iron.

Here is a conclusion that can be drawn:

- Mary's intake of iron for one day was marginal.

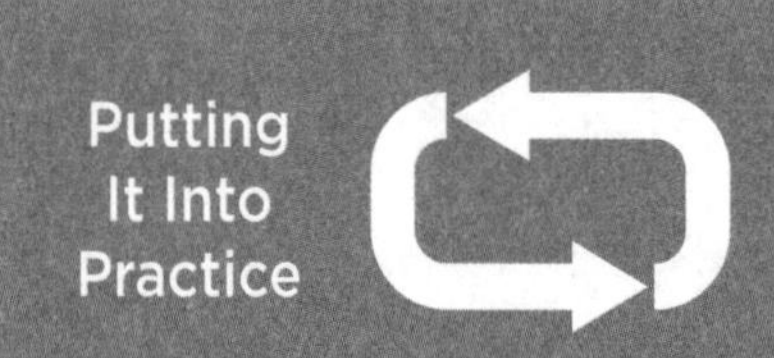

2. Many people take atorvastatin calcium, levothyroxine, and warfarin. List the potential drug-nutrient interactions associated with these drugs.

What's next? Other information that would help in evaluating Mary's iron situation includes:

- Laboratory Data. Serum hemoglobin and hematocrit will help to determine whether Mary actually has iron-deficiency anemia.
- Physician's Diagnosis. Does the physician say Mary has iron-deficiency anemia?
- Diet History. More than a single day, it could be determined to know whether Mary frequently consumes less iron than the DRI-RDA. Check food intakes for other days, calculate an average intake over many days, or instigate a calorie count/food diary to determine intake over time.
- Food Frequency. Use a food frequency questionnaire to examine how often Mary eats iron-rich foods.

In many situations, a comparison with MyPlate is a convenient and meaningful tool for evaluation. The MyPlate Super Tracker will tally the number of servings a client has consumed from each food group and compare these with recommended servings, along with the DRI-RDA data for specific nutrients, as well as a nutrient analysis.

Nutrition Data and Dietary Management

By now, it's clear that a CDM, CFPP needs to consider many factors at once to provide effective dietary care. Let's consider another example.

Case #2: Connie

Connie has Type 2 diabetes and hypertension. What information needs to be reviewed to understand her nutritional care? Here are some pieces of data that will be especially important:

- Blood Sugar Levels. By noting blood sugar levels first thing in the morning (fasting blood sugar), following meals and at bed time, a determination can be made whether Connie's diabetes is under control on a daily basis.
- Hgb Alc Lab Value. Hemoglobin A1c determines blood sugar control over the past three months.
- Medications. Drugs that may affect blood sugar levels such as oral medications, insulin, or sliding scale insulin.
- Blood Pressure Readings. Usually part of the nurse's notes, blood pressure readings over time determine whether Connie's blood pressure is under control.
- Mealtime Observation. Meal observation is critical in determining how well Connie is tolerating, consuming, and following her therapeutic diet.
- Weight, Percent Body Weight, Weight Changes. If Connie happens to be overweight, weight reduction is likely to improve management of both the diabetes and the hypertension. However, weight loss may be an indicator of poorly-controlled diabetes.

If blood sugar or blood pressure consistently run too high, team members may confer to decide on adjustments. Solutions may involve changes in medication and/or diet. It's important to recognize that these are closely intertwined. In addition, decisions are based on an understanding of the unique person receiving care. A physician makes a final decision based on input from team members. What can you offer as a CDM, CFPP? Note how well Connie understands and complies with her diet, and give professional judgment as to how effective a dietary change might be, based on the information collected. For example, if she is not tolerating her diet well, a change in diet order may be recommended by the CDM, CFPP and/or the Registered Dietitian Nutritionist. A physician may also decide to accomplish medical goals more with medications and a change in diet order.

Let's imagine Connie is a resident in a long-term care facility. Since admission six months ago, she has paid careful attention to her diet and has lost 17 pounds. Now, it is documented in her medical record that her blood sugar levels and blood pressure levels are making a gradual decline. In the past few days, she has had two episodes of hypoglycemia (very low blood sugar), and the nurse has given her juice to bring her blood sugar back up to safe levels. This could be a signal that Connie's weight loss has improved her health, and it may be time for an adjustment to her care plan. The reason is that the nutrition-related data that has been reviewed may not represent the whole clinical picture. It's always possible that there are other medical factors at play. The physician is responsible for an actual diagnosis and medical assessment. What is your role as a CDM, CFPP in this situation? Because of the background and expertise to focus on the nutrition-related information, the CDM, CFPP is the prime candidate to point out Connie's weight changes, to highlight a possible relationship between her weight and clinical changes, and alert the Registered Dietitian Nutritionist and other team members. The information provided by the CDM, CFPP may signal a need for further evaluation and possible adjustments to the overall treatment plan. The further evaluation must be completed in cooperation with the Registered Dietitian Nutritionist.

Case #3: Ricky

Let's consider another situation. Ricky is a resident of a long-term care facility and has been bedridden for more than a year. He developed two pressure ulcers (Stage I) several months ago. At the time, it was noted that he was underweight and his serum transferrin level was below normal. The CDM, CFPP and the Registered Dietitian Nutritionist agreed that Ricky was experiencing some protein-calorie malnutrition. He has been following a high-protein, high-calorie diet. What information is most pertinent to understand his nutritional needs today? Here are some ideas:

- Weight. Monitor his weight to see whether it is up, down, or remaining stable.
- Serum Transferrin (or other blood indicator of protein status preferred in your facility). Determine whether his protein status is improving in response to the diet by using serum transferrin.
- Pressure Ulcers. What is the status of the pressure ulcers? Have they improved, remained stable, or advanced to another stage? Determine if any new ulcers have developed.
- Diet Tolerance/Intake. To balance the above information with the overall nutrition care, determine if Ricky is eating his food and tolerating it comfortably and consistently.
- Calorie Count. If observations raise concerns, perform a calorie count to quantify the situation. Compare intake of calories and protein with estimated needs.

All of this information feeds into the ongoing monitoring of Ricky's nutritional status. It becomes critical to identify nutrition problems to assure that his nutritional status is raised and maintained at optimal levels. As has been determined, nutritional status is a major factor in the development and healing of pressure ulcers.

Case #4: Marilyn

Here is one more scenario. Marilyn is a client in a nursing home. She entered in excellent nutritional status, and was in the early stage of Alzheimer's disease. She was also following a diet to manage high blood cholesterol levels. Since her admission, she has experienced an advancement of Alzheimer's and has lost more than 6 percent of her body weight within the past month. Nutrition Services has been monitoring her ongoing nutritional care and may be concerned with:

- Weight. How does Marilyn's actual weight compare with her ideal body weight and usual body weight? Monitoring weight changes and determining percent weight change are key indicators of overall nutritional status.
- Serum Transferrin (or other blood indicator of protein status preferred in your facility). Evaluate protein status and find out whether she is maintaining or losing lean body mass.
- Clinical Information. Determine and evaluate what stage her Alzheimer's disease is in and whether any new symptoms have arisen.
- Diet Tolerance/Intake. Mealtime observation is essential to find out how Marilyn is eating and drinking—and whether the Alzheimer's disease is affecting her food intake. She may be inattentive to meals, or may be exhibiting behaviors that interfere with nutritional intake. Evaluate whether dietary restrictions for high blood cholesterol are affecting her nutrient intake.
- Calorie Count. If meal observations raise concern, perform a calorie count to quantify the situation. Compare her intake of calories and protein with estimated needs.

Notice that Marilyn's blood cholesterol levels are not high on the priority list. This is a matter of clinical judgment. Because of her rapid weight loss, her nutritional status has advanced to the forefront as a nutritional concern. Her protein calorie status takes priority. With a decline or threatened decline in nutritional status, it's much more important to protect her overall and immediate health. Most likely, one of the recommendations for Marilyn will be to liberalize her diet. This will provide more flexibility in offering high-fat foods to provide a diet that is dense in calories. The CDM, CFPP and/or the Registered Dietitian Nutritionist may need to contact team members and the family responsible for Marilyn. They may have historical data about the progression of the disease and the potential for further weight loss. In this case (and others), when weight loss is significant, the Certified Dietary Manager should refer and consult with the Registered Dietitian Nutritionist.

Each facility may have its own policies, regulatory concerns, and standards that influence a CDM, CFPP's actions in providing nutrition care. Some standards of practice or standards of quality management actually dictate what information will be reviewed in monitoring clinical conditions. Regulations addressing financial reimbursement to the facility may require specific monitoring and documentation. Concerns for clients' rights will affect how strong a role a client plays in making

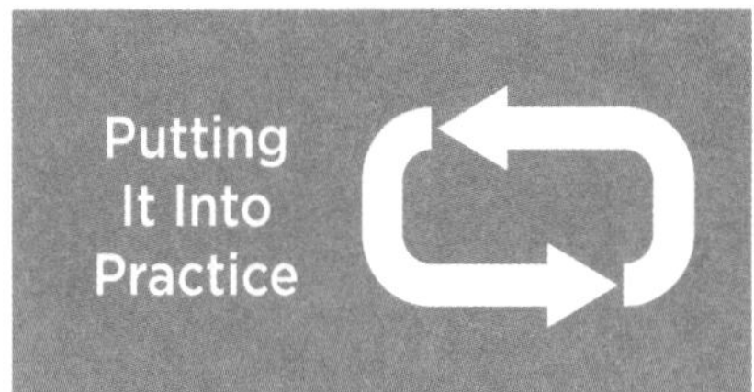

3. Explain why Ricky could be having protein-calorie malnutrition despite being ordered a high-protein, high-calorie diet.

decisions about his or her own care. An institutional policy and/or regulatory requirement may identify the role of the CDM, CFPP differently in various locales.

Honor Client's Rights While Providing Nutrition Care

HIPAA is the federal law intended to protect the privacy of healthcare clients. Besides HIPAA regulations, nursing home clients have patient rights and certain protections under the law. The nursing home must list and give all new clients a copy of these rights. Examples of these rights are in Figure 10.4. When interviewing clients, recording information from the medical record, and calculating nutritional intake, it is important to consider both HIPAA and Resident Rights. Here are some ways to put those regulations into practice:

- Actively seek dietary information from the clients.
- Liberalize the diet whenever possible to increase consumption.
- Honor and provide choices at meals and snacks.
- When visiting during their meals, get down to eye level with the client, especially if they are hard of hearing.
- Listen to the client and family regarding food choices, feeding techniques, and requests.
- When observing during their meals, keep some distance away so the client doesn't feel uncomfortable with someone standing over them while they are eating.
- Try to eliminate trays in the dining room to provide a more home-like atmosphere.
- Protect the communication of information about the clients to interdisciplinary team members. Make sure to do so in a way that protects the confidentiality of the information and the dignity of the client.

There will be further discussion of this topic as it pertains to the management of meals, nourishments, and supplements in Chapter 15.

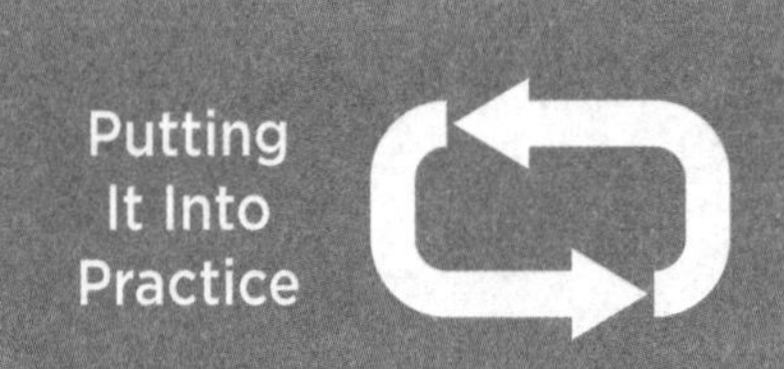

4. William has not been eating much of his meals, and his weight is decreasing undesirably. He mentions he isn't eating as much because the food tastes bland.

   What can be done to help William?

Figure 10.4
Nursing Home Resident Rights

Nursing home residents have certain rights and protections under the law. The nursing home must list and give all new residents a copy of these rights.

These resident rights include, but are not limited to:

- The right to be treated with dignity and respect.
- The right to be informed in writing about services and fees before you enter the nursing home.
- The right to manage your own money or to choose someone else you trust to do this for you.
- The right to privacy, and to keep and use your personal belongings and property as long as it doesn't interfere with the rights, health, or safety of others.
- The right to be informed about your medical condition, medications, and to see your own doctor. You also have the right to refuse medications and treatments.
- The right to have a choice over your schedule (for example, when you get up and go to sleep), your activities, and other preferences that are important to you.
- The right to an environment more like a home that maximizes your comfort and provides you with assistance to be as independent as possible.

Source: https://www.medicare.gov/what-medicare-covers/what-part-a-covers/rights-protections-in-a-nursing-home

Chapter References

RESOURCES

Bellows, L; Moore, R. Nutrient-Drug Interactions and Food—9.361. Colorado State University Extension. Published September 2013.*

Hermann J. Drug-nutrient interactions. Oklahoma State University Extension. Published October 2019.*	https://extension.okstate.edu/fact-sheets/drug-nutrient-interactions.html
Oklahoma Cooperative Extension Service: Drug-Nutrient Interactions	http://pods.dasnr.okstate.edu/docushare/dsweb/Get/Document-2458/
Policy on Weight Monitoring—Nutrition 411.com	http://www.consultant360.com/nutrition411.com
Rights & Protections in a Nursing home. Medicare.gov.*	https://downloads.cms.gov/files/MDS-30-RAI-Manual-v115-October-2017.pdf
Rights & Protections in a Nursing Home. Medicare.gov.*	https://www.medicare.gov/what-medicare-covers/what-part-a-covers/rights-protections-in-a-nursing-home

*Accessed March 21, 2020.

Modify Diet Plans

Overview and Objectives

Food and meal services are just one portion of a Certified Dietary Manager, Certified Food Protection Professional's (CDM®, CFPP®) responsibilities in supporting nutrition care. Planning menus for individuals or groups throughout the life cycle combines many of the concepts that have been learned so far. In specialized cases, a unique set of procedures and service mechanisms are required for nutrition support. A CDM, CFPP needs to understand how these concepts interact and how a diet order becomes a meal that will be consumed. Remember, food does not become nutrition until it is consumed and utilized by the person. After completing this chapter, you should be able to:

- Develop menus
- Implement nutrition plan into meals/foods to be served
- Identify menu planning needs for infants, children, and older adults
- Modify menus to meet fiber needs, texture, or feeding needs
- Identify the food components and their contribution to calorie intake
- Calculate percent of calories from carbohydrate, protein, and fat
- Calculate fluid intake
- Identify sources of nutrition information for determining nutrient intake
- Explain the uses of nutritional analysis software
- Use a Nutrition Facts label to identify nutrient intake
- Modify menus to control for calories, carbohydrates, proteins, fats, vitamins, and minerals
- Modify menus to suit various racial, cultural, and religious differences; and to accommodate medical or other personal condition(s)
- Respect client preferences, needs, and food habits

11

To be successful in helping clients attain good health, it is necessary to do more than provide healthy food. It also means investigating the factors that affect the food intake of those clients. Let's take a closer look at some of the factors that influence what foods are chosen, and how people may feel about the dietary choices they make. These factors include cultural heritage, regional trends, religious practices, social and emotional meanings, availability of food, personal taste, aesthetic influences, attitudes and values, lifestyle, and personal health. Cultural heritage, regional trends, religious practices, social and emotional meanings of food were covered previously in Chapter 8. In addition, it is important to discuss the availability of food, personal taste, and aesthetic influences on food choices before developing menus.

Availability of Food

An important factor that influences food choices is simply what is available. This relates to cash on hand and what food a person can afford to buy. It relates to the ability to go shopping. Someone who cannot go to a grocery store on a regular basis is more likely to rely on canned and dried foods that store well in a cupboard or on frozen foods. Someone who has access to a garden during the growing season may eat a great deal of fresh vegetables.

Availability also relates to local crops. Certain foods are more available in some areas than others. In coastal areas, fresh seafood may be key to the cuisine because it is caught close by. Pineapple is used extensively in Hawaii, because it is fresh and readily available. However, this trend is changing somewhat with the globalization of the United States food supply. Today, American consumers can enjoy food from anywhere in the world. However, affordability (price) may affect choices, and some imported foods may not be as fresh or as economical as local foods.

Another aspect of availability comes into play when an individual is eating away from home, or when "home" is an institution. If someone else is providing meals, the menu dictates what foods are available. Preferred foods may not be options. An individual will then choose something else. Over time, this can significantly change a person's dietary habits and nutrition status. In particular, if preferred foods are not available, some individuals simply will not eat adequately.

Personal Taste

Personal taste is really a combination of biology and preferences that are developed in each person. The biological sense of taste arises from contact of food with the mouth (tongue and soft palate), where taste buds sense five types of tastes—bitter, sweet, sour, salty, and umami (savory).

From the tongue and soft palate, taste sensations transfer to the brain, where they are processed. One misconception is that certain parts of the tongue sense certain tastes—such as the tip of the tongue for sweetness, or the sides of the tongue for saltiness. Actually, this is not true. Experts say that tastes buds can sense all flavors on all areas of the tongue. How the brain interprets these signals and puts them together may vary from one person to another. Taste has its basis in taste genes, which were recently identified.

Along with what the taste buds sense, other factors contribute to our sense of taste. Smell is very important. The aroma of good food enhances taste tremendously. On the other hand, someone suffering from a cold virus and stuffy nose may notice that food doesn't have much flavor. This is because sense of smell is reduced. An unpleasant smell can ruin a meal. Another part of taste is called mouthfeel. This describes how food feels in the mouth as we eat it. Mouthfeel can be crunchy or smooth, creamy or lumpy. This has a strong impact on what we describe as the taste of food.

In general, all people tend to select foods that taste good to them. Preferences vary considerably. Many develop from habit, as well as from individual variations in how we sense the flavors of foods. While cultural influences and food habits are part of the picture, biology is another part.

Aesthetic Influences

Sometimes, for holiday fun, people change the color of food. Think of St. Patrick's Day and green food. Green milkshakes are commonly available at this time. Many people enjoy green shakes because they taste like mint. We think of "green" and "mint" as belonging together. But what happens when we color mashed potatoes or cheese sauce green? These foods may not be appealing. Why? Because they just don't look right. Some people may even associate green in these foods with mold. Clearly, all people have expectations about how food should look. Most of the time, there isn't a thought about these expectations.

The way food is presented or its "visual impact" can be quite powerful. For example, maybe a person really enjoys beef stew. The colorful assortment of shapes and flavors can be very attractive—brown chunks of meat, creamy-white potatoes, orange carrot slices, and light-green celery bits. Now, what happens if that stew was blenderized and put in a cup? Will the same person be able to enjoy the food in the same way? It may now look like a medium brown-colored sludge. The flavors, though, haven't changed. Most will say this doesn't look or sound appealing.

Again, this example demonstrates the need for visual appeal when eating. As it turns out, this example represents a key challenge in providing dietary care. Sometimes, clients are unable to chew or swallow well and need to receive blenderized food. A CDM, CFPP may be called upon to overcome this aesthetic disadvantage when serving pureed food.

In addition, some people will respond strongly to whether foods are mixed together or presented separately. This can be personal choice, but can also have cultural influences. For example, a person raised in traditional Appalachian culture may never have seen a casserole. A person influenced by traditional Japanese culinary practices might expect to see each food separate from others, and may feel uncomfortable with mixed dishes.

Color of food is just one factor in the aesthetic impression food conveys. Presentation is also significant. How food looks on a plate—or in a bowl—influences how we believe it will taste. How is meat sliced? How are fruit pieces cut? Does the food have appealing shapes? What sauces and garnishes are present? What kind of dishware, trays, and table settings provide the backdrop for the meal? The finest chefs give tremendous attention to these details. Much like the first impressions that are formed of people upon meeting, the visual first impressions of meals affect how much they are enjoyed.

Aesthetic Concerns

As previously learned, nutrition is not just a matter of nutrients. Creating menus to meet diet orders alone is not enough. A CDM, CFPP also needs to ensure that menus are planned, served, and are enjoyable, appealing, and satisfying to clients. Ultimately, the appeal of a menu can have a great effect on nutritional well-being of clients. Many therapeutic diet restrictions make this a special challenge. As was discussed above, simply puréeing foods and spooning them into dishes does not make for an appealing meal.

CDM, CFPPs can use a number of approaches to improve the aesthetic value of pureed foods. For example: puree whole entrees (rather than individual components) to provide appealing flavors; form pureed foods into molds; add a thickening agent to pureed foods to form a soufflé; or layer pureed meats, sauces, and noodles to form lasagna. This can be sliced and presented on a plate, offering a more eye-appealing presentation. Add garnishes, gravies, and sauces to make them look pleasing and interesting.

A mechanical soft diet is another meal type in which modified consistency may require attention to look attractive. Some foods appropriate for this diet are easy to handle, such as a tuna noodle casserole or ground beef pie. However, a roast meat that is chopped for a mechanical soft diet may need a sauce, a gravy, and/or a garnish to make it more appealing.

Another diet that presents challenges is a sodium-controlled diet. Anyone who is accustomed to high-sodium foods and table salt may have difficulty adjusting to the blandness of this diet. Once again, it is not enough to simply prepare recipes without salt. For flavor, other seasonings need to take the place of salt. A CDM, CFPP can incorporate seasonings such as herbal blends, spices, lemon juice, low-sodium sauces, and other low-sodium seasonings to improve enjoyment. Garnishes, such as the simple parsley sprig, lemon wedge, or carved vegetable, can cast a very positive impression of food.

All menus should provide variety in color, shapes, and texture (as appropriate) to create a positive presentation on a plate or tray. Theme meals, special events involving food, and the dining environment itself contribute greatly to enjoyment of meals. It is up to a CDM, CFPP to think creatively and apply culinary skills to assure that special diets do not look and feel like deprivation to clients. Instead, all meals should be able to hold their own with respect to aesthetic value.

In any facility, a menu drives every activity in the kitchen and is the fundamental tool for planning diets. The menu is the blueprint or map for what clients will be served. A menu must meet the nutrition needs of each client. It must supply adequate calories, protein, carbohydrate, fat, vitamins, minerals, and fluid. It is up to the Certified Dietary Manager, Certified Food Protection Professional to acknowledge and address the specialized nutrition needs of each client group.

Menu Planning: Respecting Personal Preferences and Cultural Practices

As was discussed in Chapter 8, personal beliefs and preferences, along with religious beliefs, customs and rituals, can have a strong influence on eating habits. Fasting is one practice that some religions observe. The length of time one fasts varies with his/her religion and can range from one day to a month. Restrictions based on dietary practices may need to be accommodated in meal service as previously reviewed in Chapter 8 (Figure 8.7).

As the nutrition screening and assessment reveal information regarding food choices based on religious practices and beliefs, accommodation may be needed in menus. The CDM, CFPP will want to work with the Registered Dietitian Nutritionist to make the appropriate substitution to honor these food choices and practices.

Overall Menu Planning Guidelines

A menu must meet the nutritional needs of the clients, regardless of their growth stage or wellness stage. It must supply adequate calories, protein, carbohydrate, fat, vitamins, minerals, and fluid. There may be specific nutritional standards for meal programs which will be covered later in this chapter. These include:

- The National School Lunch Program and School Breakfast Program
- The Child and Adult Care Food Program (CACFP)
    - Child Care Centers
    - Home Day Cares
    - Senior Feeding Sites (Senior Congregate Feeding Sites and Home-Delivered Meals)
- Correctional Facilities

In most of these settings, as well as in many healthcare facilities, a common standard for nutritional evaluation are the Dietary Reference Intake (DRI) and the Recommended Dietary Allowance (RDA). An analysis of the DRI-RDA is most effective when it spans a period of days. For example, if there is a seven-day cycle menu, the menu can be analyzed for the percent of DRI-RDAs met for key nutrients, including vitamins and minerals, as averaged over seven days. This is a cumbersome task, and is best accomplished with the help of computer software designed for nutrient analysis. DRI-RDAs are designed for application to groups of people. However, DRI-RDA values vary based on age and gender. It is best to select the standards most representative of the group being served.

Another tool that will help you know if your menus comply with the Dietary Guidelines for Americans is MyPlate. There are MyPlate nutrition recommendations for ethnic groups, preschoolers and kids, and older adults. To verify the menu for compliance, simply total the number of servings in each group and compare it with the MyPlate recommendations. With certain therapeutic diets, it is not always possible to meet all nutrition needs. For example, a typical clear liquid diet is lacking in protein and calories, as well as major vitamins and minerals. Unless liquid nutrition supplements are incorporated, a full liquid menu may be inadequate in key nutrients.

Many other factors are involved with the menu planning process. This textbook only addresses the nutrition factors. See the chapter in *Foodservice Management—By Design* that addresses menu planning.

Types of Menus

There are three common types of menus: Cycle, Fixed, and Single-Use. The most common menu planning tool in the institutional setting is called a **cycle menu**. It is a menu that repeats itself over a certain period of time. Different menu cycles may be used for different facilities. For instance, in a hospital, because the client doesn't stay as long as in a long-term care setting, there might be a four, five, six, or seven-day cycle menu. In a long-term care setting or a school food service, a longer cycle menu such as a four, five, or six-week cycle may be better. An odd-week cycle, such as five days or five weeks, often works better so the client doesn't notice that roast turkey is served every fourth day or week.

A **fixed menu** (the menu is the same every day) is often found in restaurants. Some healthcare facilities have adopted the fixed menu and provide room service style dining where the client orders off this menu. A **single-use menu** is a menu planned for a special occasion or a specific day, such as a Mother's Day Brunch or a Chinese New Year. These are often called monotony breakers to help break up the monotony of a cycle menu.

In order to meet the varied needs of clients today, many healthcare facilities are adopting a **selective menu**. This is an adaptation of the cycle menu where clients have the opportunity to make choices or selections in advance of meal service.

GLOSSARY

Cycle Menu
A menu that repeats itself over a certain period of time

Fixed Menu
A menu that offers the same foods every day

Single-Use Menu
A menu designed to be used once, usually for a special occasion

Selective Menu
An adaptation of a cycle menu that allows clients to choose foods in advance of meal service

Menu Options

A selective menu is the way to implement current federal regulations and, more importantly, enhance the quality of life and quality of care for clients. A selective menu provides two or more choices from which the client can choose. For example, a selective menu usually offers at least two choices for an entrée, and multiple choices for most items on the menu. Typically, a selective menu is distributed to clients in advance of the meal (about a day or half a day before service, depending on the system). Clients note their selections, which are retrieved and used in the kitchen as trays or meals are prepared. Computer-based selective menu systems may use handheld computers and/or telephone systems for entry of choices into an automated system. Refer to *Foodservice Management—By Design* for further information.

In healthcare facilities, or in any environment where the foodservice department is responsible for honoring therapeutic diets, it is standard practice to review menu choices before they are served. If clients make choices on a selective menu, a member of the foodservice staff then reviews these choices and compares them to the diet order to ensure compliance with the prescribed order. Common adjustments on selective menus that might need to be made include:

- Portion sizes of products that count as fluid, for a fluid-restricted diet
- Portion sizes of high-carbohydrate foods, for a carbohydrate counting diet
- Consistency of foods and liquids, for specific dysphagia diets
- Special adjustments for diets with multiple restrictions
- Adjustments to incorporate a standing order, such as the addition of a liquid nutrition supplement to meals

What happens if the client does not request enough food on a selective menu? What if the client selects food that is not on his/her diet? Foodservice staff should be trained to address a client's diet when the foodservice staff drops off the menu. (E.g. "Good morning, Mrs. Smith. I know that you are on a sodium-restricted diet. Here are your menu selections for today.") This helps remind the client of his/her diet and sets the stage for the menu choices. If they see that the client has not selected very much food, the foodservice staff might say, "Oh, Mrs. Smith, our roast chicken is very tender and moist today. May I add that to your selection?"

On a selective menu, there may also be items a client writes in as a special request. How this is handled depends on the facility policy. In general, health facilities attempt to honor write-in requests if they are practical. Many facilities develop a standardized list of write-in options to provide greater choice for clients.

A nonselective menu is one in which clients do not have the opportunity to make choices for main dishes. Instead, they receive a standard, predefined menu. This is more common in a group dining experience, such as a nursing home or assisted living facility. Even with a nonselective menu, the focus should still be on the clients and honoring their individualized food preferences with appropriate substitutions. It is important to work with the medical staff to implement more liberalized diets so that all clients receive the general diet except for when texture modifications are necessary.

In a nonselective menu system, it is also important to review and modify standard menu choices to accommodate specific diet orders. If the facility has implemented a liberalized diet, there may be very few diet orders, other than texture modifications. In this case, allowing for individual food preferences is still very important, which may mean substituting a food item. Menu substitutions *must* be of equal nutritional value. For instance, if someone doesn't like cabbage, the substitute should be a food with similar nutrient content, such as broccoli or cauliflower. Since menus are planned to incorporate color, try to replace a food with a similar or additional color. For example, if a client dislikes broccoli, a romaine lettuce salad may be a good substitute. The facility should have a list of approved substitutes for your menu cycle. See Figure 11.1 for general food substitution choices.

Service Options

Restaurant style service is another way of implementing culture change in a nursing home, even with a nonselective menu. The regular cycle menu entrée can be the daily special with an option of sandwiches, grilled items, vegetables, and salads. Restaurant style dining might include the following:

- Foodservice staff waiting on tables
- Food ordered and delivered in courses
- Food plated in the dining room
- Specials such as sandwiches, salads, or desserts offered tableside from a cart

Buffet Style Service

Buffet style service is offered in some long-term care facilities to improve the dining experience. Be prepared to provide extra help for clients who are not able to serve themselves. Buffet style service offers the same number of choices as restaurant style service, only clients serve themselves. Establish procedures and provide adequate staffing to assist with person-centered dining.

Menu Planning Throughout the Lifecycle

Menu planning is different depending on the lifecycle stage of a person or population. The next section of this chapter will discuss the different menu planning considerations for pregnancy, infancy/toddler, preschool, children and adolescents, and the aging population/elderly.

Figure 11.1
Examples of Food Substitutions

FOOD ITEM	FOOD CHOICES	VITAMIN A CONTENT (per 1/2 cup serving) IU	VITAMIN C CONTENT (per 1/2 cup serving) mg
Dark Green Vegetables	Asparagus, boiled	905	7
	Broccoli, frozen, boiled	1208	50
	Brussels sprouts, frozen, boiled	1435	70
	Green beans, canned	54	8
	Green peppers, boiled	194	28
	Kale (use in soups)	8853	265
	Mixed vegetables, frozen	1944	1.5
	Pea pods, boiled	532	17
	Peas, frozen, boiled	824	38
	Romaine lettuce, 1 cup	2098	1
Bright Orange Vegetables	Carrots, frozen	9094	1.6
	Sweet potatoes, boiled, mashed	1444	8
	Winter squash, baked	793	7
White Vegetables	Cabbage, boiled	60	28
	Cauliflower	7	27
	Celery	226	1.5
	Rutabaga	1.5	16
	Turnips	0	10

Source: U.S. Department of Agriculture—National Nutrient Database for Standard Reference

Menu Planning for Pregnancy

Although many CDM, CFPPs work with an aging population, others may be employed in various maternal and child health programs such as the Special Supplemental Nutrition Program for Women, Infants, and Children (WIC), which is a federal assistance program of the Food and Nutrition Service (FNS) of the U.S. Department of Agriculture. Nutrition needs of these populations are unique.

It is recommended that all women planning to become pregnant consider a visit with the healthcare provider to discuss preconception planning. Preconception planning often includes the use of a prenatal vitamin, as well as potential behavior, dietary, and lifestyle modifications. The goal for all pregnancies, whether planned or unplanned, is to work towards optimal nutrition.

Current recommendations for weight gain during pregnancy are based on pre-pregnancy weight and BMI, as well as individualized factors related to the health of mom and infant. See Figure 11.2 for suggested weight gain amounts from the National Institute of Child Health and Human Development.

Optimal weight gain supports healthy outcomes for both mother and infant. Both underweight and overweight women may be at increased risk for pregnancy-related

Figure 11.2
Recommended Weight Gain for Pregnancy

PREGNANCY BMI	RECOMMENDED WEIGHT GAIN RANGES
Underweight: BMI < 18.5	28-40 lbs.
Normal Weight: BMI 18.5-24.9	25-35 lbs.
Overweight: BMI 25-29.9	15-25 lbs.
Obese: BMI ≥ 30	11-20 lbs.

Source: National Institute of Child Health and Human Development. 2013. Recent NICHD Research Reveals that Gaining More Than the Recommended Weight During Pregnancy Increases the Risk for Complications

complications. Most women should gain one to four pounds total during the first trimester, and approximately two to four pounds per month during the second and third trimesters.

The developing infant is called a fetus. The placenta is a new organ that develops in the first month of pregnancy and provides an exchange of nutrients and waste between the fetus and the mother. The amniotic fluid is the fluid surrounding the fetus. This stage of development does require increased amounts of some nutrients. A woman's weight gain is generally distributed as follows:

Fetus .... 6-1/2 to 9 lbs.
Placenta .... 1-1/2 lbs.
Amniotic Fluid .... 2 lbs.
Increase in Size of Uterus, Breasts, and Blood Volume .... 9 lbs.
Pounds, Fat. .... 2-8 lbs.

Energy, Protein, and Fat

Energy needs increase during pregnancy, but pregnancy is not really the time to "eat for two." During the second and third trimesters, women should eat an additional 300 calories per day, based on weight gain/loss goals. It is important to encourage women to consume nutrient-rich foods. Protein needs should be assessed, as the RDA increases from non-pregnant needs plus 10-15 grams per day. A woman who follows a vegetarian diet or eats limited meat and dairy products may need to increase protein variety in the diet. Fats are important for infant brain and eye development. Encourage women to consume up to 25-35% of their total calories from polyunsaturated and monounsaturated fats (salmon, nuts, seeds, avocado, olive and canola oils). Polyunsaturated fats are a source of omega-3 fatty acids.

Minerals of Special Interest

Most micronutrient needs are also higher for pregnant women. Prenatal vitamins are recommended to help supplement nutrition during pregnancy, and a healthcare provider can help determine which vitamins/minerals are best for each woman.

Iron needs increase during pregnancy from 18 mg to 27 mg per day, and may increase much more if diagnosed with anemia. Iron is essential for producing the extra blood volume required to nourish a developing fetus. In addition, the fetus stores the extra iron during development, so that after birth, an infant has adequate iron stores to last about four to six months. Depending on lab values, an additional iron supplement may be necessary.

Calcium is an important mineral throughout one's lifecycle. Adequate calcium intake of 1000-1300 milligrams per day promotes fluid regulation, fetal bone development, and inhibits bone loss in women. If adequate calcium is not present in the diet, additional calcium supplementation may be necessary.

Vitamins of Special Interest

It is recommended that women of childbearing age add at least 400 micrograms of folic acid daily, which can come from foods and/or supplements. Folate is necessary to sustain the growth of new cells and the increase in blood volume during pregnancy. It is critical to have sufficient amounts prior to and during the first trimester to prevent neural tube defects, such as spina bifida. In spina bifida, parts of the spinal cord are not fused together properly, so gaps are present. Because of the importance of folate during pregnancy and the difficulty most women encounter trying to get adequate folate through the diet, the Food and Drug Administration (FDA) has required manufacturers of certain foods to fortify them with folate. Vitamin B12 works with folate to create new cells. Women who are vegans and exclude animal products should consume foods fortified with vitamin B12 or take a vitamin supplement containing vitamin B12.

Both vitamin A and vitamin C needs increase slightly during pregnancy. Women should consume extra servings of fruit and vegetables during pregnancy. Figure 11.3 provides a daily food guide for pregnant and lactating women. The increased demand for some nutrients can be met through a balanced diet of fruits, vegetables, whole grains, lean meats, and low-fat dairy products. A simple approach is to add one extra serving from each food group to account for increased nutrient needs.

Here are some tips to plan menus for pregnant women:

- Offer a varied and balanced selection of nutrient-dense foods. When there is such an increased need for so many nutrients, empty calories are rarely an adequate choice.
- Avoid cold, luncheon (deli) meats. If consumed, heat them to an adequate internal temperature in order to prevent Listeria. Heat deli meats to a temperature of 165 degrees Fahrenheit.
- In addition to traditional meat entrees, provide some entrees based on legumes and/or grains and dairy products.
- Avoid frying foods and using rich sauces.
- Use low-fat milk and milk products.
- Include fruits and vegetables in all areas of the menu, including appetizers, salads, entrees, and desserts.
- Use iodized salt to provide adequate iodine.
- Offer iron-rich foods such as meats, egg yolks, seafood, green leafy vegetables, legumes, dried fruits, and whole grain and enriched breads and cereals.
- Offer foods rich in fiber such as legumes, whole grains, fruits, and vegetables.
- Use folate-fortified breads and cereals.
- Include a variety of fish choices that are lower in mercury such as shrimp, canned light tuna, salmon, or catfish. Offer no more than 6 ounces of albacore tuna weekly; and avoid shark, swordfish, mackerel, and *tilefish* (deep-sea fish) as these are highest in mercury.

Figure 11.3
Daily Food Guide for Pregnancy and Lactation

FOOD GROUP MYPLATE MESSAGE	# OF SERVINGS PER DAY	WHAT COUNTS AS A SERVING?
Protein Food Go lean with protein	5-1/2 - 6-1/2 oz. per day	• 1 egg • 1/4 cup of dried beans or peas* • 1 Tbsp. of nut butter • 1/2 oz. of nuts • 1 oz. of meat, poultry, or seafood
Grains Make half of your grains whole grains	6 - 8 oz. per day	• 1 slice of whole grain bread • 1 oz. of ready-to-eat cereal • 1 oz. roll • 1-6 inch corn or flour tortilla • 1/2 cup cooked pasta, rice, or hot cereal
Dairy Switch to fat-free or low-fat (1%)	3 cups per day	• 1 cup of milk (1% or skim) • 1 cup yogurt (1% or skim) • 1-1/2 oz. of natural cheese • 2 oz. of processed cheese
Fruit Focus on fruits	2 cups per day	• 1 cup of fruit • 1 cup of 100% fruit juice • 1/2 cup dried fruit
Vegetables Vary your veggies	2-1/2 - 3 cups per day	• 1 cup raw vegetables • 1 cup of cooked vegetables • 2 cups of raw leafy vegetables • 1 cup of 100% vegetable juice • 1 cup dried beans or peas*
Oils**	5 - 6 tsp. per day	• Vegetable oil (canola, corn, olive, soybean, sunflower, safflower, and blends) • Margarine, soft • Salad dressing • Nuts and seeds • Other fat-containing foods

Source: Center for Nutrition Policy and Promotion, U.S. Department of Agriculture. Visit www.choosemyplate.gov to create an individualized meal plan for pregnancy and/or lactation.

** Dried beans and peas are unique, in that they can be counted in the vegetable group or the protein group.*

*** Oils are not considered a MyPlate food group, however, they do provide essential nutrients. Therefore, oils are included in USDA Food Patterns.*

- Increase fluid intake when increasing fiber intake.
- Encourage intake of prenatal vitamin as prescribed.

Various medical experts, including the U.S. Surgeon General, advise pregnant women to avoid alcohol during pregnancy. Alcohol can cause fetal alcohol syndrome, which exhibits itself as facial malformations and impaired development in children.

Dieting (or food restriction) during pregnancy is not recommended as it may negatively impact nutrition status. However, certain medical conditions may require a modified diet plan. It has not been shown that caffeine and sugar substitutes adversely affect the fetus, but it is recommended to use these substances in moderation. Furthermore, use of herbal supplements can be especially hazardous during this critical time, as some may interfere with hormonal balance or affect the developing fetus. A pregnant woman considering use of herbal supplements should first seek advice from a qualified health professional.

During pregnancy, several nutrition-related symptoms and complaints are common and may require modifications in menu planning as shown in Figure 11.4.

Breastfeeding/Lactating Women

Breastfeeding or lactating women, much like pregnant women, have higher nutrient needs. Interestingly, many nutrient needs are even higher during lactation than in pregnancy. All breastfeeding and postpartum women are encouraged to continue use of the prenatal vitamin/mineral supplements and maintain proper nutrition. During lactation, women may need 300-500 extra calories per day and hydration needs may increase. Small amounts of caffeine are acceptable. Very little or no alcohol is advised. Review Figure 11.3 for menu planning considerations.

Feeding and Menu Planning for Infants

Infant growth is directly linked to nutrition status. Adequate nutrition is vital to growth and development, especially during the first year, when infants can double their weight in the first four months and can triple their weight by the end of the first year of life.

Weight, length, and head circumference are anthropometrics used to measure infant growth; and the National Center for Health Statistics (NCHS) growth charts are used to monitor the growth patterns.

Infant feeding schedules are based on developmental stages and age progression. Breast milk and iron-fortified formula are recommended for the first year of life.

Figure 11.4
Pregnancy Nutrition-Related Conditions that May Affect Menu Planning

CONDITION	MENU ADJUSTMENT
Nausea and Vomiting *May be due to hormonal changes during pregnancy.*	Dietary advice in the past has concentrated on frequent, small, carbohydrate-rich meals. Recent advice allows women to eat whatever food they think will stay down.
Taste Changes and Cravings *May result from hormonal changes.*	Some women may develop an aversion to certain foods such as meats, strong smelling vegetables, or caffeinated drinks, or they may request salty or sweet foods.
Constipation *The GI tract slows down and begins relaxing during pregnancy.*	Some women may need to increase their fiber and fluid intake.
Indigestion *Is caused by the growing fetus crowding the stomach. The muscle that controls the passage of food into the stomach also relaxes.*	Some women may need small, frequent meals, avoiding caffeine, or not lying down after eating. They may need to sleep with their head elevated.

Breastfeeding

Breastfeeding provides optimal nutrition for infants and is also deemed an important global health initiative for Healthy People 2030. It has been shown that breastfeeding is advantageous and provides emotional and physical benefits. Breastfeeding can promote normal tooth and jaw alignment, decrease risk of ear infections, and may reduce the risk of sudden infant death syndrome (SIDS). In addition, data suggests that breastfeeding may decrease the risk of chronic health problems like obesity and some allergies. Healthcare professionals should provide support, encouragement, and education on breastfeeding during pregnancy and beyond, to dispel myths and barriers to successful breastfeeding. Education should be provided for mothers pumping and storing milk to ensure proper food safety practices.

Formula

Iron-fortified infant formula is an alternative choice for mothers who cannot or choose not to breastfeed.

All formulas must meet nutrient standards set by the Food and Drug Administration (FDA); formulas come in three different forms: ready-to-feed, liquid concentrate, and powdered varieties. Education should be provided on proper mixing, storing, and handling to prevent contamination and foodborne illness. If an infant is allergic to the protein in milk-based commercial formulas or does not tolerate the formula, other variations and specialty formulas are available on the market.

Regardless of infant feeding choice, healthcare professionals should respect the mother's choice for feeding an infant. Hunger and fullness cues, as well as growth spurts, should be discussed for both breastfed and formula fed infants.

Nutrients of Concern

A qualified healthcare professional will assess the need for vitamin and mineral supplementation related to rapid growth, and turnover supplementation is often recommended for some nutrients.

Data confirms many infants may not consume optimal amounts of vitamin D. The American Academy of Pediatrics (AAP) recommends 400 IU of vitamin D for infants beginning in the first few days of life. Oral vitamin D supplementation is suggested for infants who are either breastfed or consuming less than ~34 ounces of formula per day.

Iron stores are generally sufficient for the first 4-6 months of life for full-term infants. Certain pre-term infants or those that are not consuming sufficient iron-rich foods between 4-6 months may benefit from supplementation. Prevention of iron-deficiency anemia is a public health goal related to infant and child nutrition; and while iron-deficiency has improved through the years, it remains a public health nutrition goal for Healthy People 2030.

Supplementation of fluoride may be recommended by the pediatrician or pediatric dentist related to dental health. The American Academy of Pediatrics (AAP), the American Academy of Pediatric Dentistry (AAPD), and the Centers for Disease Control and Prevention (CDC) do not recommend a fluoride supplement for infants less than six months of age. For infants older than six months of age, water sources should be evaluated for over or under consumption of fluoride, and determine if supplementation is necessary.

Complementary Feedings

Between four and six months, many infants are developmentally ready for complementary foods. AAP does suggest delaying solids until six months, but some infants may be ready between four and six months of age. Infant developmental readiness and offering solids should be discussed with a qualified healthcare provider. Solids should not be introduced later than eight months of age.

Signs of developmental readiness:

- Shows good head control and sits in chair with support
- Opens mouth or grabs for food
- Moves food easily from the front to the back of the mouth and swallows

The food guide for infants in Figure 11.5 shows various stages of feeding an infant. The first solid food provided is often infant rice cereal, by spoon, as it is easily digestible. The mixture should be runny at first, and thicker as the infant becomes familiar with foods. Next fruits and vegetables may be added, along with some proteins. New foods should be added to the infant's diet one at a time and with several days between new offerings to monitor for intolerances or allergies. As the infant progresses, different tastes and textures may be added to the diet; and the infant may also become less interested in breast milk or formula. Infants may adjust differently to new tastes and textures, so it may take several introductions before an infant accepts a food. An infant should be seated for all meals and snacks; and also a cup may be introduced at six months with breast milk, formula, or small amounts of water.

Fruit juice is not necessary, and generally not recommended, in the infant diet as it shows no nutritional benefit over fruits and vegetables. If juice is included in the diet, the American Academy of Pediatrics (AAP) suggests that, for children 1-3 years old, it should be limited to four ounces daily. One hundred percent juice should be offered only by cup and can be diluted with water and may be offered during "snacks." In addition, other "sugary drinks and beverages" should not be offered to an infant.

Babies should never be allowed to sleep with a bottle or, at later stages, walk around with the bottle or cup in their mouths to help prevent baby bottle tooth decay. Infant gum and tooth care should be provided by an adult after feedings. Special nutrition considerations may be given when an infant is ill.

Finger Foods

Infants can begin to eat "finger foods" when they are able to crawl, grasp food with fingers, and chew food with their jaws. This developmental stage can occur between eight and 12 months as infant development continues to progress. During this stage, the foods may be chopped and have a thicker texture. Begin family meals between eight and 12 months, and offer infants three meals and three snacks daily.

Foods to Avoid

Several foods should be avoided during the first year. Honey may be contaminated with harmful bacteria and may cause *Clostridium botulinum*, a foodborne illness. In addition, all foods must be prepared, cooked, and stored properly for food safety.

Certain foods may cause choking and should be avoided. Some of these foods include nuts, raisins, hot dogs, popcorn, grapes, tough chunks of meat or cheese, popcorn, peanut butter, or hard candy. AAP recommends educating parents and caregivers on

Figure 11.5
Food Guide for Infants

AGE	FOOD	AMOUNT
Birth-4 Months An infant's stomach is quite small and requires more frequent feedings. On-demand breastfeeding is recommended. Night-time breast and formula feedings are normal and beneficial for infant growth and development. Watch for hunger and fullness cues.	Breast milk or iron-fortified formula	On-demand breastfeeding, 14-42 oz. formula, smaller more frequent feedings daily, varied based upon age and growth spurts.
4-6 Months Infants have growth spurts at various stages and may require more frequent feedings during these times.	Breast milk or iron-fortified formula	Breastfeed 5+ times daily or 26-40 oz. formula over 4-6 feedings daily.
Solids may be offered from a spoon when baby is developmentally ready.	Iron-fortified infant cereal by spoon	Give 1 Tbsp. with breast milk or formula to start (runny consistency), start with rice cereal, work up to 1-2 Tbsp. twice daily.
	Puréed/strained, cooked fruits and vegetables (plain)	Give 1-2 tsp. once or twice daily, slowly increase to 2 Tbsp. twice daily. Caution with home-prepared, high-nitrate vegetables such as carrots and spinach.
6-8 Months Offer foods one at a time and several days between new offerings.	Breast milk or iron-fortified formula	Breastfeed 3-6 times daily, 24-32 oz. formula over 3-5 feedings daily.
Begin offering a cup with breastmilk, formula, and small amounts of water.	Iron-fortified infant cereal	Cereal can be prepared to a thicker consistency.
Juice has no nutritional benefit over fruits and vegetables and is not necessary.	Puréed/strained fruits and vegetables	3 Tbsp. twice daily
If juice is provided, offer only 4 oz. daily in a cup and consider diluting with water.	Puréed/strained proteins, meats, egg yolks, mashed legumes/beans (plain)	1 to 2 Tbsp. twice daily
8-12 Months Begin finger foods and larger pieces of foods, but watch for choking hazards.	Breast milk or iron-fortified formula	Breastfeed 3-5 times daily, 24-32 oz. formula over 3-4 feedings daily.
Continue to offer the cup more often.	Iron-fortified infant cereal	4-6 Tbsp. daily
Baby should be weaned from the bottle by one-year.	Other grains: bread, dry cereal, other finger foods	4-6 Tbsp. daily
Allergens should be discussed with the qualified healthcare provider.	Vegetables: puréed, mashed, cut up (plain)	3-4 Tbsp. daily
No cow's milk should be offered until 12 months.	Fruits: puréed, mashed, cut up (plain)	3-4 Tbsp. daily
Honey should never be offered to an infant due to risk of *Clostridium botulinum*.	Proteins puréed or chopped lean meat, poultry, beans/legumes, yogurt, cheese, egg yolk (plain)	2-3 Tbsp. twice daily

Notes: Every baby develops differently and diet patterns should be individualized. Talk with the healthcare provider regarding specific questions.

Source: U.S. Department of Agriculture

the infant and child choking risks.

Certain foods are known to be potential allergens: milk, eggs, wheat, peanuts, tree nuts, chocolate, shellfish, and soy. AAP reports that some evidence suggests early introduction of "known allergen foods" may make the child less likely to become allergic; but a full family history should be discussed with the healthcare provider to determine when these foods should be introduced to the infant.

Cow's milk is not recommended until age one due to poor digestion, and potentially causing internal bleeding and iron-deficiency anemia. At one year, 16-24 ounces of whole milk may be offered at meals and snacks.

Changing Nutrient Needs for Toddlers and Children

Growth, of course, increases the demand for all nutrients, as does a child's activity level. Protein, calcium, phosphorus, magnesium, and zinc are important, as are other dietary sources of nutrients. Some of the nutrients consumed during childhood will actually be stored and used for upcoming growth spurts. Foods that are not nutrient-rich, such as cookies, candy, and soda, should not be consumed as a regular part of the diet. Children may fill up on these foods leaving less room for healthful options, and high consumption of these foods may contribute to poor nutrition status.

Menu Planning for Preschoolers

Preschoolers exhibit some food-related behaviors that may alarm parents. For example, many toddlers go through food jags, when they want to eat just one food continually. Preschoolers also often pick at foods or refuse to eat vegetables or drink milk. Lack of variety and varying appetites are typical of this age group. These menu planning tips deal with preschoolers' food habits:

- Offer meals and snacks on a regular schedule.
- Offer food in child-friendly portions. For a preschooler, the USDA suggests a typical portion size is about 2/3 of the usual adult portion. An even smaller portion may encourage a child to try a new food.
- Let the child participate in food selection and preparation.
- Make sure the child has appropriately-sized utensils and can reach the table comfortably.
- Offer foods in a variety of ways such as raw, cooked, individually, or mixed.

Several factors make planning a menu for preschoolers challenging. Modified textures and strong tastes and flavors may impact acceptance. Also, mixed dishes may not be accepted. Consider offering a plate with dividers and single foods.

Try to make sure each meal includes:

- One softer food that is easy to chew
- One crisp or chewy food (important for developing chewing skills, but beware of choking hazards)
- One colorful food, like a fruit or vegetable
- Two finger foods

Cook vegetables until they are soft enough to easily cut with a fork and then cut them into smaller pieces. If carrots are served, they should be cooked to just softened and/ or cut into thin slices or "matchsticks." For children who will not eat vegetables, you can also include them in tomato sauce on spaghetti, on pizza, and in chili. Soups, casseroles, and even smoothies are great places to add vegetables. Child development professionals have stated that children need to be offered a new food seven to 10 times before they will attempt to try that food. It may take many more tries until they "like" a food. Use different preparation methods to help them accept new foods.

Most preschoolers prefer carbohydrate-rich foods, including cereals, breads, and crackers, as they are easy to hold and chew; nutritious ones are good to use as snack foods. Cut fruits and vegetables also make good snacks. Allow the child to explore new foods as snacks, and make them fun. Snacks are important to preschoolers because they need to eat more often than adults to get the nutrients they need. They may enjoy smoothies made with yogurt and fresh or frozen fruit. You can even add a few baby carrots when blending smoothies to boost vitamin A. Cottage cheese with fruit is another balanced snack option.

Before the age of four, at which time their skills to chew cut up food start to develop, serve foods in bite-size pieces that are either eaten as finger foods or with utensil. For example, cut meat into strips or use ground meat, cut fruit into wedges or slices, cut sandwiches into quarters, and serve pieces of raw vegetables instead of a mixed salad.

Menu Planning for School-Age Children

Among elementary school-age children, a few more nutrition principles should be considered. Energy needs vary, depending on a child's age, size, activity, and pattern of growth. In general, it's important to understand that the entire growth process involves building new tissue at a rapid rate. This places many key nutrients in high demand, including protein, calcium, and iron. As a child grows, total protein requirements grow, too. The need for calcium remains stable at 800 mg per day from one year of age until 11 years of age, when it increases again. Consuming an adequate amount of calcium is very important at this time (and beyond), as it is essential for healthy bone growth. Adequate calcium in the early years may also prevent osteoporosis in later years. The need for iron is actually highest in children ages 4-8, and adolescents ages 14-18. Iron is essential for brain development, behavior, and growth in children.

Balanced snack choices are important for school-age children as well, as they do not always have the desire or the time to sit down and eat. Snacks can include fresh fruits and vegetables, juices, breads, unsweetened cereals, popcorn, tortillas, muffins, milk, yogurt, cheese, pudding, custard, sliced meats and poultry, eggs, or peanut butter.

The *Dietary Guidelines for Americans* emphasizes the fact that there has been a dramatic and significant increase in the incidence of overweight and obese children in the last 40 years, and with this, a concern for the associated risk in nutrition-related chronic disease. Some evidence suggests that adolescents and school-age children should consume nutrient-dense, minimally processed foods and eat a healthy breakfast to combat this obesity trend.

Another concern in childhood years is the prevalence of hyperactivity, or Attention Deficit Hyperactivity Disorder (ADHD). This is characterized by difficulty in paying attention and a certain amount of impulsive behavior. The condition is poorly understood, and both parents and educators find cause for concern when a child is diagnosed with ADHD. While pharmaceutical treatments are common, perceived dietary interventions are becoming more prevalent. It should be noted that research has not supported the value of dietary treatments for this condition.

Nutrition for Adolescents

The beginning of adolescence is marked by a growth spurt that results in physically mature adults. Most girls are in this rapid growth spurt by age 11. For boys, this spurt starts later, usually between 12 and 13 years of age. The growth spurt ends at about age 15 for girls and age 19 for boys. Both boys and girls grow in height and weight. Boys put on twice as much muscle as girls, while girls tend to deposit more fat. During the adolescent growth spurt, they may grow to approximately 20 percent of their adult height and have a gain of 50 percent of ideal body weight.

Whereas parents are the main providers of food for young children, adolescents make many of their own food decisions. Of course, it helps to have healthy foods available to them to eat at home. Eating patterns of adolescents can be influenced by peers, lifestyles, body image, popular media, and food preferences. Meal skipping (usually breakfast and/or lunch) and snacking are common. Although snack foods can be nutritious and make a contribution to the overall diet, popular teen snack foods may gravitate towards choices such as chips, cookies, candies, soft drinks, caffeinated energy drinks, and ice cream. Eating disorders often start during adolescence. **Anorexia nervosa**, self-induced starvation and highly distorted body image, has been noted as particularly common among adolescent girls. Another disorder called **bulimia nervosa** involves binge eating and forced purging, such as by vomiting or excessive use of laxatives. **Binge eating disorder** (BED) involves eating a large amount of food in a short period of time and exhibits a "lack of control" over eating. All are unhealthy approaches to controlling weight and require intensive, long-term treatment.

GLOSSARY

Anorexia Nervosa
An eating disorder with symptoms including self-induced starvation and highly distorted body image

Bulimia Nervosa
An eating disorder characterized by binge eating and forced purging—usually by vomiting, the use of laxatives, or other means of getting rid of the food

Binge Eating Disorder (BED)
Eating a large amount of food in a short period of time and exhibiting a "lack of control" over eating

While disordered eating patterns are of concern for adolescents, another concern is obesity. According to the *Dietary Guidelines for Americans*, children and adolescents ages 2 through 19 years, 11.9 percent are at or above the 97th percentile of the body mass index (BMI) for age growth charts, 16.9 percent are at or above the 95th percentile, and 31.7 percent are at or above the 85th percentile. Minority children have a higher prevalence of both overweight and obesity.

Healthy eating habits are important for all adolescents. Adolescents need four glasses of milk (or equivalent) daily and high-iron foods such as meats, egg yolk, seafood, green leafy vegetables, legumes, dried fruits, whole grain and enriched breads and cereals. Teenagers often drink empty-calorie beverages, such as soft drinks and caffeinated energy drinks, instead of more nutritious choices such as milk or juice. Nutrients that may be lacking in an adolescent's diet include calcium, iron, vitamin A, vitamin C, and sometimes even nutrient-rich calories and protein. Adolescent girls are at higher risk

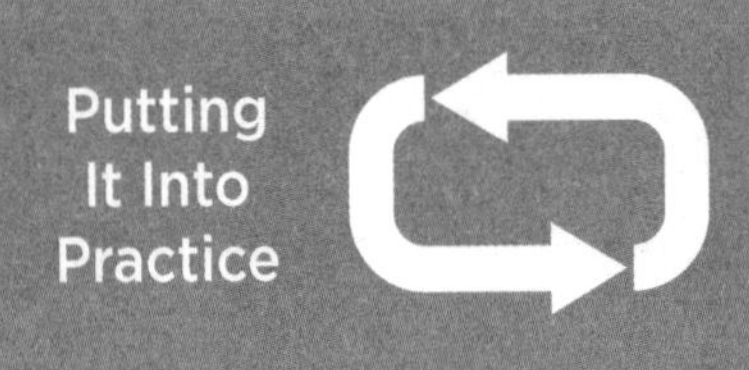

1. Should an overweight child or adolescent be on a calorie-restricted diet? Explain.

for nutritional deficiencies than boys because girls must obtain more nutrients in fewer calories than boys.

Menu Planning for Adolescents

In planning menus for adolescents, it is a good idea to include nutritious snack choices that are portable and can be eaten on-the-run, such as:

- Small packages of nuts or sunflower seeds
- Fresh fruit
- Individually packaged unsweetened cereals
- Mini muffins
- Mini bagels
- Yogurt
- Popcorn
- Fig bars
- Oatmeal raisin cookies

To meet the increased nutrient needs consider offering the following:

- Fiber—whole grain pancakes or waffles with fruit, whole grain toast or muffins, cereals with fresh fruit, whole grain bagels with peanut butter
- Protein and iron—lean meats or fish
- Vitamins A and C—yellow/orange vegetables, citrus fruits, tomatoes and leafy greens combined in whole wheat tortillas with low-fat cheese
- Calories—Emphasize additional nutrient/calorie-dense foods such as nuts and seeds

National School Lunch Program (NSLP) and School Breakfast Program

Legislation that established the National School Lunch Program was signed by President Harry Truman in 1946. The School Breakfast Program began as a pilot program in 1966, and was made permanent in 1975. Through these programs, the USDA supports nutritious, low-cost, reduced price or free breakfasts and lunches to more than 25 million children each school day. School districts and independent schools that choose to take part in the programs receive cash subsidies and donated commodities from the USDA for each meal served. Participating school districts must serve meals that meet federal requirements. They must offer free or reduced price meals to eligible children, and also at an established price for paid students. Schools can also be reimbursed for after-school snacks served to children through age 18 in after-school educational or enrichment programs. In addition, the Fresh Fruit and Vegetable Program offers a snack during the elementary school day, but also exposes students to a variety of fresh fruits and vegetables.

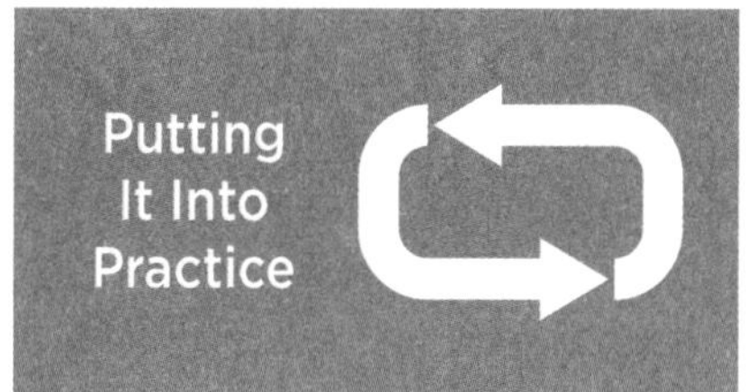

2. Modify the following snack to contain adequate protein, fiber, vitamins, and minerals:
    - Saltines with peanut butter
    - A glass of soda

School meals must meet the recommendations of the *Dietary Guidelines for Americans*, with no more than 30 percent of calories from fat, and less than 10 percent from saturated fat. Regulations also establish a standard for school meals to provide whole grains, fruits and vegetables, lean meats, and low-fat milk within an established calorie range (based on grade). There are also sodium restrictions, rules on competitive foods, and a focus on providing opportunities to make healthy choices during the school day. School meals must meet federal nutrition requirements, but decisions about what specific foods to serve and how they are prepared are up to school foodservice administrators.

In 2010, with the passage of the Healthy, Hunger-Free Kids Act, the USDA implemented changes that reflect the recommendations for school-age children: more fruits and vegetables, whole grain products, and less fat and sodium. Changes have also included a slight increase in the reimbursement rates and changes in the commodity products to meet the suggested menu changes (whole grains, lean meats, low-fat cheese, fruits and vegetables, etc.).

Nutrition for the Elderly

Among the U.S. population, the number of older Americans is growing most quickly. The population of older Americans will continue to escalate between the present time and 2030, when the baby boom generation reaches age 65. With advances in medicine, average life spans are increasing. What does all this mean for a CDM, CFPP? Among other things, it means that a typical foodservice operation is likely to be serving more older adults. The number of elderly individuals in nursing homes is expected to triple within the next few decades. The eldercare foodservice industry, providing nutrition to older Americans through a variety of models (not just nursing homes), is growing quickly. To serve this population well, it's essential to understand a number of changes that occur during the aging process—and the impact they have on nutrition.

"Elderly" is a loose term, and there is no defined age at which the body undergoes dramatic aging-related changes. What happens with aging? The metabolism changes and body systems and organs lose their peak efficiency. The rate of decline is typically very gradual, and shows great individual variation, including both genetic and environmental factors. Changes brought about by the aging process affect nutrition status. Of particular importance are changes that affect digestion, absorption, and metabolism of nutrients.

The basal metabolic rate (baseline energy requirement) decreases an average of 2.9 and 2.0 percent per decade, respectively, for men and women of normal weight, and is accompanied by a 25 to 30 percent loss in muscle mass. A general decrease in activity level and reduced caloric intake may further accelerate a decline in nutrition status.

However, the elderly can work towards preserving muscle mass and inhibiting bone loss or osteoporosis. Studies have shown that consuming optimal amounts of protein and completing weight training exercises may increase muscular strength and basal metabolism, and improve appetite and blood flow to the brain.

Overall, the functioning of the cardiovascular system declines with age. The workload of the heart increases due to atherosclerotic deposits and less elasticity in the arteries. The heart does not pump as hard as before, and cardiac output is reduced in elderly people who do not remain physically active. Blood pressure increases normally with age. Lung capacity decreases throughout life. This decrease does not restrict the normal activity of healthy older persons, but may limit vigorous exercise. Kidney function deteriorates over time, and the aging kidney is less able to excrete waste. Adequate fluid intake is very important, as is avoiding mega-doses of water-soluble vitamins because they put a strain on the kidneys to excrete them.

Factors Affecting Nutrition Status

The nutrition status of an elderly person is greatly influenced by many variables, such as physiological, psychosocial, and socioeconomic factors, as outlined below.

Physiological Factors:

Illness. The presence of illness, both acute and chronic, and use of modified diets can affect nutrition status. The most prevalent nutrition-related problems in the elderly are chronic conditions that usually require therapeutic diets. Certain chronic diseases are associated with anorexia or loss of appetite. Examples include gastrointestinal disease, congestive heart failure, renal disease, neurological impairment, depression, and cancer. Other medical events, such as stroke, may not be associated with anorexia, but can affect one's ability to eat.

Caloric intake. An individual who adjusts caloric intake downwards to accompany decline in basal energy expenditure and muscle mass faces a new challenge: that of nutrient density. With even fewer calories, nutrient-dense food choices become increasingly crucial.

Dentition. Approximately 50 percent of Americans have lost their teeth by age 65. Poor or compromised oral health or ill-fitting dentures may cause chewing problems for many elderly people. According to the American Heart Association, poor oral health is also linked to coronary heart disease.

Functional disabilities. Functional disabilities interfere with the ability of the elderly to perform daily tasks, such as the purchasing and preparing of food and eating. These disabilities may be due to arthritis/rheumatism, stroke, visual impairment, diminished heart function, or dementia (deterioration in mental functioning, such as thinking and memory).

Taste and smell. Around age 60, there is a decline in the ability to taste and smell. Taste buds in the tongue are less sensitive, and the nerves in the nose that detect aromas need extra stimulation to perceive smells. Seniors may find ordinarily seasoned foods too bland related to these changes.

Changes in the gastrointestinal tract. The movement of food through the gastrointestinal tract slows down over the years causing constipation, a frequent complaint of older people. Constipation may also be related to low fiber and fluid intake, medications, or lack of exercise. Other frequent complaints include nausea, indigestion, and heartburn. Intestinal changes typical of aging also reduce absorption of the vitamin B12 produced in the body.

Medications. More than half of seniors take at least one medication daily and many take six or more a day. Medications often alter appetite, taste, or the digestion, absorption, or metabolism of nutrients. This has been discussed in previous chapters.

Thirst and dehydration. Many elderly people have a diminished perception of thirst that can cause problems. In addition, medications and medical conditions can also cause dehydration. Because the aging kidney is less able to concentrate the urine, more fluid is lost, further setting the stage for dehydration.

Psychosocial Factors:

Cognition. Functions such as attention and memory may be affected by declining cognition. Deficiencies in this area affect nutrition status. Examples could include forgetting to eat or not recognizing how long a food has been in the refrigerator or pantry.

Social support. An individual's nutritional health results in part from a series of social acts. Purchasing, preparing, and eating foods are social events for most people. For example, elderly people may rely on each other for a ride to the supermarket, cooking, or sharing meals. The benefits of social support are largely due to the companionship and emotional support they provide. This support can have a positive effect on appetite and dietary intake; likewise, losing that support can negatively impact appetite and dietary intake.

Socioeconomic Factors:

Education and income. Higher levels of education are positively associated with increased nutrient intakes. Money spent on food is a significant predictor of dietary quality. Many elderly are often faced with financial insecurity and may have to choose between food, medications, or other household or medical bills.

Living arrangements. The elderly, particularly women, are more likely to be widowed. The trend has been for widows and widowers in the United States to live alone after their spouse dies. Research indicates that living alone is a risk factor for dietary inadequacy.

Availability of federally-funded meals. The availability of nutritious meals through federal programs, such as Meals on Wheels and Senior Congregate Feeding Sites, are critical to the nutritional health and independence of the aging population. Many communities also have Senior Centers that provide meals, as well as educational and social programs.

Menu Planning for the Elderly

Basic guidelines for menu planning for older adults need to address a range of factors. Menu choices need to stimulate eating through aroma, taste, and visual appeal. They need to provide nutrient-dense choices, and adapt comfortably to any physical limitations. If chewing is a problem, menus must offer softer foods. Chapter 5 presents guidelines for offering a mechanical soft diet, which may be helpful. Figure 11.6 includes some other useful techniques and ideas for meal planning.

At-Risk Populations

Individuals in various states of illness are at risk for developing nutritional problems. For example, a client who has cancer may experience a loss of appetite along with increased nutrient needs due to the demands of a growing tumor. A recent study (Lazemi, et al.) showed that 10.3% of the elderly residents in nursing homes were malnourished. A client of a nursing home who is unable to move about may be at risk for developing pressure ulcers. Sound nutrition is crucial for protecting against this common problem. An individual who has difficulty swallowing, or one who is afflicted with Alzheimer's disease, may not be able to consume adequate amounts of food. Some clients need to follow sodium restrictions. Others are following diets that are controlled for saturated fat and cholesterol. Others are following portion-controlled diets for management of diabetes, and others may be eating pureed foods.

Figure 11.6
Menu Planning Techniques for the Elderly

TECHNIQUE	SPECIAL CONSIDERATIONS
Serve Moderately Sized Meals	Healthy older adults have a slower metabolism and need to reduce calories. They also hate to see food wasted.
Add Complex Carbohydrate and High-Fiber Foods	Older people requiring softer diets will prefer high-fiber foods that are soft in texture such as cooked beans and peas, bran cereals soaked in milk, oatmeal, canned fruits, and cooked vegetables.
Use Fat Sparingly	Use lean meats and low-fat dairy products.
Offer Adequate Protein	To help balance the budget, offer lower-cost protein sources such as dried beans and peas, cottage cheese, macaroni and cheese, eggs, liver, Greek yogurt. Add nonfat dry milk to gravies.
Use Herbs and Spices to Make Foods Flavorful	The sense of taste decreases with age so adding herbs and spices will make food more appealing.
Provide Variety	Include traditional menu items as well as ethnic and regional cuisine.
Encourage Fluid Intake	Offer a variety of beverages such as flavored coffees and teas or liquid foods such as soup, ices, and gelatin desserts or fruit-flavored water. Limit caffeine intake, which may be dehydrating.
Make Sure Foods are Nutrient-Dense	Older people need fewer calories but the same or added nutrients such as vitamin D, calcium, and zinc. Make sure snacks and desserts are nutrient-dense by reducing fat and sugar, and adding complex carbohydrates.

Another type of food-related risk of concern is food-borne illness. The FDA identifies certain populations as being more susceptible to contracting food-borne illness. These include pre-school age children and older adults. Within these groups, immune response may not be as strong as it is during other phases of the life cycle. Sound food safety and sanitation practices become even more crucial when serving these populations.

Regulatory Issues

In long-term care facilities subject to Centers for Medicare & Medicaid Services (CMS) regulations, some specific advice applies to menu planning. The menu planning considerations include the following:

- Each client receives, and facility provides, at least three meals daily, at regular times comparable to normal mealtimes in the community.
- There must be no more than 14 hours between a substantial evening meal and breakfast the following day (or 16 hours if a nourishing snack is provided at bedtime).
- An evening meal should provide at least 20 percent of the day's total nutritional requirements.
- The facility must offer snacks at bedtime daily.

- Food is attractive and palatable, incorporating needs as identified through observation, client and staff interviews, and review of client council minutes.
- If a food group is missing from the client's daily diet, the facility has an alternative means of satisfying the client's nutrient needs.
- Substitutes of similar nutritive value are offered to clients who refuse food served.

CMS regulations emphasize clients' rights—their options to exert control over their own care. This certainly extends to meals and menus. Both the menu as planned and the manner in which CDM, CFPPs implement it must address these rights. If a client specifically refuses a food or requests a substitute, it is up to the CDM, CFPP to be of service in every way that is practical. If the facility uses a nonselective menu, it is especially important to make alternates available upon request. A client also has the right to refuse treatment, including a therapeutic diet. In making choices, a client should be well informed. It is up to the CDM, CFPP to work with other members of the healthcare team, as needed, to review any diet-related concerns and assure that clients' rights are being honored. In long-term care, a client council is a committee composed of clients who provide feedback and suggestions about care— including dietary services. In other institutional settings, there may be a similar body of clients. In a university, for example, there may be a council of students and/or other patrons who provide comments and suggestions for menu planning. A CDM, CFPP must solicit and respond to input from client groups such as these when planning menus and serving meals.

Diet Spreadsheets

In a facility serving clients who follow a variety of therapeutic diets, a menu must be versatile enough to provide nutritious, satisfying meals for every diet. This detail is mapped out on a diet spreadsheet. A diet spreadsheet displays the menu offerings and portion sizes for each diet, for each meal, and for each day of the cycle menu. Figure 11.7 shows a segment of a diet spreadsheet for a lunch meal. With the trend in liberalization of therapeutic diets in health care, diet spreadsheets should be developed to be as simple as possible, with no more restriction than is therapeutically necessary. At the same time, the strategy of making all menus "healthy" means that menu planners strive to limit total fat, saturated fat, cholesterol, and sodium in even a general (unrestricted) diet. Implementing healthful guidelines may also mean providing a variety of fruits and vegetables, including high-fiber foods in a menu, and more. Thus, a healthy "general" diet emerges that may be suitable for certain therapeutic needs as well.

In all, the goal is to keep a list of therapeutic diets reasonably short. This can lead to optimal health for all clients, while providing the best possible range of choices for each client. Management considerations apply, too. It is ideal to plan a menu in which many products are common to all diets. This minimizes the need to produce many different products at once, and also minimizes food waste, which is essential to controlling food costs. Sometimes, portion sizes vary among diets. Unique portion sizes are specified on the menus. A foodservice operation must be able to produce foods on a given menu in a manner that meets standards for quality and budget, while accommodating the unique therapeutic and nutritional needs of each client.

Another consideration in menu planning is providing thickened liquids for some therapeutic diets. For example, including chilled, thickened water at bedside may increase hydration. Work with others in your facility to make sure that your clients are

Figure 11.7
Segment of a Diet Spreadsheet—Lunch for Cycle Day 3

GENERAL DIET	SODIUM-CONTROLLED DIET	CARB-CONTROLLED DIET	RENAL DIET	PURÉED DIET	FULL LIQUID DIET
Tossed salad with low-fat dressing	Tossed salad with low-fat, low-sodium dressing	Tossed salad with low-fat dressing	Tossed salad with low-sodium dressing x 2	1/2 cup puréed vegetable medley	1 cup strained cream of chicken soup
Roast turkey sandwich. 3 oz. turkey on wheat bun with lettuce and tomato	Roast turkey sandwich. 3 oz. turkey on wheat bun with lettuce and tomato	Roast turkey sandwich. 3 oz. turkey on wheat bun with lettuce and tomato	Roast turkey sandwich. 3 oz. turkey on wheat bun with lettuce and low-sodium mayonnaise	Puréed turkey and noodle portion with parsley flakes	
Assorted fresh fruit	Assorted fresh fruit	Assorted fresh fruit	Fresh apple	1/2 cup pink applesauce	1 cup strained fruit juice
Cookie	Cookie	1/2 cup sugar-free gelatin	1/2 cup regular gelatin (count in fluid restriction)	1/2 cup regular gelatin	1/2 cup regular gelatin
Coffee, tea, or beverage of choice	Coffee, tea, or beverage of choice	Coffee, tea, or beverage of choice	1/2 cup fruit punch (count in fluid restriction)	Coffee, tea, or beverage of choice	Coffee, tea, or beverage of choice
Skim or low-fat milk	Skim or low-fat milk	Skim or low-fat milk	Potassium and sodium-free candy as desired (e.g. gum drops)	Skim or low-fat milk	1 cup milkshake
Condiments as desired	Mayo, sugar, pepper, herb-based sodium-free seasoning as desired (No potassium-based salt substitute without a physician's order)	Sugar substitute, salt, pepper as desired	Mayo, sugar, pepper, herb-based sodium-free seasoning as desired (No potassium-based salt substitute without a physician's order)	Condiments as desired	Condiments as desired
Notes	Note that if a fresh roast turkey product low in sodium is used, the same meat is appropriate on sodium-controlled menus.	Adjust portion sizes of bread, fruit, and milk if needed for specific meal pattern or carbohydrate count.	Mayonnaise is not reduced for fat, as fat is an important source of calories in a renal diet. Omit tomato because it is high in potassium, add low-sodium mayonnaise for extra fat calories.	Adjust consistency of products as needed to meet individualized orders for IDDSI.	

receiving liquids at the appropriate IDDSI level of thickness throughout the day.

Using Nutrition Analysis Data to Modify Menus

Thinking back to nutrition screening and assessment, the nutrition services team (the Certified Dietary Manager, Certified Food Protection Professional, Nutrition and Dietetic Technician, Registered; and the Registered Dietitian Nutritionist) completes the nutrition screening and nutrition assessment as the first step in the nutrition care process. It is now the job of the nutrition services team to translate the nutritional needs into food choices for the client. It is understood that the percent of calories from nutrients (carbohydrate, protein, and fat) can make a difference in overall health. Recommendations for a healthy diet often use guidelines based on percentages of these nutrients. In addition, guidelines for percentages of carbohydrates, protein, and fat in diets to treat high blood cholesterol, diabetes, and other conditions are well documented. Therefore, it is important for a CDM, CFPP to be able to determine how many calories are in food.

Let's do a quick review. Three macronutrients provide calories. These are:

- Carbohydrate (CHO): 4 calories per gram
- Fat: 9 calories per gram
- Protein (PRO): 4 calories per gram

Remember that alcohol also provides calories (seven calories per gram), and when applicable, this should be included in calorie calculations. Knowing this, calculate calories and percent calories of any food or diet, as long as the grams of carbohydrate, fat, and protein (and alcohol, if applicable) are known. Figure 11.8 shows the formula for calculating total calories. Once total calories are calculated for any food, meal or food record, it is possible to calculate the percent of calories contributed by each component. Percent of calories is simply a way to express the proportions, or how much each macronutrient (and alcohol, if applicable) is contributing to the total calories. This is also called caloric distribution. Figure 11.9 shows the math for calculating percent calories. Figure 11.10 shows a sample calculation of calories and percent of calories.

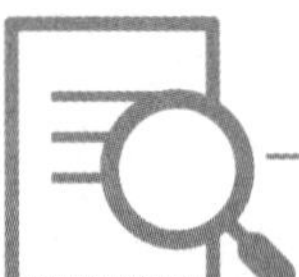

View the Supplemental Material to see Calorie Exchange and Fluid Intake Focus on Formulas

To calculate caloric distribution for a meal, a one-day menu, or a food record, use the same formulas shown in Figures 11.8, 11.9, and 11.10. For the Figure 11.10 calculation, simply total grams of carbohydrate, fat, protein, and alcohol from all the foods in the diet for Step 1. Here are a few words of caution about interpreting the percent of calories information: Do not compare the caloric distribution of each individual food in a diet to the *Dietary Guidelines for Americans* or other standards. Let's say that the menu is aiming to achieve a caloric distribution of 50 percent of calories from carbohydrate, 20 percent of calories from protein, and 30 percent of calories from fat. Is it all right to eat the two graham crackers we examined in Figure 11.10? View the sample calculation in Figure 11.9 to determine the answer. The answer is: they exceed the caloric distribution of 50 percent of the calories from carbohydrate. When applying caloric distribution guidelines, don't worry about individual foods. Simply review the total for the day.

However, if daily totals are not balanced, it can be helpful to look at the caloric distribution of individual foods. For example, if the daily total is too high in fat, look at which individual food(s) provided the highest percentage of fat, and reduce portion sizes of these foods to bring the diet into balance.

Figure 11.8
Calculating Total Calories

This formula works for a single food, a meal, or any food record. To calculate a calorie distribution:

STEP 1: Find out how many grams of carbohydrate, fat, protein, and alcohol are present.

____ grams of carbohydrate
____ grams of fat
____ grams of protein
____ grams of alcohol (remember calories from alcohol are non-nutritious)

STEP 2: Multiply each by its calorie contribution.

____ grams of carbohydrate........ x 4 cal/gm = ____ calories from carbohydrate
____ grams of fat........ x 9 cal/gm = ____ calories from fat
____ grams of protein........ x 4 cal/gm = ____ calories from protein
____ grams of alcohol........ x 7 cal/gm = ____ calories from alcohol

STEP 3: Add the subtotals you obtained in Step 2.

____ calories from carbohydrate
____ calories from fat
____ calories from protein
____ calories from alcohol
____ = TOTAL CALORIES

Calculating Fluid Intake

Water/fluid is also an essential nutrient. Managing fluids is a critical part of clinical care. It is important when there is a concern about dehydration—a common condition among those who are elderly, those who are eating poorly, those who are taking certain medications, and those who are undergoing various forms of medical stress. Certain conditions may require a diet order that includes an instruction to push fluids. Conversely, there are times when the body cannot rid itself of water adequately. For example, a person experiencing end-stage renal failure is not able to excrete water. As water builds up in the bloodstream, it dilutes the rest of the blood's contents. It often raises blood pressure and disrupts the sensitive balance of electrolytes (chemicals) in the blood. Fluid restriction may be required to avoid potentially life-threatening conditions. Other conditions that may require fluid restriction include advanced liver failure, congestive heart failure, and certain hormonal disorders.

When a fluid restriction is needed, a physician specifies the restriction along with the rest of the diet order. Fluid restrictions are expressed in milliliters (mL) or cubic centimeters (cc). Although these are equivalent, mL is the preferred term by The Joint Commission. They recommend that "mL" is less likely to be misread in a medical record. (It is important to note that the Centers for Medicare & Medicaid Services (CMS) prefers the use of cc's.) A number indicates how many mL's (or cc's) should be consumed per day.

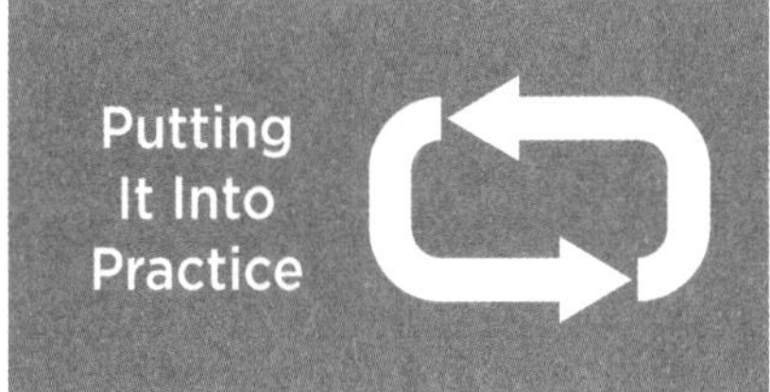

3. Calculate the calories in a meal with 20 grams of protein, 45 grams of carbohydrate, and 10 grams of fat.

For example, a diet for an individual in renal failure may read:

60 gm protein, 2 gm Na, 2 gm K, 1000 mL fluids.

This means the diet is limited to 60 grams of protein, 2 grams of sodium, 2 grams of potassium, and 1000 mL of fluid per day.

To honor an order such as this one, nursing and food service staff must communicate and work together. Some of the fluid may be served with meals. Other fluid may take the form of a drink offered by the direct care staff, e.g. with medications. Thus, the first step in implementing a fluid-restricted diet order is to find out the amount that should be provided by food service. The facility may have a universal standard—80 percent from food service and 20 percent from nursing services, for instance. That would be 800 mL from foodservice and 200 mL from nursing services. If there is no standard, it is necessary to meet with the interdisciplinary team to specify and agree upon a split in fluids. Then document the distribution for the dietary allowance of fluid on the nutrition care plan and in the health record. Keep the fluids from foodservice consistent. For example, a 1200 mL fluid restriction, with 400 mL provided by nursing. Distribution of the remaining 800 mL may include the following: 240 mL—breakfast; 240 mL—lunch; 240 mL—dinner; 80 mL—snack. Be sure to manage menus and trays meticulously to stay in compliance.

When planning a day's worth of menus, how are fluids counted? First, a conversion factor is needed (e.g. One cup or 8 fluid ounces = 240 mL). Figure 11.11 lists some related fluid conversions. Next, decide what menu items count as fluids. This is specified in the diet manual, so use the manual as a reference, and again, document. Generally, anything that looks like a liquid at room temperature counts as fluid. Examples include: broth, juice, soft drinks, milk, shakes, coffee, tea, fruit ices, ice cream, sherbet, liquid nutritional supplements, gelatin, and popsicles. Pudding, custard, yogurt, hot cereal, and gravy do NOT count as fluid. Like calorie counting and carbohydrate counting, fluid counting is not 100 percent precise. For example, many fruits and vegetables contain water, but most systems do not count that as fluid.

As a practical matter, most foodservice departments also provide a message on menus or tray tickets for fluid-restricted meals. One facility may use a red stamp to mark "Fluid Restriction." Another may generate a special message through a software program that prints tray tickets. Usually, nursing staff also post an alert near a client's bed. To protect a client's privacy, many facilities use only color-coding to signal special restrictions.

Sources of Nutrient Information

Be prepared to calculate the amount of calories and fluid in the diet, as well as other pertinent nutrient information. Where can information be obtained for these calculations? Nutrient information is available from several sources. We will examine three: USDA Nutrient Database, nutrient analysis software, and Nutrition Facts Labels.

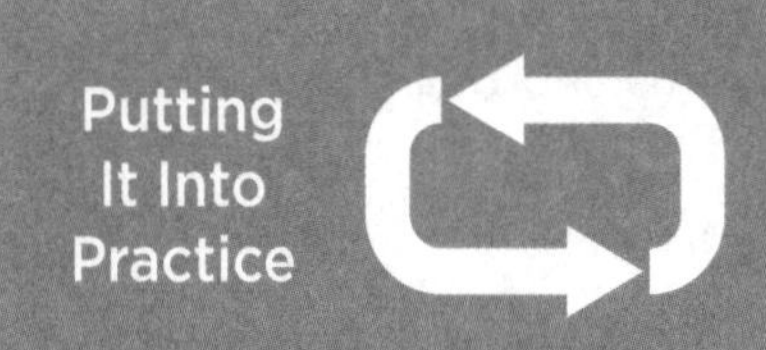

4. How many cups is a beverage that is 360 milliliters?

Figure 11.9
Calculating Percent of Calories

Take another look at Step 2 in Figure 11.8. Use the subtotals obtained in Column 1 of this calculation. Now take a look at the total calories obtained in Step 3 in Figure 11.8. Enter this figure (total calories) in Column 2 below.

COLUMN 1: Calorie Type	COLUMN 2: Total Calories	COLUMN 3: Calories from this Component
_____ Calories from carbohydrate	_________	Calories from carbohydrate ÷ Total calories = _______
_____ Calories from fat	_________	Calories from fat ÷ Total calories = _______
_____ Calories from protein	_________	Calories from protein ÷ Total calories = _______
_____ Calories from alcohol	_________	Calories from alcohol ÷ Total calories = _______

Round each figure to two decimal places. Next, remove the decimal point (or multiply by 100) to change each figure to a percentage. To check the work, add the percentages together. The total should come close to 100%. (Depending on rounding, a total like 99% or 101% might be found. This is okay.)

Figure 11.10
Sample Calculation: Calories and Percent of Calories of a Specific Food

Determining calories for 2 full graham crackers. So far, it is known that this serving contains 24 gm of carbohydrate, 3 gm of fat, and 2 gm of protein.

24 gm of carbohydrate x 4 calories/gm = 96 calories from carbohydrate
+
3 gm of fat x 9 calories/gm = 27 calories from fat
+
2 gm of protein x 4 calories/gm = 8 calories from protein

Total calories = 131 calories

COLUMN 1: Calorie Type	COLUMN 2: Total Calories	COLUMN 3: Calories from this Component
96 calories from carbohydrate	131	96 ÷ 131 = 0.73 or 73%
27 calories from fat	131	27 ÷ 131 = 0.21 or 21%
8 calories from protein	131	8 ÷ 131 = 0.06 or 6%

To check the calculation, we can add the three percentages, and see if they total close to 100%:
73% + 21% + 6% = 100%

Figure 11.11
Fluid Conversions

VOLUME	FLUID OUNCES (fl. oz.)	MILLILITERS (mL)
1 cup	8	240
3/4 cup	6	180
1/2 cup	4	120
1/3 cup	2.7	80
1/4 cup	2	60
2 Tbsp.	1	30

USDA Nutrient Database

Historically, almost all nutrient data came from laboratory research conducted by the USDA. Over the years, the USDA has vastly augmented its information, adding nutrients such as dietary fiber and trace minerals—and now, caffeine, lycopene, isoflavones (a food component in soybeans), trans-fatty acids, and many others. For the most part, nutrient data in other books and software programs comes from the USDA database. Following are six points to keep in mind with USDA data.

1. Much of the USDA data is available per 100 gram portion. For a small serving of meat, this might be realistic (100 grams is just over 3 ounces). However, for some foods, it is not a "usual fit" with dietary habits. For instance, one cup of circular-shaped oat cereal is only 30 grams. When using USDA data, be sure to check units of measure carefully and select a unit that applies to the amount needed. Also, it may be necessary to convert weights to volume measurements. If the data is not available in the format needed, use a conversion table from another source, such as *Food for Fifty*, a quantity food production cookbook.
2. Using the USDA nutrient data requires careful attention to edible portion and/or product yield. *Edible* portion is the amount of a food that one can actually eat after preparation is complete; product yield is the final volume of the cooked food. Consider that meat shrinks when it is cooked, and grain products like rice and pasta expand. If the nutrient values for a ground beef patty are needed, first determine the final weight of the cooked patty, and match it to "cooked" ground beef in the database. Imagine starting with a six-ounce patty, and it cooks down to four ounces. If nutrients are calculated based on the USDA data for six ounces of cooked ground beef, it will result in an over-estimate of nutrients. Be sure to match "ounces" and "cooked" to the nutrient database. Now consider macaroni. Nutrients for one cup of uncooked macaroni may be about three times higher than nutrients for one cup of cooked macaroni. Again, match macaroni to a weight or volume and then carefully select "dry" or "cooked." Weight and volume can be confusing, for example one cup of dry rice is 7 oz.
3. When calculations of total calories based on grams of carbohydrate, fat, and protein (as in Figure 11.8) are made, the calorie total calculated when compared to the USDA database information may not match perfectly. That is OK. The USDA uses more highly refined techniques for determining calorie information.

4. The USDA data is primarily built on individual foods. Each time a recipe or combination dish (e.g., lasagna) is made up of individual foods, the most accurate way to determine nutrients is to calculate them based on individual ingredients. This is a cumbersome process. However, the USDA data does include some combination dishes (e.g., lasagna). It will need to be determined and a decision made as to how closely a USDA item matches the recipes or sources for foods used in the facility.
5. Historically, USDA nutrient data was all for generic foods. Today, the USDA maintains quite a bit of information by brand name. This is useful, as many people eat not only brand-name foods, but also packaged and convenience foods that would be difficult to calculate any other way.
6. Some data simply is not available. Despite the massive research conducted by the USDA, the task of determining nutrient values for thousands of foods is no small feat! As a result, certain nutrient values may be absent. This can lead to *false zeroes*. A false zero is a report that a nutrient is absent in food, when in fact it is not available.

Nutrient Analysis Software

Because calculating nutrients in a recipe, meal, or menu can be a great deal of work, many dietary professionals use software for the job. Nutrient analysis software is readily available within a range of budgets. Some programs are built into foodservice management software packages. This can be convenient because they draw on lists of foods and recipes that are already in the system. Be aware, though, that any software does initially require data entry, such as an inventory list, individual recipes, and menus.

When selecting a program for nutrient analysis, look carefully at the sources of nutrient data. Generally, nutrient databases are built on USDA data, which is freely available.

Some packages use the USDA database in its entirety; others use a small proportion of USDA data. So, look at the number of foods contained in a program's database. Also check whether foods can be added to the database locally (by the CDM, CFPP or other nutrition services staff) using Nutrition Facts Labels.

In addition, some software developers invest immense effort into expanding the database by adding nutrient data available from food manufacturers, restaurants, and other sources. A database offering significantly more foods than USDA has most likely undergone development to list more brand-name and convenience foods. Some developers use sources beyond the USDA to eliminate false zeroes in the database through mathematical calculations and estimations. This eliminates the problem of under-reporting certain nutrients. Which nutrients and food components are included varies by software package.

Another consideration with software is portion sizes or units of measure. Some packages offer more choices for portion sizes and units of measure, as compared with the USDA database. This can improve accuracy and efficiency for a program user. When evaluating options, also look at how it is recommended to find and enter foods. This should be a straightforward and convenient process. Finally, review the types of reports available. Most software will compare calculated totals with nutrient standards, such as MyPlate, RDAs, diabetic exchanges, and/or many others. Some reports are graphic and easy to read. Reports may be available for individual foods, recipes, menus, or averages for a series of days.

Let's look at how a computer may be used to get a nutrient analysis for one portion of a recipe.

- First, type the name of an ingredient (or part of the name), and the computer lists choices so that a match can be chosen.
- Then type in how much of that ingredient is needed to be used in the analysis, such as one cup—or select a measurement from a drop-down list.
- After entering all the ingredients, the computer will divide the results by the yield, such as 12 portions.
- Then the computer will indicate exactly how much of each nutrient (and the percent of the RDA) is contained in one portion.

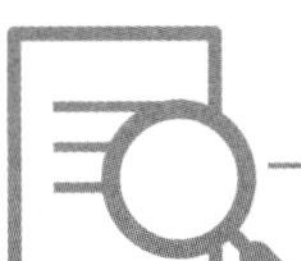

View the Supplemental Material to see Figure 11.12 Sample Nutrient Analysis.

Most computer analysis programs can also give you a percentage breakdown of calories from protein, fats, carbohydrate, and alcohol. Of course, these figures can be printed on a printer and/or stored in the computer. A sample nutrient analysis for a recipe appears in Figure 11.12.

Nutrition Facts Labels

The Nutrition Labeling and Education Act of 1990 requires labeling for most foods, except meat and poultry. The FDA notes that Nutrition Facts labels are designed to offer consumers the following:

- Nutrition information about almost every food in the grocery store
- Distinctive, easy-to-read formats that enable consumers to find the information they need to make healthful food choices
- Information about the amount of nutrients per serving
- Standardized serving sizes, which make nutritional comparisons of similar products easier
- Nutrient reference values, expressed as Percent Daily Values, that help consumers see how a food fits into an overall daily diet
- Uniform definitions for terms that describe a food's nutrient content such as "light," "low-fat," and "high-fiber"—to ensure that such terms mean the same for any product on which they appear
- Claims about the relationship between a nutrient or food and a disease or health-related condition, such as calcium and osteoporosis, or fat and cancer. These are helpful for people who are concerned about eating foods that may help keep them healthy.
- Declaration of total percentage of actual juice in juice drinks

A Nutrition Facts label (Figure 11.13) must include information about: total calories, calories from fat, total fat, saturated fat, trans fat, cholesterol, sodium, total carbohydrate, dietary fiber, sugars, protein, vitamin A, vitamin C, calcium, and iron. Optionally, a label may include: calories from saturated fat, polyunsaturated fat, monounsaturated fat, potassium, soluble fiber, insoluble fiber, sugar alcohols, other carbohydrate, percent of vitamin A present as beta-carotene, and other essential vitamins and minerals. If a label makes a claim regarding one of these optional items, then it must provide the nutrition facts for the item. For instance, if the label claims "high fiber," it must list the fiber content and meet the definition for "high fiber" as described above.

Let's review each section of the Nutrition Facts label. Figure 11.13 is labeled with the sections that will be reviewed.

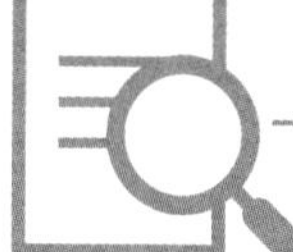

View the Supplemental Material to see Figure 11.13 Nutrition Facts Label for Macaroni & Cheese.

1. Serving Size

This is the first place to look on a nutrition label and one that is extremely important because it can be very misleading for your clients. Serving sizes are standardized and are provided in standard units such as cups or pieces. The most important part of this section is the Servings Per Container. One might assume that the information on the label is the total for the package or container. For instance, they might assume that a 12 ounce bottle of juice is one serving, when in reality it is three servings. Since the serving size listed is what influences the nutrition data, including the calories, the client could be consuming three times as many calories as the client thought.

Another fact to watch is the number of individual food items (or pieces) per serving on larger packages. A good example of this is different types of snack chips. Here are three snack chips with the serving size all different, but all are a one-ounce serving:

- 1 ounce (33 chips)
- 1 ounce (12 chips)
- 1 ounce (9 chips)

2. Check Calories

If the Servings Per Container is two and the consumer wants to calculate the nutrients for the entire package, double all of the calories and other nutrient numbers, including the % Daily Values. In this example of macaroni and cheese, how many calories would be consumed if the entire package was eaten? The FDA provides the following information to help consumers judge whether the calories per serving is low, moderate, or high:

General Guide to Calories

- 40 calories is low
- 100 calories is moderate
- 400 calories or more is high

3. Limit These Nutrients

This section lists key nutrients and macronutrients: Total Fat including Saturated Fat, Trans Fat, Cholesterol; Sodium; Total Carbohydrate, including Dietary Fiber and Sugars; and Protein. The first nutrients, Total Fat (Saturated and Trans Fats), Cholesterol, and Sodium (all highlighted in yellow) are the ones consumers generally eat too much of according to the Dietary Guidelines, so these nutrients should be limited. Please note that these are not highlighted on the actual Nutrition Facts label.

This section of the label, along with Total Carbohydrates and the micronutrients, expresses each nutrient as a percentage of the *Daily Value*. **Daily Values** (DVs) are reference intake levels devised specifically for nutrition facts labeling. They allow the food manufacturer to compare the amount of a nutrient (e.g., iron) in a food to the amount that a consumer would need. By using the % Daily Values column, it can be determined if a food is high or low in a nutrient. These are generalized figures for a nutrient, which can be applied to healthy people as a single group. Think of them as a generic set of "one-size-fits-all" nutrient recommendations for consumers. These differences from the Recommended Dietary Allowances were learned about previously, since the RDAs are broken down by age. For labeling purposes, when there is variation

GLOSSARY

Daily Values (DVs)
Reference intake levels devised specifically for Nutrition Facts labeling based on a standard 2,000 calorie reference diet

in actual RDAs, Daily Values reflect the higher values within ranges. This section also contains Total Carbohydrates, with sugars and dietary fiber broken out separately. Dietary fiber is highlighted in blue because, according to the Dietary Guidelines, most Americans should add more fiber to their diets. Use the dietary fiber information to help increase fiber intake by looking for foods with more grams of dietary fiber. A word of caution: dietary fiber needs to be increased gradually, and should also include adequate intake of water.

4. Get Enough of These Nutrients

These are micronutrients Americans should generally consume more of: vitamin A, vitamin C, calcium, and iron. They are expressed as a percentage of Reference Daily Intakes (RDIs). Obviously, not all of the essential nutrients are listed on the Nutrition Facts label. For Nutrition Facts labeling, the FDA has selected some key nutrients that relate to common health concerns.

5. Footnote

The footnote section highlights the fact that the label data is based on a 2,000 calorie diet. The remaining information will only be on the label if there is room on the package. The optional data represents general information for all Americans and is not specific to the food product. As can be seen, it tells what the recommended total fat grams, as well as other nutrients, should be for a 2,000 calorie diet. This information can be very useful when comparing the label data to this information. This food product has no dietary fiber, yet the % Daily Value indicates that 25 g each day should be consumed. If following the dietary advice, increasing fiber intake throughout the remaining meals of the day is warranted.

As can be seen, Daily Values used for Nutrition Facts labeling are less precise than RDAs. In fact, they are quite generalized. If a detailed nutrient evaluation is needed for an individual, the first choice of reference should be RDAs. However, Nutrition Facts labels do provide an excellent educational tool for consumers. They offer consistency and give consumers a way to compare nutritional values of foods.

Note that many labels also provide a set of nutrient information based on common serving or preparation practices. For cereal, the nutrition label values are generally for the values for the cereal alone and for the cereal plus milk. For a bakery mix, the label may list values for the mix alone (the contents of the package), and also for the mix prepared with added ingredients, according to preparation instructions on the package. Some labels vary based on intended use.

Finally, labeling standards govern the use of special terminology to describe foods. For the most up-to-date information on the Nutrition Facts label, search www.fda.gov. Foods must meet specific criteria to make certain labeling claims. In addition, many terms have legal definitions when it comes to labeling statements. Just like the Nutrition Facts, these claims are based on per-serving information.

Now, let's consider the Nutrition Facts label as a source of nutrient information. When planning a menu, the menu should follow certain dietary recommendations and be adequate in key nutrients. For example, the foodservice department would like to include a frozen casserole—a convenience item—on the menu. How can the nutrients be identified? If this product is not available in the USDA nutrient database (or in a nutrient analysis software system used), identify the nutrients from the Nutrition Facts label. Here are some pointers:

- First, compare the serving size. Determine whether the label-defined serving size is the same as on the menu plan. If not, use an adjustment factor. For example, imagine a product shows a serving size of 1/2 cup, but the planned amount to be served is 3/4 cup. Adjust all the nutrients by a factor of 1.5. Multiply each nutrient value by 1.5 to get the nutrients needed for the serving size.
- Next, use the label to obtain calories and any of the following: fat, saturated fat, cholesterol, sodium, carbohydrate, fiber, sugars, and protein.
- Note: To determine the adjustment factor, divide the new amount (3/4 cup or .75) by the old amount (1/2 cup or .5). .75 ÷ .50 = 1.5

In addition, nutrient information is available from a book called *Bowes & Church's Food Values of Portions Commonly Used*, or the USDA *Nutrient Database for Standard Reference*. The USDA nutrient data is available in the form of free downloads from the Internet. Conduct an online search of any food to retrieve its nutrient information. Or, display lists of foods containing a selected nutrient. The web address for searching USDA data appears in Appendix A.

As indicated earlier, there is no actual amount of vitamin A, vitamin C, iron, and calcium, only the percent of RDIs. Generally, if the food provides a minimum of 20 percent of the Daily Value for these four nutrients, it can be considered an adequate source of that nutrient.

Exchange Lists

Due to its flexibility to accommodate patient food preferences, carbohydrate counting has gained popularity. However, it is important to understand the basics of the Exchange System.

Figure 11.14 shows the overall exchange groups with the grams of carbohydrate, protein, fat, and calories. Within the exchange lists are foods grouped together because they are alike. Each serving of a food has about the same amount of carbohydrates (CHO), protein, fat, and calories. Foods within each list can be exchanged or traded for each other without affecting the CHO, protein, fat, or calories of a meal. The steps below provide a quick overview and method of estimating the amount of CHO, protein, fat, and calories in a meal.

Step 1: Compare the food(s) that need to be analyzed to the exchange lists. Assign an exchange group. Identify how many exchanges it represents. For mixed dishes, it may be necessary to list more than one exchange group. Do not count any of the foods in the "free foods" exchange list.

Step 2: After all of the foods have been compared to the exchange lists, total the exchanges for each group.

Step 3: For each exchange group, multiply the total number of exchanges by the standard carbohydrate, fat, protein, and calorie figures for that exchange group.

Figure 11.14
Exchange Groups

GROUP	CARBOHYDRATE	PROTEIN	FAT	CALORIES
Carbohydrate Group				
Starch	15 grams	3 grams	0-1 grams	80
Fruit	15 grams	—	—	60
Milk				
Fat-free	12 grams	8 grams	0-3 grams	90
Reduced-fat	12 grams	8 grams	5 grams	120
Whole	12 grams	8 grams	8 grams	150
Other				
Other Carbohydrates	15 grams	Varies	Varies	Varies
Non-starchy Vegetables	5 grams	2 grams	—	25
Meat and Meat Substitutes Group				
Very lean	—	7 grams	0-1 grams	35
Lean	—	7 grams	3 grams	55
Medium-fat	—	7 grams	5 grams	75
High-fat	—	7 grams	8 grams	100
Fat				
Fat group	—	—	5 grams	45

When obtaining a calorie count or calculating intake from a food record, the estimates will be only as good as the original records. Again, be sure to document. Calorie counts in facilities can be challenging. To collect the best records possible:

- Inform everyone who may be involved in care that a calorie count is in progress. This includes the client, visitors, nurses, and other caregivers.
- Post a notice or make another visible reminder (as permitted by your policies and procedures).
- Keep printed menus or try a ticket from meal trays. Ask each person to record the percent consumed next to each menu item. Percents (rather than actual measurements) are useful. They do not require others to guesstimate portion sizes. Then refer to the actual menu and food production information to determine what the portion size was.
- If possible, review records frequently throughout the day. If a meal has not been recorded, check with the caregiver or, if appropriate, with the client directly.

- Ask all caregivers to record any additional items the resident consumes, even if they are not printed on the menu. Examples: A resident asks for a can of ginger ale; a nurse offers a patient a cup of apple juice for taking medications; or a visitor brings in a cookie.

Obtaining a valid calorie count requires excellent communication, as well as vigilance and monitoring.

Carbohydrate Counting

Carbohydrate counting is a method of managing dietary concerns for an individual who has diabetes. This system is based on one simple idea: Foods that contain carbohydrate become glucose in the body. Glucose is blood sugar. (Note that fiber does not become blood sugar because it is not digested.) In a diet for managing diabetes, the bottom line is often how much glucose enters the body and how often.

Carbohydrate counting is based on a prescribed level of carbohydrate intake. For example, one client may be aiming for 220 grams of carbohydrate per day; another may be aiming for 185 grams. Generally, this carbohydrate intake needs to be distributed throughout the day to prevent surges in blood glucose levels. How rigid this distribution needs to be is determined by a patient's diabetic condition itself and medication regimens. It varies tremendously among individuals. Carbohydrate counting is done in conjunction with blood glucose monitoring, and members of the healthcare team evaluate any necessary fine-tuning in carbohydrate totals and distribution.

To count carbohydrates, simply tally grams of carbohydrate in each food consumed. It is necessary to count the carbohydrate in starches as well as sugars. Starchy foods include grain products, potatoes, dried beans, peas, and corn.

Foods with sugar include fruit, sweets, soft drinks, and milk. (Milk contains lactose, or milk sugar.)

Nutrition Facts labels can be useful. Check the product label for grams of carbohydrate. Count every 15 grams of carbohydrate shown as one carbohydrate choice. Or, simply add the grams of carbohydrate from product labels to the tally.

Understanding carbohydrate counting can seem complex at first, but with care and practice, this important skill is easy to master. If you use carbohydrate counting in your facility, check with your Registered Dietitian Nutritionist to determine how they calculate this for clients you work with.

Summary

The Certified Dietary Manager, Certified Food Protection Professional has many important responsibilities in supporting nutrition care. It is vital to understand the steps and procedures involved in order to provide the client with the best care possible.

Chapter References

RESOURCES	
Academy of Nutrition and Dietetics. Accessed September 18, 2019.	https://www.eatright.org
American Academy of Pediatrics Institute for Healthy Childhood Weight. Infant Feeding. Nestlé.*	https://ihcw.aap.org/Pages/infantfeeding.aspx
American Academy of Pediatrics. Professional Resources.*	https://www.aap.org/en-us/professional-resources/Pages/Professional-Resources.aspx
American Academy of Pediatrics. Where We Stand: Fruit Juice. Healthychildren.org. Updated May 19, 2017.*	https://www.healthychildren.org/English/healthy-living/nutrition/Pages/Where-We-Stand-Fruit-Juice.aspx
Ansel K. How Much Protein Do You Need, Really? Food & Nutrition. Published July 17, 2017.*	https://foodandnutrition.org/blogs/stone-soup/much-protein-need-really/
Centers for Disease Control and Prevention. Before Pregnancy. Updated February 26, 2020.*	https://www.cdc.gov/preconception/index.html
Department of Nutrition and Dietetics. Isha Hospital.*	http://www.ishahospital.com/department-of-nutrition-dietetics/
Guidelines for Feeding Healthy Infants. WIC Learning Online. Updated June 2017.*	https://wicworks.fns.usda.gov/wicworks/WIC_Learning_Online/support/job_aids/guide.pdf
Healthline Editorial Team. Nutritional Needs During Pregnancy. Healthline. Published May 24, 2017.*	https://www.healthline.com/health/pregnancy/nutrition
Legvold D, Salisbury K. Foodservice Management—by Design. 2nd Edition. Association of Nutrition & Foodservice Professionals; 2018	
Stang J, Story M. Nutrition Screening, Assessment, and Intervention. In: Stang J, Story M. *Guidelines for Adolescent Nutrition Services*. University of Minnesota: Center for Leadership, Education and Training in Maternal and Child Nutrition; 2005: 35-54.*	https://pdfs.semanticscholar.org/8fc2/97a0c9f9120247785d421ab139fbb89673e7.pdf
U.S. Department of Agriculture. Food Data Central. Agricultural Research Service.*	https://fdc.nal.usda.gov
U.S. Department of Agriculture. Food and Human Nutrition. National Agricultural Library. Accessed September 18, 2019.*	https://www.nal.usda.gov/food-and-human-nutrition
U.S. Department of Agriculture. MyPlate. Accessed September 18, 2020.*	https://www.choosemyplate.gov
US Food & Drug Administration. How to Understand and Use the Nutrition Facts Label. Updated March 11, 2020.*	https://www.fda.gov/food/new-nutrition-facts-label/how-understand-and-use-nutrition-facts-label

**Accessed March 21, 2020*

Chapter References (Continued)

RESOURCES	
U.S. Food and Drug Administration. Nutrition Labeling and Education Act (NLEA) Requirements – Attachment 1. Updated November 24, 2014.*	https://www.fda.gov/nutrition-labeling-and-education-act-nlea-requirements-attachment-1
U.S. Food and Drug Administration. Using the Nutrition Facts Label: For Older Adults. Updated March 11, 2020.*	https://www.fda.gov/food/new-nutrition-facts-label/using-nutrition-facts-label-older-adults
Waibel RA. Religion and Dietary Practices. Faqs.org.*	http://www.faqs.org/nutrition/Pre-Sma/Religion-and-Dietary-Practices.html
World Health Organization. Breastfeeding.*	https://www.who.int/health-topics/breastfeeding#tab=tab_1

**Accessed March 21, 2020.*

Implement Physician's Dietary Orders

Overview and Objectives

Like the menu in the kitchen, the physician's dietary orders drive the clinical activities in the foodservice department. After completing this chapter, you should be able to:

- Recognize medical and nutrition terminology
- Demonstrate sensitivity to client needs and food habits
- Provide needed diets from the Foodservice Department
- Determine availability of foods from the kitchen
- Exhibit competency in suggesting the correct diet orders for clients
- Include patient input on diet prescribed by physician
- Recognize appropriateness of diet order for diagnosis
- Explain the importance of adhering to the written diet orders

Remember the discussion about the diet manual that the facility adopts which was covered in Chapter 9? Once there is a physician's diet order, the next step is making sure the diet is translated into food on a plate based on the recommendations from the approved diet manual. The diet manual will assist the Certified Dietary Manager®, Certified Food Protection Professional® (CDM®, CFPP®) and other healthcare professionals to interpret the diet order. The purpose of the diet manual is to establish a common resource with practice guidelines for all healthcare professionals to use as a guide when providing nutrition care for clients. The decision on which diet manual will be used should be made by the interdisciplinary team, recommended with input from the Registered Dietitian Nutritionist, and approved by the medical director at the facility. Here are some guidelines to use to evaluate the diet manual:

1. Make sure the manual includes the most current information on diets based on research findings.
2. Choose a manual that uses a standard such as the Dietary Reference Intakes (DRIs).
3. Look for manuals that include diets routinely ordered in the facility.
4. Use only as a guide.

When a decision has been made on a diet manual, it may need some customization for the facility. This discussion should be led by the Registered Dietitian Nutritionist along with the rest of the interdisciplinary team to ensure clarity in diet orders:

- Add standard diet terminology from the facility to assist in providing a common language.
- Have a sign-off sheet so that each member of the interdisciplinary team and the physician has approved the diet manual. The sign-off sheet should be updated annually.
- Place the manual on all floors, at each nursing station, or each unit, in the diet office, and in the kitchen. Another option is to have the diet manual available electronically.
- Make sure everyone knows where it is and how to use it.

View the Supplemental Material to see Figure 12.1 Sample Diet Order.

Obtaining a Physician's Diet Order

How the physician's diet order is received may vary depending upon the type of facility. For instance, in the hospital, it may be received via a phone call from the floor nurse giving the diet order information for a new client. At this point, it is important to ask for written documentation of the diet order to assure accuracy. Each facility should have a policy and procedure as to how diet orders are communicated. Many facilities use standardized forms. See Figure 12.1 in the Supplemental Material for a sample diet order notification/communication form. Many facilities use communication forms like this as a trackable way for nursing to communicate to the foodservice department any new diet orders for patients or residents who are newly admitted or have a change in their diet order.

Another method of obtaining the diet order is to review the health record. There is often a section in the record called Physician's Orders, which will include the diet order. With the advent of electronic health records, physicians may issue their orders electronically. No matter how the order is received, it must be interpreted and implemented for each client.

To interpret the Physician's Diet Order, it is important to know standard medical terminology such as CHF, Dx, NPO, and others. Review the terminology chart in

Chapter 9 and keep it handy when reading the physician's orders. If ever in doubt about how an order reads, be sure to consult with the Registered Dietitian Nutritionist or Registered Nurse for clarification.

Interpreting the Diet Order

The CDM, CFPP assists the client to translate their clinical treatment (physician's diet order) into appropriate food choices. As part of the nutrition screening process, the interview will help communicate and clarify the diet order with the client. An important part of the process is to demonstrate sensitivity to patient needs and food habits and translate them into food that will be consumed. What response might be given to a client who doesn't want to follow their diet order? Is this an issue?

A movement or paradigm shift is occurring in institutional care: To involve clients in choices about their diet, their meal times, and their dining locations. Centers for Medicare & Medicaid Services (CMS) guidelines have an increased focus on providing person-centered care (also called person-directed culture), giving client/family/guardians more voice about desires and will of the client.

CMS and the Pioneer Network

CMS notes that the most frequent questions and concerns received by their staff focus on the physical environment and dining/food policies in nursing homes. Therefore, in 2010 Pioneer Network and CMS held their second co-sponsored national symposium, Creating Home II National Symposium on Culture Change and the Food and Dining Requirements, sponsored by the Hulda B. & Maurice L. Rothschild Foundation. The Symposium brought together a wide group of stakeholders, including nursing home staff, regulators, provider leadership, researchers, Registered Dietitian Nutritionists, vendors, and advocates for culture change.

In August 2011, Pioneer Network announced the **New Dining Practice Standards**. The Pioneer Network promotes culture change in long-term care to meet the needs of clients. The New Dining Practice Standards were established by convening a group of stakeholders/organizations with a vested interest in this topic.

Organizations that participated in and now endorse/agree to the New Dining Practice Standards include: Long Term Care Nurses Assocation (LTCNA), American Association of Nurse Assessment Coordination (AANAC), Academy of Nutrition and Dietetics (Academy), American Medical Directors Association (AMDA), American Occupational Therapy Association (AOTA), American Society of Consultant Pharmacists (ASCP), American Speech-Language-Hearing Association (ASHA), Association of Nutrition & Foodservice Professionals (ANFP), Gerontological Advanced Practice Nurses Association (GAPNA), Hartford Institute for Geriatric Nursing (HIGN), National Association of Directors of Nursing Administration in Long Term Care (NADONA/LTC), and the National Gerontological Nursing Association (NGNA).

According to the Pioneer Network, "These nationally agreed upon new food and dining standards of practice support individualized care and self-directed living versus traditional diagnosis-focused treatment for people living in nursing homes. The Food and Dining Clinical Standards Task Force made a significant effort to obtain evidence and thus the New Dining Practice Standards document reflects evidence-based research available to-date." (2011)

GLOSSARY

New Dining Practice Standards
Standards for resident dining as developed by the Pioneer Network to enhance person-centered care at mealtime and support the use of liberalized diets in long-term care

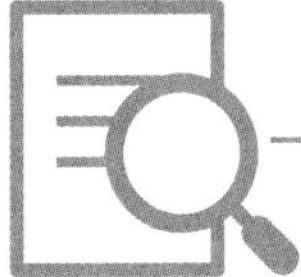

Updates to revised Pioneer Network Dining Standards can be found in the Supplemental Material when available.

The document includes the following new Standards of Practice:

- Individualized Nutrition Approaches/Diet Liberalizations
- Individualized Diabetic/Calorie Controlled Diet
- Individualized Low Sodium Diet
- Individualized Cardiac Diet
- Individualized Altered Consistency Diet
- Individualized Tube Feeding
- Individualized Real Food First
- Individualized Honoring Choices
- Shifting Traditional Professional Control to Individualized Support of Self Directed Living
- New Negative Outcome

"Food and dining are an integral part of individualized care and self-directed living for several reasons, including: (1) the complexity of food and dining requirements when advancing models of culture change; (2) the importance of food and dining as a significant element of daily living; and (3) the most frequent questions and concerns CMS receives from regulators and providers consistently focus on dining and food policies in nursing homes. Therefore, this area is one most in need of national dialogue to improve the quality of life for persons living in nursing homes while maintaining safety and quality of care." Let's examine how to improve a client's quality of life through food in a long-term care facility.

Implementing the Diet Order

In long-term care facilities, preventing weight loss and malnutrition may override the need for clients to follow a strict therapeutic diet. Healthcare professionals are finding that general diets may improve outcomes because clients are more willing to eat foods that have not been modified for therapeutic diets.

According to documents included in the New Dining Standards from the Pioneer Network, the Centers for Medicare & Medicaid Services (CMS) states "Liberalized diets should be the norm, restricted diets should be the exception. Generally weight stabilization and adequate nutrition are promoted by serving the residents a "regular" or minimally restricted diet. Research suggests that a liberalized diet can enhance the quality of life and nutritional status of older adults in long-term care facilities. Thus, it is often beneficial to minimize restrictions, consistent with a resident's condition, prognosis, and choices before using supplementation. It may also be helpful to provide the residents their food preferences, before using supplementation. This pertains to newly-developed meal plans as well as to the review of existing diets.

Dietary restrictions, therapeutic (e.g., low fat or sodium restricted) diets and mechanically altered diets may help in selected situations. At other times, they may impair adequate nutrition and lead to further decline in nutritional status, especially in already undernourished or at-risk individuals. When a resident is not eating well or is losing weight, the interdisciplinary team may temporarily discontinue dietary restrictions and liberalize the diet to improve the resident's food intake to try to stabilize their weight. Sometimes, a resident or resident's representative decides to decline recommended dietary restrictions and MNT. In such circumstances, the client, facility, and practitioner work together to identify alternatives for care (CMS Tag F 325 Nutrition).

The current thinking is given that most nursing home residents are at risk for malnutrition and may in fact have different, therapeutic targets for blood pressure, blood sugar, and cholesterol, a regular or liberalized diet which allows for resident choice is most often the preferred initial choice. As with any medical issue, residents should be monitored for desired outcomes as well as for potential adverse effects. Some homes have actually made the "regular" diet with ranges of consistency modifications such as "puree to mechanical soft" their only available option, then honored the resident's choice to eliminate "not recommended" foods by his/her choice, then monitored his/her clinical outcomes and made changes as necessary. That being said, homes with transitional care units or that serve younger disabled people may choose to offer the more restrictive diets as an option for long-term health.

All persons moving into a nursing home should receive a regular diet unless there is a strong medical historical reason to initiate/continue a restricted diet. Those who require modified diets can be assessed by the dietitian or physician, and if necessary the speech therapist or interdisciplinary team members. There needs to be continuous monitoring when using modified diets to ensure that they continue to be medically indicated, much the same way using other medical devices is monitored. When potential interventions have the ability to both help and harm, such as modified diets and thickened liquids, the interventions should be reviewed by the interdisciplinary team and discussed with the client and/or their family/power of attorney prior to their implementation. Clients and/or their families/power of attorney should be educated regarding these interventions and the care plan monitored for both safety and effectiveness. The physician and interdisciplinary team should treat disease *provided* it is consistent with the client's goals for care, is *supported* by the literature, and *does not decrease quality of life.*"

Let's use the example of an elderly client with diabetes and her physician's diet order of Consistent Carbohydrate Diabetic Diet. How does the CDM, CFPP implement this diet order to comply with CMS guidelines and current recommendations for diabetic diets? The first step is to meet with the Registered Dietitian Nutritionist to determine a calorie level and discuss how many carbohydrates might be used for meals and snacks. In this process, the diet manual is key in determining what the physician's order may be and how it may differ from what is written. What happens if the diet order received doesn't match the standard diets offered by the facility? Who is responsible to request the change should be determined by the facility's policies and procedures. If no policy exists, confer with your Registered Dietitian Nutritionist.

The second step is to work on menu modifications. Look at the regular menu and decide if any changes need to be made to the regular menu to offer a carbohydrate counting diet. Look at foods containing carbohydrates such as dairy products, vegetables, fruits, and bread. It is helpful to keep in mind that about 15 grams of carbohydrate is equal to one carb choice or "exchange." Count one carbohydrate exchange as one 'carb' on a carbohydrate counting diet. For a regular diet that also complies with a carbohydrate counting diet, it is typical to offer about three to five 'carb choices' at each meal and to provide 1500–2000 calories per day. If there are desserts on the menu that are more than three 'CHO choices,' it might be wise to consider eliminating them from the regular menu. The menu will be more in line with the Dietary Guidelines and MyPlate.

By making the regular menu fit the carbohydrate counting diet, it eliminates the need for a menu extension. Each time a diet extension can be eliminated, it will save food budget dollars and staff preparation time. By developing a regular menu that also meets other therapeutic diet needs, it results in serving a less complex and healthier menu. Better yet, the client with diabetes (and other medical conditions) will be more satisfied with their diet.

View the Supplemental Material to see Figure 12.2 Training Handout.

The third step is education for clients, staff, and family members. They may not understand why the client/family member is being served a piece of pumpkin pie instead of a gelatin dessert. For staff, make use of training sessions or in-service training time to educate the interdisciplinary team about implementing diet orders. The CDM, CFPP and Registered Dietitian Nutritionist may want to develop handouts for physicians, nurses, and foodservice staff. See Figure 12.2 in the Supplemental Material for an example of a training handout.

The fourth step is to follow-up with clients. How do they like the diet? Do they understand the diet? The client may still prefer diabetic/sugar-free jellies and syrups. It will be important to monitor the amount of food consumed for clients with diabetes, as well as their fasting blood glucose, to make sure that the consistent carbohydrate regular diet is appropriate.

In acute care hospitals/facilities, some of the same steps for implementing the physician's diet orders apply. Using the scenario above, the first step would be meeting with the Registered Dietitian Nutritionist and other appropriate staff members to promote the idea of using a carbohydrate counting menu.

The second step, menu modification, will be a little different than in long-term care, particularly if clients select their own food choices. If a room service-style menu is used, it is important to identify all the carbohydrate foods and label them either with the number of 'carbs' or the grams of carbohydrate for each food. Include directions at the top of the menu to explain that the client should select, for example, three to five 'carbs' or 45 to 75 grams of carbohydrate for each meal.

Again, the third step is the same as in long-term care—providing education to clients, staff, physicians, and families. Provision of the education may change for the clients. For instance, the CDM, CFPP or the Registered Dietitian Nutritionist might be preparing them for reading food labels because they will be going home in the near future. Because this is acute care, understanding counting carbohydrates will be critical for floor nurses that might be providing food substitutions for pediatric clients.

Follow-up, or the fourth step, will also be a different process. In the acute care setting, the clientele may not stay for more than a few days. Nutrition follow-up may be part of a quality survey that is handled by the facility. If they return for an outpatient visit because they are having trouble balancing their carbohydrate choices and insulin doses, it may mean they need additional nutrition education provided by the Registered Dietitian Nutritionist.

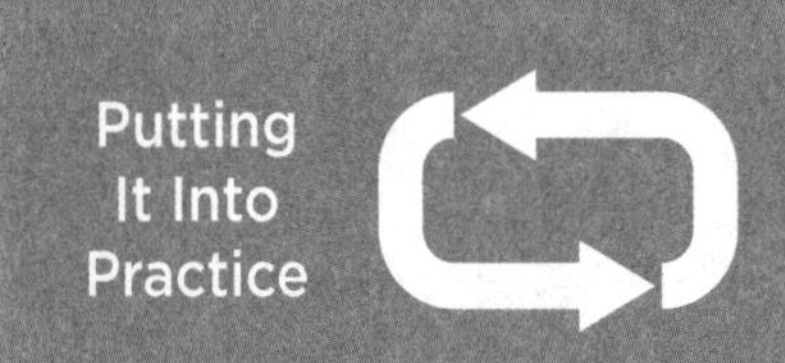

1. At lunch time, regular pumpkin pie is served to a elderly patient with diabetes who has not been eating well and she is on a liberalized regular diet. The patient enjoys the pie, however her husband feels she should not get dessert because of her diagnosis of diabetes. What should you do?

Provision of Diets from the Foodservice Department

Part of implementing the physician's dietary orders is providing the needed diets from the Foodservice Department. The CDM, CFPP will have the opportunity to respond to client requests to have foods that may not be on their diet order. For example, a client with diabetes may want potatoes for supper and it is not on the diet extension for a diabetic diet. This is another reason why moving to a carbohydrate counting diet will benefit the client. With a carbohydrate counting diet, the Certified Dietary Manager can honor this client request by providing this reasonable substitution.

In addition, the CDM, CFPP may also have to comply with other diet orders such as a 2-gm sodium diet or a restricted fat diet. Depending on the facility's menu extensions, it may be necessary to provide the client more information about meeting the diet order. For example, if the regular menu has glazed ham as an entrée, the menu extension would have a different entrée selection for a 2-gm sodium diet, such as roast pork. What if the client who is on the 2-gm sodium diet asks for glazed ham? What can be done to implement the physician's dietary orders and satisfy the client's request? Remember, according to the CMS guidelines, there is an increased focus on providing person-centered care. The response should be an explanation to the client what their diet order is and why, and if they still insist on having glazed ham, provide them with the glazed ham. Then, it is very important to document this conversation with the client and his/her menu choice in the health record (See Figure 12.3).

Appropriateness of the Diet Order

Not only is it important to provide the needed diets from the Foodservice Department, it is also essential to recognize the appropriateness of the diet order for the diagnosis. To determine if the diet order is appropriate for the diagnosis, begin with the health record. The record provides both the diet order and the diagnosis. This is when the application of all of the information learned in previous chapters comes into play. For instance, when conducting the nutrition screening, compare the information gathered to all of the medical diagnoses and determine the appropriate diet order. Then compare the information from what has been gathered to the diet order and see if they are in agreement.

Figure 12.3
When Clients Request a Food Not on Their Prescribed Diet

1. A client requests a food not on their prescribed diet.
2. Meet with the client and briefly discuss what their diet is and why, and listen to their request.
3. Relay the information to the RDN and the RN.
4. Discuss liberalizing the diet order with the physician. Follow up with the client.
5. Document the conversation and response in the medical record, include client input on the diet, and what was discussed/decided by the MD. Make changes as ordered by physician.

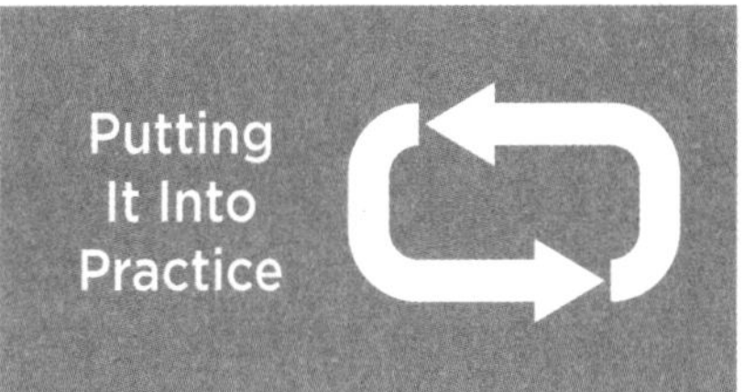

2. According to your estimate, how many 'carbs' are in this breakfast? 1 serving orange juice, 1 serving 2% milk, 1 serving oatmeal, 1 medium banana, and 1 hard-boiled egg?

Here is an example to consider: The nutrition screening for a new client, Herbert, shows the following information:

- Age at Admission: 80
- Height: 5'9"
- Weight: 117 lbs
- BUN: 97 g/sL
- Creatinine: 7.9 mg/dL
- Albumin: 2.9 mg/dL
- Potassium: elevated
- Blood Pressure: 150/92 mm Hg
- History: Herbert has had only one kidney since he was a child. Last year, after prostate surgery, he went into acute renal failure. Tests show his only kidney is declining in function. Herbert does not want dialysis or a transplant.
- Diet Order: 40 gm protein, 2 gm NA, and 2 gm K (potassium)

Is this diet order appropriate for Herbert? This may not be appropriate, as this diet order is a strict renal diet. Herbert does not want dialysis or a transplant and putting him on a strict renal diet will not improve his kidney function. He is already very underweight. In keeping with the CMS and Pioneer Network New Dining Practice Standards, Herbert might benefit from a regular diet to encourage him to eat and enjoy the time he has left. Refer your findings to the Registered Dietitian Nutritionist or contact the Director of Nursing with your concerns.

The interpretation and implementation of the diet order is a key component of nutrition care. The role of the CDM, CFPP is to translate the order into foods that are provided and consumed by the client.

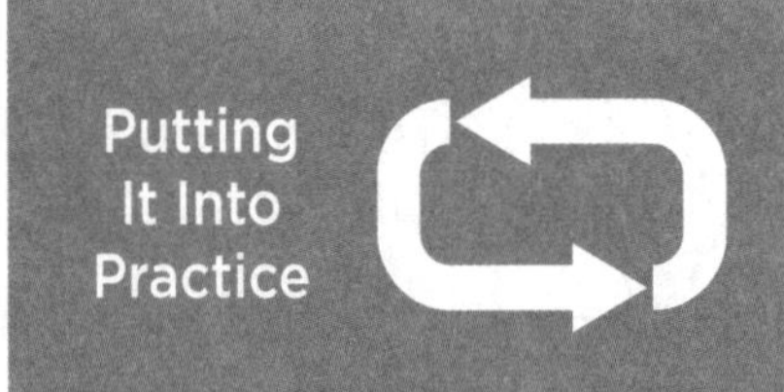

3. What steps should you take if a patient who is on the 2-gm sodium diet asks to have bacon with breakfast?

Chapter References

RESOURCES	
MED-PASS—Diet Order and Communication. Accessed March 30, 2020.	www.med-pass.com
Pioneer Network. Accessed March 27, 2020.	https://www.pioneernetwork.net/wp-content/uploads/2016/10/The-New-Dining-Practice-Standards.pdf.
Resources for Culture Change. Centers for Medicare & Medicaid Services (CMS). Accessed March 27, 2020.	https://partnershipforpatients.cms.gov/p4p_resources/tsp-culturechange/toolculturechange.html

Apply Standard Nutrition Care

Overview and Objectives

In order to apply standard nutrition care, the Certified Dietary Manager®, Certified Food Protection Professional® (CDM®, CFPP®) will need to use many tools. There are regulations and standards governing the healthcare industry that require planning, documentation, and ongoing clinical care following prescribed models. A CDM, CFPP plays a role in compliance to provide optimal care. After completing this chapter, you should be able to:

- Review the client's nutrition needs based on guidelines provided
- Assess and apply the nutrient content of foods to the foods delivered and consumed by the client
- Explain the purpose of the care plan
- List the steps involved in developing a nutrition care plan
- Identify sources to consult to assist in implementing nutrition care plans

Clinical care revolves around a care plan. Every good outcome hinges on advanced planning. Imagine a simple everyday task, such as going to the grocery store. Making a menu and a list of items to purchase will make a trip to the grocery store more effective. Let's say a client wanted to buy food to prepare dinner this evening. If that person goes to the grocery store unprepared (no idea of what to have), they won't know what is needed and what to buy. Upon arriving home, they might not be able to complete dinner preparation, perhaps due to missing ingredients needed for the dinner. Meanwhile, grocery aisles may tempt a person with things not needed. Money may be spent on impulse items instead of the items needed to cook a meal. Planning is needed and useful for a mundane task like grocery shopping, so imagine how critical it can be to provide medical care, where the stakes are high and the outcomes affect the quality of clients' lives profoundly.

Previous chapters discussed how the CDM, CFPP and the Registered Dietitian Nutritionist determine client needs based on established guidelines. Chapters 1 and 2 discussed the Dietary Guidelines for Americans, the USDA Food Patterns and MyPlate and nutrient needs for the population (based on the DRIs and the RDAs).Chapter 4 discussed modifications that need to be made if a client has a food allergy. In Chapters 5 and 6, the concepts and the appropriate medical nutrition therapy interventions for specific disease states were discussed. Chapter 7 outlined the process of obtaining nutrition screening data and how it is used to determine needs based on individual client data. In addition, it discussed how nutrient needs are determined based on this clinical data. Finally, Chapter 11 outlined how to determine the nutrient content in foods and how it is calculated. Please refer to these chapters for a review of this information.

Developing Comprehensive Care Plans

A care plan is a written plan of medical care for a client. It involves identifying the client's interests, preferences, abilities, and personal goals. It identifies objectives for helping a client reach the best possible physical, mental, social, spiritual well-being and other wellness goals. It describes steps that members of the healthcare team will take to assist the client in meeting goals and identifies the disciplines that will carry out the approaches. Each client has their own unique set of needs; thus they need a unique, individualized care plan. A care plan essentially charts the course for actions that members of the healthcare team will take to support and improve an individual's well-being. All members of the team use it as a focal point and driving force in their routine of care for clients. The care plan assures that team members' actions contribute toward assessed clinical needs and objectives that are entirely customized to each unique client. A care plan actually makes the work that each team member performs more effective. Let's examine the idea of a comprehensive care plan, and then examine the steps involved in developing a plan of care that specifically addresses nutrition.

The focus of Centers for Medicare & Medicaid Services (CMS) guidelines is client-centered care. CMS expects each facility to interview its clients so interdisciplinary team (IDT) members can "know the individual and what is meaningful to that person." In the past, "quality often reflected a judgment made by others" in developing a comprehensive care plan. By striving to include the client, CMS hopes to have less judgment by others and more input from the client. In today's healthcare environment, emphasis on teamwork is primary. That team begins with the client and includes interdisciplinary contributions to the care planning process. There has to be coordination among members of the team and ongoing communication among team members, including the client, in order to improve a client's quality of life.

Care planning is part of the RAI (Resident Assessment Instrument) process as shown in Figure 13.1.

Figure 13.1
Overview of the Resident Assessment Instrument (RAI) and Care Area Assessments (CAAs)

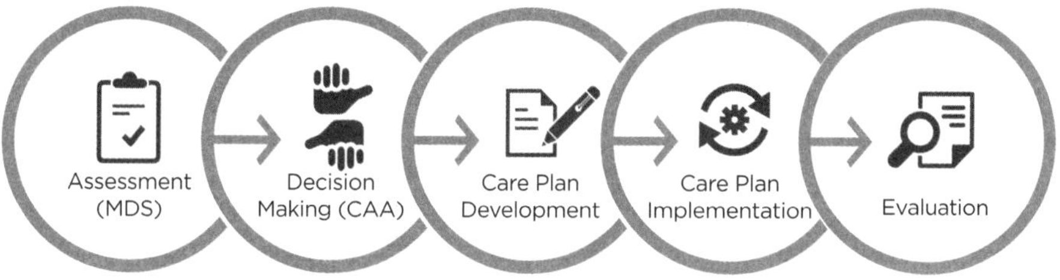

As team members develop a care plan together, it becomes a master plan that drives client-centered work carried out by individual professionals. A care plan developed by members of a coordinated healthcare team and that addresses the multi-faceted needs of a client is called a **comprehensive care plan**.

Per the RAI Manual 2019, it is important to note that for an Admission assessment, the resident enters the nursing home with a set of physician-based treatment orders. Nursing home staff should review these orders and begin to assess the resident and to identify potential care issues/problems. Within 48 hours of admission to the facility, the facility must develop and implement a Baseline Care Plan for the resident that includes the instructions needed to provide effective and person-centered care of the resident that meets professional standards of care (42 CFR §483.21(a)). After this the facility must develop a comprehensive care plan for each client that includes measurable objectives and timetables to meet a client's medical, mental, and psychosocial needs, which are identified in the comprehensive assessment. The plan of care must deal with both the relationship of services ordered to be provided (or withheld), and the facility's responsibility for fulfilling other requirements in these regulations.

According to the RAI Manual, Federal statute and regulations require that residents are assessed promptly upon admission (but no later than day 14) and the results are used in planning and providing appropriate care to attain or maintain the highest practicable well-being. This means it is imperative for nursing homes to assess a resident upon the individual's admission. The IDT may choose to start and complete the Admission comprehensive assessment at any time prior to the end of day 14. Nursing homes may find early completion of the MDS and **Care Area Assessments (CAAs)** beneficial to providing appropriate care, particularly for individuals with short lengths of stay when the assessment and care planning process is often accelerated.

CMS regulations further stipulate that an interdisciplinary team—in conjunction with the client, client's family, surrogate, or representative, as appropriate—should develop quantifiable objectives for the highest level of functioning the client may be expected to attain, based on the comprehensive assessment.

GLOSSARY

Care Planning
Establishing a course of action with input from the resident (resident's family and/or guardian or other legally authorized representative), resident's physician, and interdisciplinary team that moves a resident toward resident-specific goals utilizing individual resident strengths and interdisciplinary expertise; crafting the "how" of resident care

Comprehensive Care Plan
42 CFR 483.21(b)(2) A comprehensive care plan must be (ii) Prepared by an interdisciplinary team, that includes—but is not limited to—the attending physician, a registered nurse with responsibility for the resident, a nurse aide with responsibility for the resident, a member of food and nutrition services staff, and other appropriate staff or professionals in disciplines as determined by the resident's needs or as requested by the resident, and, to the extent practicable, the participation of the resident and the resident's representative(s)

Care Area Assessment (CAA)
A process designed to assist the assessor to systematically interpret the information recorded on the MDS and guide the clinician to focus on key issues identified during the assessment process

GLOSSARY

Care Area Triggers (CATs)
Specific resident responses for one or a combination of MDS elements that identify residents who have or are at risk for developing specific functional problems and require further assessment

According to the CMS interpretive guidelines, "the interdisciplinary team should show evidence in the CAA summary or clinical record of the following:

The client's status in triggered CAA areas (called **Care Area Triggers** [CATs]);

- The facility's rationale for deciding whether to proceed with care planning; and
- Evidence that the facility considered the development of care planning interventions for all CAAs triggered by the MDS."

The care plan must reflect intermediate steps for each outcome objective if identification of those steps will enhance the client's ability to meet his/her objectives. Staff will use these objectives to monitor client progress. Facilities may, for some clients, need to prioritize their care plan interventions. This should be noted in the health record or on the plan of care.

The requirements reflect the facility's responsibility to provide necessary care and services to attain or maintain the highest practicable physical, mental, and psychosocial well-being, in accordance with the comprehensive assessment and plan of care. However, in some cases, a client may refuse certain services or treatments that professional staff believe may be indicated. Desires of the client should be documented in the comprehensive assessment and reflected in the plan of care.

Following are some questions to consider when preparing a care plan:

- Does the care plan address the needs, strengths, and preferences identified in the client assessment, including the CAAs?
- Is the care plan oriented toward preventing avoidable declines in functioning or functioning levels?
- How does the care plan try to manage risk factors?
- Does the care plan build on the client's strengths?
- Does the care plan reflect standards of current dietetic practice?
- If the client refuses treatment, does the care plan explain alternatives to address the problem?
- Is the care plan evaluated and revised as the client's status changes?
- Does the care plan identify the healthcare professional that will carry out the approaches?
- Do treatment objectives have measurable outcomes?
- Does the care plan corroborate information regarding the client's goals and wishes for treatment?

Developing a comprehensive care plan is the responsibility of the interdisciplinary team. Although the physician must participate as part of the interdisciplinary team, he or she may arrange with the facility for alternative methods, other than attending care planning conferences, such as one-on-one discussions and conference calls.

Although the MDS and supplemental assessments give much information about the client's problems, they won't always identify or trigger them all. One purpose of the care plan conference is to help identify additional approaches for care. The Registered Dietitian Nutritionist and/or CDM, CFPP needs to identify a client's nutrition-related problems, set measurable goals with time limits, and determine appropriate interventions.

In long-term care, the care plan, which is part of the client's health record or electronic health record, is updated at least quarterly and as the client's condition changes. The date of the quarterly review is entered on the care plan. When a problem is no longer a problem, this needs to be noted on the care plan by highlighting it "Resolved" with the date of resolution next to it, or noting resolution in a computerized system.

Steps in Developing a Nutrition Care Plan

The nutrition care process involves screening clients for nutrition risk, nutritional assessment of clients, and development of a nutrition care plan addressing the clients' risks or identified problems. To learn more about the CAA, CAT, and Care Planning process please review RAI Manual Chapter 4 and MDS Assessments timing Chapter 2.

All care planning relates to a list of specified problems. These problems are pinpointed by various members of the healthcare team as they complete their respective assessments. As described above, members of the team tackle this list together. Aspects of the care plan are tightly interwoven among disciplines, and many plans require the efforts of multiple disciplines to succeed. Completing the detail of a plan is often up to the individual professionals involved. Once a plan is developed, the specifics of how it will be implemented follow. Afterwards, it is important to evaluate the effectiveness of care.

For clients who are not new admissions, be alert for significant changes in the client's health. Those changes can be either a decline or an improvement. Not all changes in a client's health status require a new care plan. If a client has the flu for a week and then recovers, a care plan isn't required. If the decline or improvement is consistent over two weeks and it covers two or more areas of decline or improvement, begin a comprehensive reassessment as soon as possible. Refer to Figure 13.2 for characteristics of decline or improvement according to MDS 3.0. For clients with no significant changes, a comprehensive reassessment including care planning is required every quarter or every 90 days.

For new clients, an admission MDS assessment must be completed within 14 days of their stay, with a baseline care plan developed within 48 hours of admission. Whether for a new client or a current client, the overall care plan should focus on the following:

- Preventing avoidable declines in functioning or functional levels, or clarifying why another goal takes precedence
- Managing risk factors to the extent possible or indicating the limits of the interventions
- Addressing ways to try to preserve and build upon client strengths
- Applying current standards of practice in the care planning process
- Evaluating treatment of measurable objectives, timetables, and outcomes of care
- Respecting the client's right to decline treatment, such as deciding to take a nourishment by mouth or tube feeding

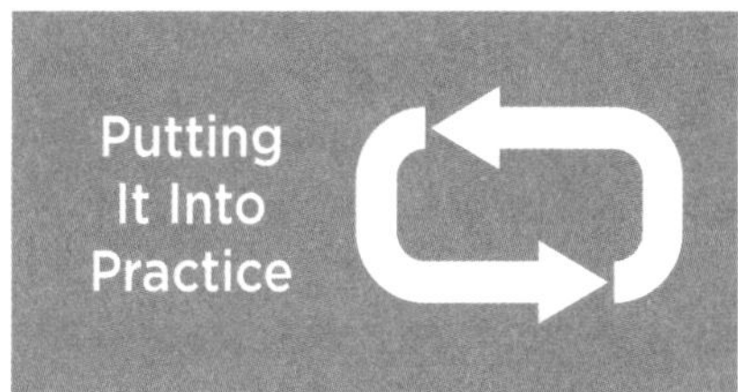

1. What are some ways to develop a person-centered care plan for your clients?

- Offering alternative treatments as applicable
- Using an appropriate interdisciplinary approach to develop a care plan that will improve the client's functional abilities
- Involving client, client's family, and other client representatives as appropriate
- Assessing and planning for care to meet the client's medical, physical, mental, and psychosocial needs
- Addressing additional care planning areas that are relevant to meeting the client's needs in the long-term care setting

Here are some basic steps for the nutrition care planning process:

Step 1. Gather Nutrition Screening Data/Identify Nutrition Problems

To determine the need for care planning, CAAs are developed from items coded on the Minimum Data Set (MDS). The MDS is a preliminary assessment to identify potential client problems, strengths, and preferences. Care areas are triggered by MDS item responses that indicate the need for additional assessment based on problem identification. There are 20 CAAs in Version 3.0 of the Resident Assessment Instrument (RAI) (refer to Figure 9.10 in Chapter 9). Ideally, the RAI is completed by the Interdisciplinary Team (IDT) that will develop the client's care plan. The following guidelines can help the team develop a meaningful statement of the problem:

- Be as specific as possible.
- State the problem as it relates to the client.
- Identify possible reasons for the problem, including the client's perspective.
- Identify any strength the client has that will help in overcoming the problem.

IDT role. The IDT uses clinical problem-solving and decision-making steps (see Figure 13.3) to make decisions. The team may find several problems/issues/conditions that have a related cause or they might be unrelated. Goals and approaches for each issue/

Figure 13.2
Characteristics of Decline or Improvement

CHARACTERISTIC OF DECLINE	CHARACTERISTIC OF IMPROVEMENT
• Client's ability to make decisions for themselves declines • Change in client's mood or an increase in the symptom frequency • Any change in ADL physical functioning area such as from limited assistance to extensive assistance • Client's incontinence pattern changes or there is placement of a catheter • Unplanned weight loss (5% change in 30 days or 10% change in 180 days) • Client begins to use trunk restraint or a chair that prevents rising when it was not used before • Overall deterioration of resident's condition	• Any improvement in an ADL physical functioning area such as a change from limited assistance to independent • Decrease in the number of areas where behavioral symptoms are coded as being present and/or the frequency of a symptom decreases • Client's ability to make decisions for themselves improves • Client's incontinence pattern improves • Overall improvement of client's condition

Source: CMS's RAI Version 3.0, Chapter 3

Figure 13.3
Clinical Problem-Solving and Decision-Making Process Steps and Objectives

PROCESS STEP/OBJECTIVES	KEY TASKS
Recognition/Assessment *Gather essential information about the individual*	• Identify and collect information that is needed to identify an individual's condition that enables proper definition of their conditions, strengths, needs, risks, problems, and prognosis • Obtain a personal and medical history • Perform a physical assessment
Problem Definition *Define the individual's problems, risks, and issues*	• Identify any current consequences and complications of the individual's situation, underlying condition, and illnesses, etc. • Clearly state the individual's issues and physical functions, psychosocial strengths, problems, needs, and deficits and concerns
Diagnosis/Cause-and-Effect Analysis *Identify physical, functional, and psychosocial causes of risks, problems, and other issues, and relate to one another and to their consequences*	• Identify causes of, and factors contributing to, the individual's current dysfunctions, disabilities, impairments, and risks • Identify pertinent evaluations and diagnostic tests • Identify how existing symptoms, signs, diagnoses, test results, dysfunctions, impairments, disabilities, and other findings relate to one another • Identify how addressing those causes is likely to affect consequences
Identifying Goals and Objectives of Care *Clarify purpose of providing care and of specific interventions and the criteria that will be used to determine whether the objectives are being met*	• Clarify prognosis • Define overall goals for the individual • Identify criteria for meeting goals
Selecting Interventions/Planning Care *Identify and implement interventions and treatments to address the individual's physical, functional, and psychosocial needs, concerns, problems, and risks*	• Identify specific symptomatic and cause-specific interventions (physical, functional, and psychosocial) • Identify how current and proposed treatment and services are expected to address causes, consequences, and risk factors, and help attain overall goals for the individual • Define anticipated benefits and risks of various interventions • Clarify how specific treatments and services will be evaluated for their effectiveness

Source: CMS's RAI Version 3.0, Chapter 4

condition may overlap and the IDT may decide to address those areas collectively in the care plan. The care planning issue is documented as part of the Care Area Assessment (CAA) review.

CDM, CFPP/Registered Dietitian Nutritionist role. Conduct nutrition screening, collect and verify data needed to determine nutrition problems. Care Area Triggers (CATs) of greatest interest to the CDM, CFPP and Registered Dietitian Nutritionist include falls, nutritional status, feeding tube, change in dentition or dental condition, dehydration/fluid maintenance, and pressure ulcers. Care planning should include provisions for monitoring the client during mealtimes and during activities that include the consumption of food. Consider the following:

- What risk factors for decline of eating skills were identified?
  - > Decrease in the ability to chew and swallow food
  - > Deficit in the ability to move food onto a utensil and into the mouth
  - > Changes in oral health status affecting eating/chewing ability
  - > Depression or confused mental state
- What care is the client receiving to address risk factors to maintain eating abilities?
  - > Assistive devices to improve client's ability to grasp or coordination
  - > Seating arrangement to improve sociability
  - > Seating in a calm, quiet setting for clients with dementia

Step 2. Assess the Client

Interview the client to determine if the triggered condition affects the client's functioning or well-being. If it isn't a concern for the client, it should not be addressed on the care plan. Make sure to address issues such as the timing of the meals with the client. For instance, the client may request a late breakfast. In this case, the client's wishes should be honored and documented in the health record and alternatives should be offered and documented in the care plan.

Step 3. Complete Nutrition Screening/Assessment and Complete MDS/Care Plan

IDT role. Gather data for their respective areas. The IDT will want to document how identified conditions are a problem for the client or how the condition affects the client's well-being.

CDM, CFPP role. The CDM, CFPP provides nutrition screening data for use by the Registered Dietitian Nutritionist in the assessment of a client's nutrition needs, and is familiar with standardized calculations of calories, protein, and fluid needs. Refer to Chapter 7 for methods of estimating needs for these nutrients.

Also, be aware that the healthcare facility or the Registered Dietitian Nutritionist may provide alternate methodologies. Calculation schemes may also be part of policies and procedures, **nutrition care protocols, standards of practice,** and/or regulations. Standards of practice are documents that define what constitutes quality in practice. They are standards addressing the role of the CDM, CFPP. For example, a standard of practice will outline how a CDM, CFPP documents in the health record. In standardized terminology developed by the Academy of Nutrition and Dietetics there are 62 specific phrases to describe nutrition diagnoses. **Care protocols** are documents that outline a care process related to a specific medical condition. For example, a facility may have a care protocol for pressure ulcers that lists some standard steps that must be taken and describes how each member of the healthcare team will contribute. The Academy of Nutrition and Dietetics has developed a systematic process to describe care for clients. This process is called the Nutrition Care Process. As the CDM, CFPP, become familiar with the standards that apply in the facility, and work with the Registered Dietitian Nutritionist to apply them consistently.

A copy of the ANFP Standards of Practice for the CDM, CFPP and the Scope of Practice for the CDM, CFPP can be found in the Supplemental Nutrition Textbook Materials.

GLOSSARY

Standards of Practice
Documents that define what constitutes quality of practice

Nutrition Care Protocols
Detailed written set of instructions to guide the care of a patient or to assist the practitioner in the performance of a procedure related to specific medical conditions

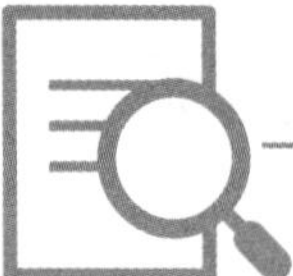

Please see the Supplemental Material for a copy of the ANFP Standard of Practice for the CDM, CFPP and the Scope of Practice for the CDM, CFPP.

Figure 13.4
Example of Care Planning Goal Statement

Subject	Verb	Modifiers	Time Frame	Goal
Mr. Jones	will consume	72 oz. liquid daily	the next 30 days	to maintain hydration and prevent UTIs.

Step 4. Determine and Agree on Goal(s)

IDT role. Agrees upon goal(s) that will lead to outcome objectives. The goal(s) and objectives must be pertinent to the client's condition and situation, be measurable, and have a time frame for completion or evaluation. Parts of the goal statement should include: The subject [first or third person, the verb, the modifiers, the time frame, and the goal(s)]. (See Figure 13.4 for example.) Types of goals may include improvement, prevention, treatment to alleviate disease symptoms, or maintenance of current status. Goals should be prioritized based on client preferences if possible.

CDM, CFPP role. If the Registered Dietitian Nutritionist is not present, the CDM, CFPP is responsible for understanding and relaying any nutrition diagnoses and care standards that the Registered Dietitian Nutritionist has identified to the IDT team and the MDS Nurse/Care Plan Coordinator. Be sure to confirm that the nutrition goal is feasible and can be served/produced/monitored.

Step 5. Identify Specific Steps or Approaches

IDT role. Using input from the client, family, and/or client representative, the IDT identifies specific steps, approaches, or tasks that will be taken to help the client achieve his or her goal(s). These approaches serve as instructions for client care and provide for continuity of care by all staff. They should include precise and concise instructions to help staff understand and implement interventions.

The client has the right to participate in care planning and the right to refuse treatment. The final care plan should be agreed to and discussed with the client or the representative.

CDM, CFPP role. Writing the goal(s) and specific steps/approaches may be an electronic process in the facility. Become familiar with the documentation process for care planning (may vary from facility to facility) and apply this information to that process. The Registered Dietitian Nutritionist may be responsible for writing the care plan. The nutrition care documentation should comply with the regulations and document the steps taken to meet the client's requests/needs/strengths.

Some examples of approaches for a goal to increase food intake might be: enhancing the taste and presentation of food; assisting the client to eat; addressing food preferences; and increasing finger foods and snacks for individuals with dementia.

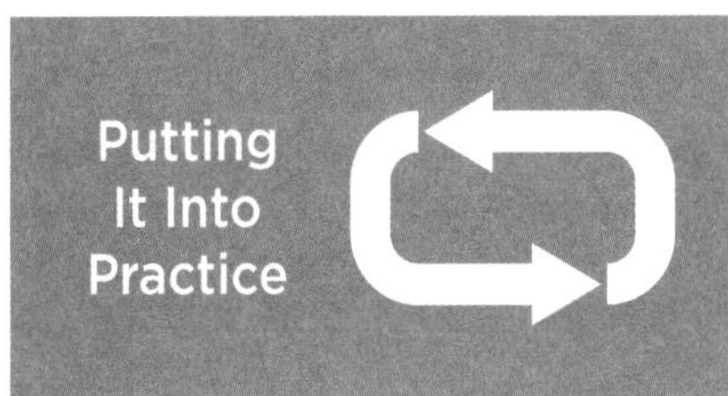

2. Write a goal statement for Mr. Bravard, who is having more difficulty feeding himself and has been eating an average of about 50% of his meals in the past 30 days. He has also lost 2 pounds this week.

Step 6. Communicate the Goal(s) and Objectives

DT role. The goals and objectives/approaches should be communicated to other direct care staff who were not directly involved in developing the care plan. Changes to the care plan should occur as needed in accordance with professional standards of practice and documentation (e.g., signing and dating entries to the care plan). IDT members should communicate as needed about changes to the care plan.

CDM, CFPP role. Communicate the goal(s) and objectives/approaches to the nutrition care staff and participate in care plan meetings/client care conferences. Be responsible for alerting the Registered Dietitian Nutritionist to any changes in the client's condition, especially significant changes that may require a reassessment. Follow the facility's policy and procedures for communicating with the Registered Dietitian Nutritionist and the IDT. It may be necessary to schedule staff training, depending upon the goal(s) and objectives/approaches.

Step 7. Evaluate the Effectiveness of the Care Plan

This final step will be addressed in Chapter 14.

Evaluating the effectiveness of the care plan will be addressed in the next chapter (Chapter 14). The CDM, CFPP's role in the development, monitoring, and evaluation is critical.

Chapter References

RESOURCES	
Academy of Nutrition and Dietetics: Position Paper. "Position of the Academy of Nutrition and Dietetics: Individualized Nutrition Approaches for Older Adults in Health Care Communities": 2010. Accessed March 30, 2020.	eatrightpro.org. https://www.eatrightpro.org/news-center/nutrition-trends/foodservice-and-food-safety/individualized-nutrition-approaches-for-older-adults-in-health-care-communities
Care Area Assessment Summary—AANAC. MDS 3.0—Centers for Medicare & Medicaid Services (CMS). Accessed March 30, 2020.	https://www.leadingage.org/nursing-home-rop-tools-and-resources-0
Centers for Medicare & Medicaid Services (CMS)	http://www.cms.gov
LeadingAge	http://www.leadingage.org/
LeadingAge California	http://communities.leadingageca.org/home
Long Term Care Minimum Data Set—Centers for Medicare & Medicaid Services (CMS). Accessed March 30, 2020.	https://www .cms .gov/Research-Statistics-Data-and-Systems/Files-for-Order/IdentifiableDataFiles/LongTermCareMinimumDataSetMDS .html
MDS 3.0 Training - Centers for Medicare & Medicaid Services (CMS). Accessed March 30, 2020.	https://www .cms .gov/Medicare/Quality-Initiatives-Patient-Assessment-Instruments/NursingHomeQualityInits/NHQIMDS30TrainingMaterials .html
Programs for Elderly. Accessed March 30, 2020.	Programsforelderly.com
RAI Manual - Centers for Medicare & Medicaid Services (CMS). Accessed March 30, 2020.	https://www.cms.gov/Medicare/Quality-Initiatives-Patient-Assessment-Instruments/NursingHomeQualityInits/MDS30RAIManual

Review Effectiveness of Nutrition Care and Manage Professional Communication

Overview and Objectives

To be effective, nutrition care must be dynamic. A Certified Dietary Manager®, Certified Food Protection Professional® (CDM®, CFPP®) and the interdisciplinary team must routinely assess new information and apply findings to ongoing plans for quality care. Effective communication is key to the work of the interdisciplinary team. After completing this chapter, you should be able to:

- Describe interdisciplinary relationships
- Communicate client information to the interdisciplinary team members
- Prepare and participate in client care conferences
- Identify effectiveness of the nutrition care plan
- Identify what client information needs to be communicated
- Evaluate care plans for individual needs
- Implement goals and approaches with appropriate follow-up
- Identify the need for client referrals
- Implement consultant recommendations as appropriate
- Honor clients' rights and confidentiality
- Work with the interdisciplinary team to develop solutions

14

The interdisciplinary team (IDT) is a group of professionals, each with unique training and expertise, who contribute to the overall care of a client. Thus, a CDM, CFPP works closely with the other team members to provide care to the client. Communication is the key that allows all of these professionals to work together and coordinate care. Let's take a look at communication channels, care conference communication, and typical roles and responsibilities, particularly as they relate to nutrition care.

As was discussed in Chapter 8, communication is not only important when interviewing the client, but also when coordinating care for the client. Communicating clearly is the key to success when working with the client, the family, and the interdisciplinary team. Remember, communication is a two-way process in order to be effective. In this discussion about effective interdisciplinary team communication, let's briefly review the basics of good communication.

There are three types of communication: written, verbal, and nonverbal. The CDM, CFPP uses all three types of communication to interact with the interdisciplinary team, or IDT. Written communication is generally done as part of documentation in the health record. The health record acts as the pivotal point for medical information. As was learned in Chapter 9, the health record contains information regarding the client. It is a document of the client's medical history, which is utilized by all of the interdisciplinary team members. In previous chapters, the health record was used to gather data relating to the client as well, as a place for the nutrition care team to document the medical nutrition therapy that is provided. Written communication can also be performed via memorandum and by email. Verbal and nonverbal communication are used daily by the CDM, CFPP. Who interacts with the nutrition care team and members of the IDT. More formal communication regarding a client's status takes place at the client care conference.

The client care conference is a time for the client, family, and interdisciplinary team to gather and discuss the progress and status of the client. It is important for the client and the family to be present if they are able. At the care conference, the team (including the client and family) discusses the current status of the client and the plan for the future. It is a time set aside to focus solely on the care of each individual client. During the care conference, each of the IDT members is given the opportunity to speak about the specifics of the care that is given by each medical discipline (MD, RN, OT, etc.). In many cases, the CDM, CFPP is the one to represent the work of the nutrition care team. This care conference provides an opportunity for the CDM, CFPP to discuss the nutrition care and intervention plan with the client, the family, and the rest of the IDT.

How does the CDM, CFPP prepare for and participate in the care conference? Below are some basic steps that are important to follow when communicating at the care conference:

- Prepare for the care conference.
  - Review the nutrition screening, nutrition assessment, and nutrition care plan to become familiar with the information.
  - Identify what client information needs to be communicated.
  - Talk with the Registered Dietitian Nutritionist if there is a question about what needs to be communicated.
  - Review nutrition progress notes to update the dietary records and the nutrition screening/assessment, if necessary.
  - Review the nutrition care plan and document any changes to the care plan.

  - Review progress made towards the goals of the nutrition care plan.
  - Review goals with the Registered Dietitian Nutritionist and prioritize nutrition goals.
  - Prepare for what will be said regarding the status of the client—a bulleted list of facts may be useful to guide what will be communicated.
  - If the Registered Dietitian Nutritionist is not available to attend the care conference, it may be necessary to report on his/her behalf.
  - Anticipate how the client and/or family might react or respond to the nutrition care plan and be prepared to answer questions.
  - Convey the message to the IDT in regards to the nutrition care plan.
  - Report on referrals made to other IDT members.
  - Report the progress made towards the goals of the nutrition care plan and update/set new goals as warranted.
- Be actively involved during the care conference.
  - Listen and receive information from the other IDT members at the care conference.
  - Be listening for "new" information that impacts nutrition care.
  - Look for the key points and specific answers to questions regarding client care.
  - Give feedback to acknowledge understanding.
  - Ask questions for clarification.
  - Discuss issues and concerns revealed in the care conference and work with the IDT to problem-solve regarding the improvement of client care.
  - Listen intently to the client and family until there is a mutual understanding of their concerns.

The care conference is an important time to discuss the client in depth in a roundtable fashion with all of the IDT members present. This is the best time for the client and family to ask questions with all of the team members present, and to discuss the wants and needs of the client to ensure appropriate care is given. At the conclusion of the care conference, there may be more coordination needed based on the needs of the client. If that is the case, the CDM, CFPP will again need to communicate with the Registered Dietitian Nutritionist and other members of the IDT in order to develop a plan for intervention, implement goals and approaches, as well as develop a plan for appropriate evaluation and follow up.

Reflection is an important part of a care conference. Upon conclusion of the care conference, it may be valuable to think about the nutrition information and care that needed to be communicated. Here are some points to think about and review:

- After the care conference is over, evaluate the effectiveness of the communication given.
  - Were there key items that were forgotten?
  - Is there a way to more clearly convey a message or information?
  - Was the jargon used understandable by the client and family?
  - Was the message clear?
  - What follow up questions can be anticipated from participants?

If there were some barriers to communication, remember these important tips:

- Overcome the communication barriers.
  - > Message quality: If using technical terms, be sure to explain them. Even though the IDT may be familiar with the jargon, the client and the family may need more clarity. Continue to seek feedback in the care conference by asking questions such as, "Should we go through that again?" Focus clearly on what is needed and why it is needed. Ask for clarification from other IDT members, the client, and family as needed.
  - > Time: Before beginning the care conference, make sure that there is enough time to complete the care conference. Try to "free up" the time from other distractions (pager, phone, other meetings, etc.).
  - > Conflict: If there is conflict, remain factual, understanding, and professional.

The Role of the Interdisciplinary Team in Coordination of Care

Administrator (in a Nursing Home)

Roles and responsibilities:

- Ensure that a nutritional screening/assessment system exists.
- Ensure adequacy of staffing to implement and maintain the system.
- Support all staff members in performing their duties.

Coordination of care: The Administrator is responsible for the overall running of the facility and is the visionary for the coordination of care. Depending on the facility and its structure, the CDM, CFPP may or may not have much contact with the Administrator. However, the support of the Administrator is critical to overall care provided at the facility to clients. As the CDM, CFPP, it is important to understand the philosophy of the facility, how the foodservice operation supports the facility in the care of clients, the expectations for the foodservice department, including the budget, and how the nutrition care team functions in the environment.

Registered Dietitian Nutritionist

Roles and responsibilities:

- Assume primary responsibility and accountability for nutrition screening and assessment, and client nutrition care planning. (This is why the CDM, CFPP should have ongoing communication with the Registered Dietitian Nutritionist.)
- Select and set up a nutrition screening/assessment system (in coordination with the nursing service and facility administration); train facility staff as needed.
- Perform nutritional assessments; may complete the Resident Assessment Instrument (RAI) and care plan.
- Develop nutrition care plan.
- Record assessment findings, recommendations, and follow-up plans in medical record and client care plan.
- Alert other team members to any part of the nutritional care plan needing their cooperation.
- Define the role of a CDM, CFPP in clinical care and provide training.
- Provide nutrition counseling.

- Monitor the screening system.
- Monitor the accuracy of diet service.
- Participate in quality management.
- May participate in client care conferences.

Coordination of care: The CDM, CFPP and the Registered Dietitian Nutritionist work closely together to coordinate care. Depending on the facility, the RDN may only be physically present on a monthly basis (or more often). The CDM, CFPP needs to have open lines of communication with the RDN in order to effectively implement the nutrition care plan. Any significant change in client status should be referred and communicated within 24-48 hours to ensure that quality care is provided.

Certified Dietary Manager, Certified Food Protection Professional (Clinical Duties)

Roles and responsibilities:

- Interview clients for diet history.
- Conduct routine nutrition screening/collect data for assessment.
- Calculate nutrient intake.
- Implement diet plans.
- Document nutrition information in clients' health records.
- Counsel clients on basic diet restrictions; specify standards and procedures for food preparation to comply with diet restrictions.
- Review effectiveness of nutrition care plans.
- Assist in nutrition care process according to established policies and procedures.

Coordination of care: The CDM, CFPP collaborates with the Registered Dietitian Nutritionist and members of the IDT to coordinate nutrition care. Any of the other members of the IDT may contact the CDM, CFPP as needed to coordinate proper care for the client. The CDM, CFPP interfaces with the foodservice staff to provide meal service and other nourishments as prescribed by the IDT. The CDM, CFPP should be contacted if there is a new admission, change in diet order, significant weight change, ongoing refusals of meals/nourishment, changes to adaptive feeding devices, illness, etc.

Nurse

Roles and responsibilities:

- Assess client needs; develop, implement, and monitor care plan.
- Deliver direct nursing care.
- Ensure the client has the opportunity to consume food: organize the client feeding responsibilities, distribute the workload, determine need for adaptive eating devices with input from occupational therapist.
- Assist with mealtimes and feeding.
- Document progress: note meaningful information about client's food and fluid intake.
- Provide education to clients.
- Complete RAI.

Coordination of care: The nursing staff provides the daily provision of care to the client. The CDM, CFPP has close contact with the nursing staff, especially related to client feeding. If a calorie count is initiated, the CDM, CFPP will communicate the order to the appropriate staff, outline the data collection process and may even train staff in data collection procedures. The nursing staff has constant contact with the client and a good grasp of the day-to-day information regarding the client. The nursing staff also has daily contact with all other team members to coordinate care. Referrals back and forth between nutrition services and nursing are continuous.

Occupational Therapist

Roles and responsibilities:

- Evaluate needs related to fine motor skills.
- Recommend assistive eating devices and other techniques to help clients feed themselves.
- Provide therapy to develop fine motor skills.

Coordination of care: The CDM, CFPP interacts with the Occupational Therapist mainly regarding adaptive feeding devices and positioning of the client during mealtime. Adaptive feeding devices will assist the client to remain as independent as possible during mealtime. The Occupational Therapist may also be involved with the Speech Pathologist and the rest of the IDT to determine the appropriateness of diet consistency (regular, mechanical soft, pureed, thickened liquids, etc.). The CDM, CFPP will then need to relay the information to the foodservice staff for the provision of meals and nourishments.

Physician (MD)

Roles and responsibilities:

- Evaluate medical conditions and develop medical diagnoses.
- Plan, oversee, and monitor treatment.
- Possess major responsibility for the nutritional status of the client (in conformance to acceptable standards of practice).
- Write diet orders and/or approve protocol for standard orders.
- Order other treatments that affect nutritional status.
- Utilize information provided by other members of the healthcare team.

Coordination of care: The CDM, CFPP interacts with the MD in regards to the diet order. It may be the initial diet order, recommendations for changing the diet order, or modifications in nourishments and consistency. In addition, if the nutrition care team needs to monitor certain laboratory tests or medication changes, the MD is the one writing the orders. However, in some situations the Registered Dietitian Nutritionist can be the one to write orders concerning nutrition care, including lab values, supplements/nourishments, and medications with MD oversight and approval. This is not done by all facilities and would need prior approval from the facility, MD, and IDT.

Social Worker

Roles and responsibilities:

- Evaluate social and support needs.
- Assist clients and families with decision-making.
- Help clients and families plan care upon discharge from a healthcare facility.
- Assist with applying for other healthcare services, such as home-delivered meals or home care.
- Identify resources.
- Provide counseling.

Coordination of care: The CDM, CFPP interacts with the Social Worker regarding client and family wishes. If the client or family wants to discuss any changes or issues, the Social Worker tends to be the primary contact for the facility. The Social Worker and/or the Activities Director may coordinate a visit home for the client over the holidays, or arrange for additional meals to be prepared if family is coming to visit and wishes to eat with the client. The Social Worker will also connect with the IDT and client to discuss code status, Physician Orders for Life-Sustaining Treatment (POLST), living wills, advance directives, and end-of-life decisions for the client. The end-of-life decisions may include feeding concerns (dysphagia and aspiration) and enteral feeding decisions.

Speech Pathologist

Roles and responsibilities:

- Evaluate the chewing and swallowing function of clients.
- Recommend appropriate therapy for dysphagia.
- Provide evaluation and therapy for speech-related needs.

Coordination of care: The Speech Pathologist will coordinate with the CDM, CFPP regarding chewing and swallowing dysfunction for clients. If the CDM, CFPP notices coughing or pocketing of food during a meal observation, a referral should be made to the Speech Pathologist for evaluation. Any consistency changes or need for thickened liquids should be communicated to the CDM, CFPP the RDN, the nutrition care team, and the rest of the IDT.

Policies and procedures must be developed and followed for optimal nutrition care. Whether dealing with clients in a hospital, long-term care facility, or other healthcare setting, the nutrition care process uses the same methods and principles. However, depending on your facility's policies and procedures and state regulations, the CDM, CFPP's exact role in the nutrition care process will vary.

Note that in current Centers for Medicare & Medicaid Services (CMS) guidelines for client care, the client and family members or significant others also play crucial roles. The client, for example, has a great deal of information and insight to offer in developing an understanding of his condition and needs. The client also has the right to contribute to care planning, and to play a well-informed role in deciding upon care. Effectiveness of care is influenced by the client or the client's representative's participation.

Gathering and Sharing Information

As each member of the team contributes specialized training, knowledge, and experience to the care of clients, all members participate in such basic tasks as:

- Assessing client needs
- Developing a plan of care
- Evaluating a plan of care
- Providing education to clients

While the details of a nutrition care plan may differ from the details of a nursing care plan or a speech therapy care plan, the overall objectives are in unison. For example, team members may work together to improve a client's nutritional status as follows:

- A Physician orders a diet.
- A CDM, CFPP conducts a diet history to find out how the client usually eats and to determine food preferences and intolerances.
- A Speech Therapist recommends an appropriate diet for dysphagia and specifies techniques to manage a swallowing disorder.
- An Occupational Therapist helps a client develop the strength and skills to feed himself effectively.
- A Nurse or Nursing Assistant provides hands-on set-up and assistance at mealtime and encourages a client to eat—or feeds a client.
- Both a Nurse and a CDM, CFPP may help monitor diet tolerance and food intake.
- A CDM, CFPP develops a menu and manages food production to ensure that the client receives appropriate foods, and that they are appetizing and wholesome.

This chapter is about professional communication and the effectiveness of the IDT to participate in and monitor the client's plan of care. To attain the best outcomes, team members have to share information. As each views the client's needs from a unique perspective, each has observations and ideas to offer. Thus, sharing information and communicating effectively are critical to providing good clinical care. How do team members share information? As discussed previously in this chapter, one means is through the medical record itself. A good starting point is the list of problems or diagnosis list (if a problem-oriented medical record system is used). Each team member documents assessments, plans, and progress in the record. Each time any team member works with a client, the first step is to open the medical record and review the documentation provided by other members of the team.

The CDM, CFPP and the RDN have completed the comprehensive nutrition care plan with input from the nutrition care team. During the care planning meeting, each member of the IDT listens to others to understand the comprehensive clinical picture. Each member contributes ideas to help meet a client's needs.

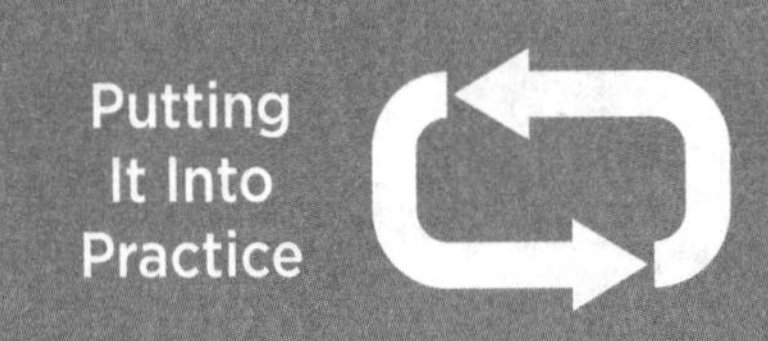

1. As you are observing a client in the dining room, you notice that Mr. H. is having trouble grasping his utensils. His coordination seems to be declining. To what member of the IDT would you refer Mr. H?

However, care does not end with a plan. The plan is only the beginning. This is particularly true in long-term care environments, in which a client may be receiving care for weeks, months, or years. After documenting and implementing the plan, the final steps in providing nutrition care are to evaluate the care by reassessing and revising the plan for the client when the need arises and at defined intervals. In reassessing a client, answer these questions: Is the nutrition care plan working? How is the effectiveness determined?

As the CDM, CFPP begins to evaluate the effectiveness of nutrition care, he/she needs to look at some of the questions that surveyors will be asking to assess the effectiveness of care:

- Has the client's ability to eat or eating skills improved, declined, or stayed the same?
- Was any deterioration or lack of improvement avoidable or unavoidable?
- If the client's eating abilities have declined, is there any evidence that the decline was unavoidable?
- What risk factors for decline of eating skills did the facility identify in the care plan?
- Is there sufficient staff time and assistance provided to maintain eating abilities (e.g., allowing clients enough time to eat independently or with limited assistance)?
- Were **Care Area Triggers (CATs)** and the Care Area Assessment (CAA) process used to assess reasons for decline, potential for decline, or lack of improvement?
- Were individual objectives of the plan of care periodically evaluated, and if the objectives were not met, were alternative approaches developed to encourage maintaining eating abilities?
- Was the care plan driven by the client's strengths identified in the comprehensive assessment?
- Was the care plan consistently implemented? What changes were made to treatment if the client failed to progress or when initial rehabilitation goals were achieved?

As can be seen from these questions, the CDM, CFPP is expected to closely monitor the implementation of the care plan. Whenever monitoring the care plan objectives, this needs to be documented in the medical record to show the other IDT members what progress is being made. Even in the follow-up period for the care plan, it will be important to communicate with the client to assess how well he/she feels the plan is working. It is also critical to communicate with the Registered Dietitian Nutritionist to see if any decline or improvement has been noted as a result of the care plan approaches.

Let's look at some specific data that will assist in monitoring the effectiveness of the nutrition care plan.

GLOSSARY

Care Area Triggers (CATs)
Specific resident responses for one or a combination of MDS elements that identify residents who have or are at risk for developing specific functional problems and require further assessment

Hydration and Dehydration

Regulations require that the facility must provide each client with sufficient fluid intake to maintain proper hydration and health. Among the most common clinical concerns in a long-term care setting is dehydration, or a lack of sufficient water in the body. As has been learned in earlier chapters, water is an essential nutrient. Inadequate water in the body can lead to a drop in blood volume, with serious consequences. In addition, older individuals may lose some of their sense of thirst, which normally protects people from becoming dehydrated. Some may even restrict their own fluid intake to avoid bathroom issues. Figure 14.1 lists possible signs of dehydration. Thirst itself is not a reliable sign of dehydration. It is possible to become dehydrated without experiencing

Figure 14.1
Possible Signs of Dehydration

- Decrease in urinary output or dark urine
- Sudden weight loss (e.g., 5 percent or more of body weight)
- Sunken eyes
- Hollow cheekbones
- Dry mucous membranes
- Cracked lips
- Skin turgor (resilience) is poor
- Change in state of alertness (in extreme dehydration)
- Deep, gasping breathing

thirst. This situation can also occur under severe heat stress. Other factors that can lead to dehydration include fever, bleeding, severe burns, vomiting, diarrhea, certain metabolic disorders, and some medications.

Consider these risk factors for the client becoming dehydrated:

- Decreased sensory ability
- Coma
- Fluid loss and increased fluid needs (e.g., diarrhea, fever, uncontrolled diabetes)
- Fluid restriction secondary to renal dialysis
- Functional impairments that make it difficult to drink, reach fluids, or communicate fluid needs
- Dementia in which the client forgets to drink or forgets how to drink
- Refusal of fluids
- Certain categories of medications

When assessing the effectiveness of the hydration care plan, consider asking/answering these questions:

- Have the staff members provided clients with adequate fluid intake to maintain proper hydration and health? How is this determined?
- What approaches were taken to ensure adequate fluid intake? (e.g., fluids were kept next to the client at all times with staff assisting or cuing the client to drink)
- Are staff members aware of the need for maintaining adequate fluid intake?
- If adequate fluid intake is difficult to maintain or the client is refusing fluids, have alternative treatment approaches been offered such as popsicles, gelatin, and other similar non-liquid foods?

Remember, too, that for clients with renal or cardiac distress, an excess of fluids can be detrimental.

Certain clinical conditions create a different kind of problem—water retention. Unhealthy water retention is called *edema*. This may occur, for example, when the heart is not functioning properly and/or kidneys are not removing excess water. Signs of edema appear in Figure 14.2. Edema is not a disease; it is a symptom. Fluid retention can make the heart and lungs work harder, and can eventually lead to a medical crisis. To manage diseases in which edema occurs, a physician may order restriction of dietary fluids. For any client following a fluid restriction, part of the follow-up evaluation will be to check on how the edema has changed.

Figure 14.2
Possible Signs of Edema

- Visible swelling in legs, ankles, feet, and/or abdomen
- Elevated blood pressure
- Sudden weight gain (e.g., more than 5 percent of body weight)

Weight is an important tool that the CDM, CFPP needs to assist in monitoring. The nutrition care team is often the first to notice changes in edema with weight monitoring.

Monitoring Diabetes

If one of the diseases that may be monitored is diabetes mellitus, there are several indicators that help the CDM, CFPP understand how well the client is doing. A goal of diabetes management is to maintain blood glucose levels at defined levels to prevent complications. What pieces of clinical data will assess this?

- Blood glucose measurements such as fasting blood glucose. Taken in the morning over a period of days.
- Measurements of glucose and ketones in the urine. Normally, both should be zero. Presence of glucose in the urine generally indicates recent high blood glucose values. Ketones can indicate that the body has gone into an abnormal type of metabolism in an attempt to nourish cells.

Ongoing management of blood glucose levels is also measured in glycosylated hemoglobin. This laboratory measurement gives a snapshot of management over time. Depending upon a client's needs and goals, blood lipid levels and total body weight may also be important.

In monitoring diabetes, it is important to talk to the client regularly to find out what concerns exist and how the dietary management is going. Check for any symptoms that indicate high glucose levels—such as thirst, excessive urination, and excessive hunger. Also check nursing notes for any reports that the client has experienced hypoglycemia (low blood sugar). In addition, observe meal intake and menu management. Consider how the client is doing with managing the form of dietary control being used, such as carbohydrate counting, or other system. Is this system proving a good match for the client? Is the client able to apply it? Is the client enjoying meals? Is the client eating any additional foods not on the menu (e.g., gifts from family or visitors)? Is the diet providing an adequate level of carbohydrates for good blood glucose control? Review the medication regimen, and note whether medicines and/or dosages have changed as well. As information is gathered and is verified by checking with other members of the healthcare team, the IDT can develop a solid picture of how the diabetes management plan is working. The information will help the CDM, CFPP make dietary suggestions to be considered and/or make a referral to the Registered Dietitian Nutritionist as appropriate. For example, a client who is having frequent episodes of hypoglycemia may need a review of medications (by the physician) and/or liberalization of diet. A client whose blood glucose levels run consistently higher than a clinical goal may need an adjustment or change in medication, an increase in exercise, and/or a more tightly controlled meal plan. As always, be sure to document observations. Monitor closely if medication and diet changes are made at the same time.

Monitoring Nutrition Status/Weight Loss

View the Supplemental Material to see Figure 14.3 101 Reasons for Weight Loss in Long-Term Care.

A variety of clinical conditions relate to nutrition status, such as protein-calorie malnutrition. There are many reasons a client may experience weight loss (see Figure 14.3 in the Supplemental Material). About one-third of these reasons are easy to correct, e.g., toileting before meals or assisting clients with dental hygiene. Any time improvement of nutrition status is one of the clinical goals, a CDM, CFPP needs to take an active role in monitoring progress. Some objective information to review (as available): weight changes, percent ideal body weight (IBW), skinfold thickness, serum transferrin, and total lymphocyte count. In monitoring weight, remember to weigh a client the same way, in the same amount of clothing, on the same scale, and at the same time of day each time for a more accurate comparison. If a calorie count has been conducted, review this information carefully, and compare it with estimated nutrient needs.

Nursing progress notes can be a helpful source of information about food intake and meal tolerance from day to day. Review them for trends and any notations of concerns or problems related to eating. Check intake and output records to find out whether the client is consuming adequate fluids.

Examine the current medication list and identify any changes. Many medications affect sense of taste; some medications also increase water loss, and may alter thirst perception. Some cause dry mouth, nausea, or other symptoms that can profoundly affect food intake.

Remember that the nutrition care plan is individualized to each client and the assessment of the effectiveness needs to be individualized as well. The following questions should be asked to the client to help assess an objective to gaining weight, eating more, or eating less:

- Are you having any problems or concerns with eating?
- Are you having any problems chewing?
- Are you having any problems swallowing?
- Are you experiencing any digestive concerns, such as nausea, vomiting, diarrhea, or constipation?
- How is your appetite?
- Are you drinking enough water?

Check carefully for tolerance of the current diet. Update food preferences, because they can change. A new medication or other condition may alter how a client tolerates a particular food. In a long-term care environment, repetition of foods may also reduce intake. A client may simply become bored with the same foods. Look for changes in dental health, and any other conditions that may affect a client's ability to feed him/herself, swallow, and maintain interest and alertness at mealtimes.

If the client is not able to communicate, look for this same information through

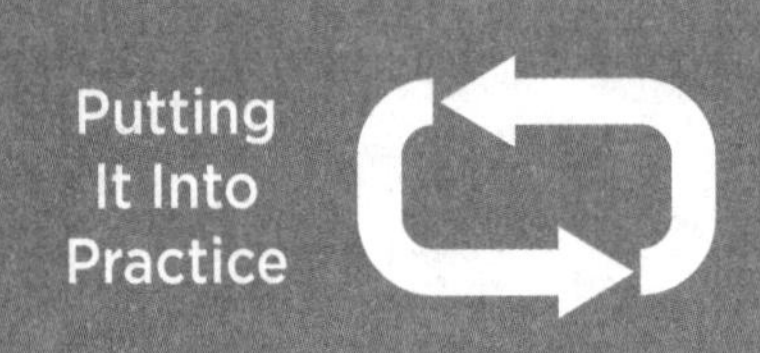

2. If your care plan goal was to have the client maintain weight, and after one month the client is continuing to lose weight, what steps should you take? What questions would you ask?

observation, asking family members, or through consultation with others who are involved in their care.

If a special dietary plan has been implemented in order to improve nutritional status, review the success of this plan. Is the client enjoying these foods? How much is the client consuming? Is there enough variety to keep meals appetizing? Nutritional supplements and/or high-calorie, high-protein foods may have been added in the daily menu. Who is responsible for ordering the supplements? How well is the client tolerating or consuming them? The bottom line, of course, is improvement in nutritional status.

Monitoring Pressure Injuries

For a client with pressure injuries, nutritional monitoring is also essential. Maintaining or improving nutritional status can contribute greatly to resolving this clinical problem. Evaluate changes in nutritional status, weight changes, percent IBW, percent usual body weight, skinfold thickness, serum transferrin, and total lymphocyte count. It is also imperative to consider protein, calorie and fluid intake, and review whether the overall diet provides a reasonable balance of other essential nutrients. Furthermore, check on the staging of a pressure injury and ask whether it has advanced, stayed the same, or improved. Note whether new pressure injuries have developed.

Documenting Progress

As with all professional activity, an evaluation of the effectiveness of care should be documented in the health record. The purpose of documentation is to summarize how the client is responding to treatment, as well as to document the degree of success in achieving goals identified in the care plan; documentation is also a way to share information with the healthcare team.

Documentation should be specific, accurate, objective, concise, and thorough. Whatever documentation method the facility uses, the CDM, CFPP may address questions such as:

- How has the client responded to treatment?
- Has there been progress in achieving the nutrition goals in the care plan?
- Are there any new nutrition-related problems?
- What has changed since the care plan and previous documentation were written, such as changes in medications, laboratory values, ability to feed self, etc.?

The timing of documentation will depend on the type of facility and its policies and procedures. Normally, in long-term care facilities documentation is completed quarterly for all clients, monthly for those at risk, and more frequently for those with special circumstances.

Summary

To help with the most effective quality nutrition care, the process needs to be dynamic. The CDM, CFPP and the entire interdisciplinary team need to routinely review, assess, modify, document, and communicate any new information and findings regarding the resident.

Chapter References

RESOURCES	
Nancarrow SA, Booth A, Ariss S, Smith T, Enderby P, Roots A. Ten principles of good interdisciplinary team work. *Hum Resour Health.* 2013;11:19.	
Peters JJ. Geriatrics, Palliative Care and Interprofessional Teamwork Curriculum; Module #2: Interdisciplinary Teamwork. Mount Sinai School of Medicine, Brookdale Department of Geriatrics and Adult Development. Accessed March 29, 2020.	https://www.nynj.va.gov/docs/Module02.pdf

Manage Selective Menus, Nourishments, and Supplemental Feedings

Overview and Objectives

Today's clients are more independent and want more choices, and the federal regulations from Centers for Medicare & Medicaid Services (CMS) are also mandating greater focus on the client. To provide exceptional nutritional care, one must think about the meals, snacks, nourishments, and supplements that are provided to the client on a daily basis. The provision of nutrition care goes hand-in-hand with the culture change in meal service systems. After completing this chapter, you should be able to:

- Review dietary requirements of client
- Determine client's knowledge and needs
- Evaluate client's food preferences
- Suggest acceptable food substitutes, based on client's preferences
- Verify substitutes in terms of availability and facility practices
- Define the culture change in feeding practices in long-term care
- Define the concept of "real food first"
- Identify clients who need nourishments/supplemental feedings
- Identify appropriate supplemental products
- Monitor the delivery of nourishments and supplements
- Audit the acceptance of nourishments and supplements

15

The choices for healthcare communities for older Americans are expanding, and the type of food and nutrition care will need to expand as well. With 2018 CMS regulations, F561 Self Determination/483.10 Residents Rights, "your facility has to demonstrate that it's allowing clients' choice and self-determination in dining." At the same time, it is important to tailor a menu to the dietary requirements of the client. Can this be accomplished? This chapter will describe the culture change movement and the provision of nutrition care via meal service, menu options, nourishments, and supplements.

Culture Change Language

Culture change in dining begins with changing some of the language used. Karen Schoeneman wrote about this in an "editorial" for the Pioneer Network Culture Change project. She asked people to come up with alternative words for 'bibs,' 'feeder,' 'elderly.' Figure 15.1 lists examples of dining terms that were suggested to help older adults maintain their dignity and healthcare facilities to become more person-centered.

Culture Change in Dining

The culture change movement in dining is driven in part by the large number of Americans who are aging and will be entering various healthcare communities as they age. It is also being driven by the change in regulations to implement more person-centered, client-driven dining programs. This is indeed an opportune time to showcase dining services and the ability to enhance the quality of life through food and dining choices.

Figure 15.1
Terminology of Culture Change

OLD TERMINOLOGY	SUGGESTED TERMINOLOGY
Elderly	Elder, older adult, individual
Wing, unit	Household, neighborhood, street
Institutional care	Individual care
Feeder table	Dining table
Feeder	Person who needs help eating
Facility, institution, nursing home	Home life center, living center
Foodservice worker, Hey You	The person's name
Dietary service, food service	Dining services
Tray line	Fine dining
Nourishment	Snack
Bib	Napkin, clothing protector
Diabetic	Person who has diabetes
Mechanical soft food	Chopped food
Trays are here	It's dinner time; dinner is served

Source: http://www.pioneernetwork.net. Used with permission.

As with any change, there is resistance based on concerns about cost, staffing, and coordinating the changes with regulations. In 2013, a group from Utah State University performed a study in skilled nursing facilities. The purpose of the study was to increase quality of service to meet the residents' expectations and meet new criteria for culture change and dining services. It was found that residents desired a home-style dining experience over the restaurant style that was generally provided. Figure 15.2 is one of the resources used for decision-making with questions that need to be answered to move forward with restaurant style dining. As the facility begins to adopt this culture change, questions need to be answered. Start with questioning the clients to help guide and decide what they want for dining services. Ask questions such as:

- What time of day do you like to eat your meals?
- Do you snack regularly?
- How frequently during the day do you want coffee, tea, or water?
- Where do you prefer to eat your meals?
- What foods do you usually eat at breakfast, lunch, and dinner?
- Where should you begin with the culture change? (expanded snack program, restaurant services, selective menu)

Next, research ways to enhance the dining experience for clients and identify appropriate resources that may be needed. Prioritize the list of ideas and choose one that could be easily accomplished to start with. Talk with, visit, or survey other facilities in the area to determine how/if they have begun to implement a culture change. Remember, the changes that are made need to reflect the client's food and dining preferences.

Once data has been gathered for implementing change, the next step is to work with all of the departments within the facility. Dining changes impact more than just the nutrition care team. This will be a change for other departments as well and they will need to support the changes. Specifically, other departments that might be affected are maintenance, financial, and nursing. Consider developing a policy and procedure that outlines every department's responsibility for each type of change initiated. Communication and training will be key steps as the facility begins to implement a culture change. It is important to note that culture change is a process that takes some time to implement.

Culture Change, Menu Planning, and Liberalized Diets

Culture change helps set the stage for providing meals in the dining area. Chapter 11 discussed the options for menus and meal service. Foodservice staff should create a "dining experience" regardless of the diet order. For example, in what way can pureed foods have more eye appeal than just to be "globs" of food on a tray? A china plate could be presented with pureed pork formed into a pork chop shape, pureed peas that are also molded, rosy applesauce, a slice of bread that has been slurried, and thickened liquids in a glass. In this way, the food looks good, smells good, and tastes good.

The type of meal service used in the facility depends on the needs and goals of the facility. There is no "one size fits all" type of meal service that is recommended. There are many different approaches to providing meals and snacks—it will depend on the needs of the clients, the facility, the foodservice equipment that is available, the budget, and other factors.

Figure 15.2

Decision-Making Tool for Culture Change to Restaurant Style Dining

- What equipment is needed for restaurant or waiter dining?
- Where will the mobile equipment be stored when not in use? Does it need to be locked?
- Is there adequate electrical and plumbing access for your plan?
- What existing equipment can be re-purposed for restaurant or waiter dining?
- Are there any physical plant changes that will be needed?
- Who will approve the expenditure?
- Can restaurant or waiter dining be operated on an interim basis with existing equipment while waiting for the capital budget?
- How many different food items can be offered?
- Will these menu food items be available to clients who do not dine in restaurant or waiter dining?
- Are there any client safety concerns such as pouring hot beverages?
- How will the menu be communicated to clients?
- Will waiters take orders at the dining table or will menus be pre-selected the day or meal before?
- Can physician-ordered diet restrictions be liberalized?
- How will items be labeled or designated for various dietary restrictions?
- Does the current facility budget cover the anticipated costs?
- How will costs be monitored or reported?
- What serving utensils or equipment will be needed?
- What glasses, dishes, or utensils will be used by the clients?
- How will condiments such as salt, pepper, sugar packets be handled for clients on "No Added Salt" and carbohydrate controlled/restricted diets?
- What disposable or reusable items, including napkins, staff uniforms, table linens, and clothing protectors, will be needed?
- How will cross-contamination be avoided when serving clients?
- How many clients will participate in restaurant or waiter dining and how long will it take to serve them?
- How will staff be assigned to restaurant or waiter dining?
- What is the cost of staffing restaurant or waiter dining?
- How will dietary restrictions be communicated and provided?
- Who will monitor and document the client choice/consumption of food?
- Will this be documented in the medical record?
- Will staff track the waste, over-production, or shortage of food?
- Do the facility policy and procedures need to be updated and approved for restaurant or waiter dining?
- Are there any forms needed for restaurants or waiter dining?
- Will you do client satisfaction surveys?
- How will you communicate about the new restaurant or waiter dining? To whom?
- Will you do a pilot test of restaurant or waiter dining?

Source: http://www.pioneernetwork.net. Used with permission.

The menu is the cornerstone for the nutrition care of the client, and the menu can be tailored to meet the needs of the facility. As was covered in Chapter 11, there are options to consider:

- Non-Selective Menu: Even though this menu does not provide choices, some facilities still use this type of menu. With a non-selective menu, the client's food preferences can still be honored and substitutions can be made for such preferences. The goal for the first round of change would be to expand the current cycle menu and perhaps even discuss implementing seasonal menus in order to increase variety. Facilities that use non-selective menus should be encouraged to form a dining committee with the residents who live there to look at implementing further culture change.
- Selective Menu: The selective menu option is the way to implement current federal regulation, but more importantly, to enhance the quality of care and quality of life for clients. Selective menus provide options from which the clients choose their meals. Selective menus are distributed and gathered in advance to help with production of food. The nutrition care team may have to be more involved with those with consistency modifications or other therapeutic nutrition needs, depending on the client. (Review this in more depth by going back to Chapter 11.)
- Restaurant Style Service and Fine Dining: With restaurant style service, the dining area is run like a restaurant with wait staff, ordering and delivering of food, and food being plated in the dining area. Fine dining would change the environment/staff to have different uniforms (chef's hats, chef's jackets, and upscale wait staff uniforms), as well as more formal food choices. When contemplating going to this style of service, staffing changes may be required and job descriptions may need to be considered. If considering this style, it might be easiest to use the non-selective menu item as the main entrée and then offer "specials" (soup and sandwich, salads, etc.) that clients can choose.
- Buffet Style Service: When using buffet style service, the dining area is run like a buffet where clients are allowed to go to the buffet, take what they choose, and eat it. Staffing changes will also be necessary. Clients who are not able to serve themselves may need extra help.
- Family Style Dining: Family style dining is the dining experience closest to that of most homes. Entrees and sides are placed into serving dishes. Clients then pass the foods around and are able to take the portion that they would like. This style may also have an impact on staffing, in that more dishes are generated. Staff would need to fill the serving dishes and distribute them. In addition, some clients may need help with scooping, dishing, and passing.
- Room Service Dining: This dining style may work best in the acute care setting. Room service uses a restaurant style or static menu with choices. When a client is hungry, he/she would order a meal based off of the menu choices. The meal is prepared and then delivered to the room, like room service ordering at a hotel. Staffing changes may include determining adequate staffing and hiring of ordering and delivery employees.

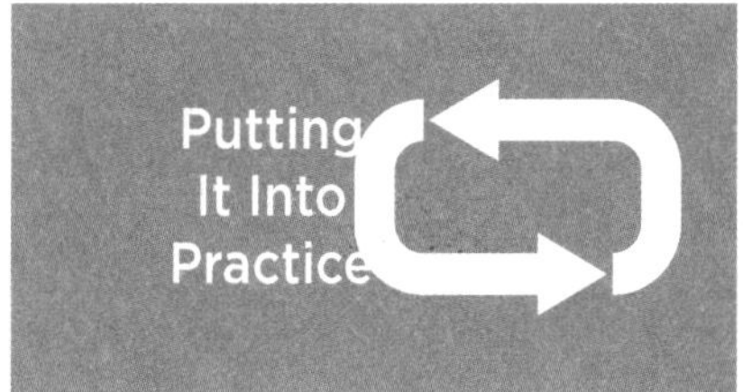

1. You are charged to increase the quality of service to residents and improve the overall dining culture and service. You are considering home-style or restaurant style service. What are some first steps to take when deciding to implement a dining culture change in your facility?

- 24-hour Dining: Food should be available to clients 24 hours a day. Since the kitchen is never really "closed" at home, some person-centered facilities have been creative so that food is available 24 hours a day. Some have accommodated this by building or remodeling kitchenettes so that foods can be stocked and available. This poses some challenges like ordering, filling these units, and keeping them stocked. Snacks could include fresh fruit and vegetables, yogurt, ice cream, cookies, sandwiches, and other snack/beverage items.

Many times, facilities offer the same number of choices regardless of the menu style (selective, restaurant style, buffet style, family style, or room service dining). All of these options are used throughout the healthcare system. It is best to carefully investigate the options, weigh pros and cons of each and, using client input, choose what system (or systems) will be most advantageous in the facility.

In each of the menu system styles, it is also important to review and modify standard menu choices to accommodate specific diet orders. If the facility has implemented a liberalized diet, there may be very few diet orders, other than texture modifications. First, follow individual food preferences, which may mean substituting a food item. Menu substitutions must be of equal nutritional value, as discussed in Chapter 11. For instance, if someone doesn't like cabbage, the substitute should be a food that replaces the vitamin C, such as tomatoes. The facility should have a list of approved substitutes for your menu cycle.

The Use of Comfort Foods in Culture Change

Food is one of the most important components in the long-term care setting. Food choices can improve quality of life for those living in LTC. Many clients look forward to their meals, especially those foods that bring back good memories of "days gone by" and connect them to their past. These items are often referred to as comfort foods. Comfort foods are foods that are familiar, can be delicious and healthy, can stimulate appetite, and create a sense of well-being and connectedness.

There are many benefits of serving comfort foods in the context of culture change. Increase the quality of life for clients is one example. Comfort foods can help with unintentional weight loss, in that they may improve a client's appetite. In turn, an increase in appetite can lead to other physical changes that may include increased energy level, wound healing, and improved overall health status. Comfort foods may also help with socialization. When clients can reminisce about nostalgic foods, that may bring back good memories and elevate mood.

Comfort foods are considered to be staples in the American diet. What comes to mind? Hamburgers? Apple pie? Roast and potatoes? Soup and sandwiches? Most comfort foods are also considered to be "home cooked" or "authentic" recipes. Offering these may be more time consuming. However, many foodservice products on the market are catering to these concepts like flavorful soups that taste homemade, frozen cookie pucks that can be baked, and breads/buns that need proofing and baking. That way the aromas are enticing to a client's senses. Finally, there may be regional and ethnic differences in what are considered comfort foods. For example, grits in the Midwest may not go over very well; however, in the southern states they will likely be more acceptable. The best way to determine what foods are considered comfort foods is to talk with clients in the facility and compile a list.

How would food service start incorporating comfort foods into the menu? Start small. It may be best to add some of these items to special event menus to see how the clients like the new food. They can easily be incorporated into these menus, since most often they require more preparation in the first place. If the recipe is a success, it could be offered again along with other menus to see if it is a comfort food that should be added to the menu. Another place to start is to seek client input into what they consider to be "comfort foods." This could be done with the client council and talk with them to start a list. Client panels or other groups that gather (coffee groups, game groups, and recreational therapy groups) could also be asked for input. A suggestion box is an easy way to get some ideas. Input from family is also helpful. Recipes are an important component in product success. Families many times can share recipes. Church cookbooks often have recipes for common comfort foods. Recipes from the staff may also be used and then expanded and tested to see if they could be duplicated in the foodservice setting. Remember, comfort foods can include both regional and ethnic preferences. A cookbook could be created based on staff, client, and family recipes, and then used by the facility, and maybe also used for a fundraising activity or contest.

The idea is not to always have comfort foods for all meals, but to incorporate them into the existing menu structure.

Comfort foods can be added to any meal or snack opportunity. There are many ways they can be added to lunch and supper, but do not forget about comfort foods that could be used at breakfast. Eggs can be made a variety of ways: scrambled, omelet, sunny-side up, hard boiled, egg bake. There are many muffin/pastry types of foods that can be added, like Danish rolls, English muffins, scones, muffins (all varieties), and coffee cake. Pancakes, French toast, and waffles are options too. Hot cereal is also a good addition. A topping bar can increase choices for hot cereal, pancakes, waffles, and French toast.

The noon and evening meals lend themselves easily to the incorporation of comfort foods. Soups could be added to the start of a meal or offered as a small snack in the afternoon. Soup as an entrée is easy to do, especially if you pair it with a sandwich or salad. Soup and sandwich or soup and salad make nice entrée options. Shown here are some soups, sandwiches, and salads to get started.

SOUP

- Chicken Noodle
- Beef Barley
- Clam Chowder
- Minestrone
- Vegetable Beef
- Vegetable
- Tomato
- Broccoli Cheddar
- French Onion

SANDWICH

- Grilled Cheese
- Grilled Ham and Cheese
- BLT (Bacon, Lettuce, and Tomato)
- Hot Roast Beef
- Hot Turkey
- Egg Salad
- Tuna Salad
- Chicken Salad
- Ham Salad

SALAD

- Caesar
- Cobb
- Three Bean
- Coleslaw
- Potato
- Pasta
- Macaroni
- Fruit

This is just a start when considering items for a menu. Many of these soups can be ordered from vendors, however, always check the Nutrition Facts label and consider the sodium that is in these pre-made soups. Maybe the vendor has access to a lower sodium version or consider making it from scratch. That way, the ingredients used can be controlled to meet the needs of the clients. Soup and sandwich could be offered in the fall/winter months, and soup and salad can be offered in the spring/summer months. A facility might also consider an ethnic food night that would include cuisine from a particular part of the country or world. Examples include: Chinese, Greek, Mexican, Italian, Thai, or any others that would add interest to the menu. This will be increasingly important as the Baby Boomer generation ages, since they have more sophisticated palates and expectations about food and dining.

Comfort foods can also be side dishes. Side dishes include pasta, bread, potatoes, rice, and vegetables. Side dishes are often paired with the main entrée.

To follow are some pasta, potatoes, rice, and vegetable examples that may be considered to be comfort foods.

PASTA	POTATOES	RICE	VEGETABLES
• Lasagna	• Mashed	• White Rice	• Cabbage
• Spaghetti	• Roasted	• Brown Rice	• Bok Choy
• Macaroni and Cheese	• Scalloped	• Wild Rice	• Kale
• Fettuccine	• Au gratin	• Fried Rice	• Collard Greens
• Orzo	• Baked	• Risotto	• Squash
• Rotini or Penne	• French Fries	• Polenta	• Asparagus
			• Whole Green Beans
			• Brussels Sprouts

Similarly, some of these food items could be added or changed, depending on the season. As spring vegetables are available (asparagus) and reasonable in price for service, they can be added to the menu for some different selections. One other side to carefully consider is bread. Is it possible to have fresh-baked buns? Yes, many come par-baked and frozen. Those products need only to be thawed and warmed in the oven. That way the aromas that are important to comfort foods are in the facility, without the challenge of bread products made from scratch.

What could be better than a wonderful ending to a great meal? Desserts are a good way to incorporate comfort foods into a menu. Dessert invokes the feelings of "old fashioned" and "made from scratch." Common dessert items include cakes, pies, pudding, custard, and fruit dishes.

Here are some desserts to consider in the menu plan:

CAKE	PIE
• Spice	• Apple
• Chocolate	• Blueberry
• White	• Peach
• Yellow	• Pecan
• Birthday	• Banana Cream
• Crumb	• Coconut Cream
• Pineapple Upside Down	• Chocolate Cream (or French Silk)
• Cupcakes	• Lemon Meringue
• Cheesecake	

Many other dessert items can be considered. Cookies, bars, pudding, custard, tarts, cobblers, crisps, and strudels could be added to the meals. Snack time is also a good time to have comfort foods. Think about offering ginger snap cookies and coffee during a speaker presentation. Is there a "movie night" at the facility where fresh, hot popcorn could be served as the snack? Get creative and consider some of these ideas to use comfort foods in the menus.

Real Food First as the First Step in Nutrition Support

The dual role of meeting nutritional needs and satisfying the personal menu requests of clients is a challenge. Some degree of protein and calorie malnutrition is strikingly prevalent in today's healthcare facilities, so the job of the Certified Dietary Manager®, Certified Food Protection Professional® (CDM®, CFPP®) is essential. Supporting sound nutrition can reduce complications and improve outcomes for nearly every medical treatment imaginable—from surgery to cancer treatment to healing of fractures and more. **Nutrition support** is a general term which describes providing foods and liquids to improve nutritional status and support good medicine.

GLOSSARY

Nutrition Support
A general term describing the provision of foods and liquids to improve nutritional status and support good medicine

In the hospital or nursing facility, there are always some clients with poor nutritional status, or with high nutrient needs, whose diets simply do not meet their nutritional requirements. The simplest form of nutritional support is a high-protein, high-calorie diet. Generally, there are two approaches to providing added protein and calories. One is to use conventional foods, selecting those that are particularly nutrient-dense. Another is to add commercial nutritional supplements to menus.

Part of the culture change that is occurring in long-term care is the notion of using real food first, before any other supplements are considered or ordered. Conventional foods have the advantage of familiarity, and are often readily accepted by clients. To make effective dietary recommendations, it is important to start with and complete a diet history and discuss food tastes, preferences, and tolerances with a client. Remember, the diet history should be client-centered and involve the family, if possible. Explore

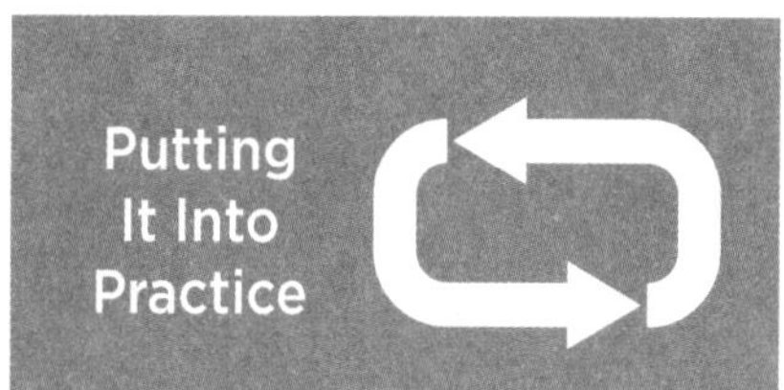

2. The administrator tells you that your department is consistently going over your supplement budget. You notice that many of the residents are on supplements. What steps could you take to reduce the use of supplements in your facility?

likes, dislikes, frequency of eating, changes to appetite, changes to taste, chewing and swallowing ability, diagnosis/diagnoses, etc. Consider liberalizing the diet if this has not been done up to this point. Liberalization may allow for more flavors, textures, and preferred foods.

There are many benefits to considering the real foods first concept:

- If the food tastes good, most people will eat it.
- There is generally an increase in appetite, which leads to an increase in consumption.
- It helps with weight maintenance. Once unintentional weight loss starts, especially in the elderly population, a decrease in functioning and health can be seen.
- Real foods can boost energy level. Well-nourished = increased energy and alertness.
- It may increase emotional and social connections with food (similar to the addition of comfort foods described above).
- It improves mood, health status, and well-being.
- It moderates stress.

Creating a "dining experience" with real food first is another important concept to consider. Making the dining room a "homey" environment is essential. Dining choices and companionship (especially the right companionship) are valued in this setting. Be sure to ask the client about where they sit and their tablemates. If they are dissatisfied with either, consider moving them to a different location or allow them to pick their own spot. Creating opportunities and giving choices are key. For snacks, real foods should be considered first. Oral supplements should only be offered after attempts at real foods first fail (see next section). Real food, again, is preferred by most people over nutrition supplements. Finally, the client's food preferences should be noted and honored at all times throughout the dining experience.

The diet history is key and identifies foods for menu enhancements. Figure 15.3 lists examples of simple menu planning techniques that can add calories, protein, and other nutrients to foods. When there is a nutritional problem, there may also be changes in appetite, taste sensation, or chewing ability. There may be mouth sores or other factors that affect nutrient intake. Consider these together to devise a workable solution. For example, a client undergoing cancer therapy may find the aromas of hot foods distressing. Here, it may be helpful to substitute chilled items for hot entrees. One client may enjoy a cottage cheese and fruit plate more than a hot meatloaf sandwich. Very large serving sizes and packed meal trays can be overwhelming to a person whose appetite or ability to eat is limited. The visual impact of a tray should feel comfortable to a client. Sometimes it might be necessary to consider six smaller feedings per day, in order to add more opportunities for eating and keeping portion sizes reasonable.

Also consider lactose tolerance when using conventional foods to boost protein and calories. Many typical choices involve dairy products. If a client is not accustomed to these or has lactose intolerance, discomfort may ensue. Increase dairy products in the diet slowly, and monitor tolerance. If lactose creates concerns, consider lactose-free alternatives.

There are many alternatives to lactose-containing foods. Alternatives may include: soy, almond and rice milks, as well as other items made with those non-dairy products. However, most are not equivalent in protein or calcium.

Figure 15.3
Techniques for Increasing Calorie and Protein Intake in Real Food

- Use spreads (hummus, nut butters, guacamole, margarine, etc.) liberally on bread, toast, vegetables, rice, pasta, and in sandwiches.
- Add gravies or sauces to entrees and side dishes.
- Add sour cream to potatoes, casseroles, and fruits.
- Use whipped cream on top of desserts and fruits.
- Add 2 tablespoons dried milk powder to each cup of whole milk. Use for drinking and when making cream soups, hot cereal, pudding, custard, hot chocolate, mashed potatoes, casseroles, milkshakes, and creamed dishes.
- Add dried milk powder to scrambled eggs, gravies, casseroles, meatloaf, and meatballs.
- Spread peanut butter on toast or English muffins, on crackers and cookies, and on apple slices and celery sticks.
- Add cheese to sandwiches, scrambled eggs, casseroles, vegetables, and sauces.
- Add chopped eggs and diced or ground meat to salads, sauces, casseroles, and sandwiches.
- Use mayonnaise liberally on sandwiches.
- Choose desserts such as custard, bread pudding, rice pudding, and fruited yogurt. Serve with whipped cream or ice cream.
- Offer whole milk products or cream in place of skim milk, or offer milkshakes as beverages.
- Cook cream soups or hot cereal with whole milk; add margarine or butter.
- Serve six small meals rather than three large ones.
- Add ice cream to enteral products to make a milkshake.
- Use enteral pudding supplements as a topping for cake desserts.
- Use olive oil or flavored oils to potatoes and vegetables.

The nutrition care team should always advocate for the use of real foods first, prior to adding any other nutrition support. It is the first line of defense. Consider fresh items, like fresh produce, when available. Create a dining experience for meals and snacks that may boost consumption. Allow adequate time for eating and make accommodations for slow eaters. Monitor frequently to assure resident satisfaction and food quality. The increased intake of food should be the priority.

The efficacy of this concept is important to share with the other interdisciplinary team members and direct care staff. The CDM, CFPP and the nutrition care team may need to assist in helping other staff with the real foods first concept. Here are some ways to assure the concept will work:

- Discuss always choosing the correct consistency and texture to ensure client safety. Make and recommend appropriate modifications when needed. If a blenderized or pureed diet is recommended, the food should not contain raw eggs. If eggs are used, they must be cooked or pasteurized egg product. Liquid or powdered milk, butter, cheese, or cream could also be added to boost protein and nutrients. Be aware of any clients who have therapeutic diet restrictions (e.g., fat and sodium) when modifying foods.
- Encourage self-feeding when possible. Verbal cueing should also be used if needed. The dining experience should be as natural and independent as possible.
- Reinforce that wholesome foods (real foods) are preferable over adding nutrition supplements.
- Offer choice, accessibility, and individualization.
- Offer choice in timing of the food. Try to follow what the routine was at home if possible or what is preferred by the client.

- Consider the rest of the schedule. Do some medications or the timing of medications change when the meal/snack is offered? Space meals and snacks evenly, when possible.

Can demands or nutritional needs always be met with oral intake? No, not always. There are some clients with poor nutrition status or high nutrient needs that cannot be met with oral feeding only. It may be that they simply cannot take in that much or that they are too sick to do so. Perhaps they have lost some ability to chew or swallow. In some cases, it is necessary to consider supplementation to the oral intake, after attempts at feeding real food first.

If after attempting the real foods first concept without any good nutrition outcomes, the next step would be to consider adding supplements. This creates a challenge for the CDM, CFPP. How does the nutrition care team, led by the Registered Dietitian Nutritionist, meet the nutrition needs of the client and satisfy the personal menu requests of the client? The first item to consider is to support sound nutrition for the client to reduce complications of disease(s) and improve the outcome for the client. It is important to add some creativity to accomplish this task. For example, a made-to-order smoothie menu may be developed with various choices for milk and yogurt, fruits, ice cream, and the addition of protein or carbohydrate powders to boost nutrition. Remember, nutrition support is defined as providing food and liquids to improve nutrition status and support good medical practices. Additional nutrition support may be needed in addition to the oral intake of the client.

Enteral Nutrition in the Role of Nutrition Support

Clients are often in need of concentrated sources of nutrition that cannot be met by meals and snacks. **Enteral nutrition** refers to the feeding, by mouth or by tube, of formulas that contain essential nutrients. It requires that the gastrointestinal tract be functioning. Specialized commercial products exist for providing nutrition support. A standard enteral formula provides one calorie per milliliter (ml); about 240 ml equals one cup. A complete enteral product contains a nutritional balance of protein, carbohydrates, fat, vitamins, and minerals. Some products are modified in carbohydrate content for routine use by individuals with diabetes. Highly specialized enteral formulas exist for patients in liver failure, renal failure, or pancreatic illness.

> **GLOSSARY**
>
> **Enteral Nutrition**
> Feeding of formula by mouth or by tube into the gastrointestinal tract

Many formulas are flavored so they can be taken orally to supplement intake of ordinary food. This is helpful for an individual who needs a high-calorie, high-protein diet and is not able to eat enough food to provide these nutrients. Commercial nutritional supplements offer some advantages over conventional foods. Complete nutritional supplements provide controlled and measured amounts of nutrients. When a client is not able to consume a variety of foods, these products offer one means of assuring adequate nutrition. In addition, they are available with key dietary modifications, such as lactose-free formulations, high-fiber formulations, and so forth. Commercial products are available in calorically dense concentrations, in ranges from one to two calories per ml of liquid product. This means an eight-ounce glass of a supplement may provide about 240-480 calories—a significant nutritional addition to a diet.

Disadvantages of commercial supplements include acceptance and cost. Client acceptance may vary, as clients might perceive a flavor described as "medicinal" or tasting "like vitamin supplements." On the other hand, these products are available in a variety of flavors and textures that may help to overcome this drawback. When offering commercial supplements, it's helpful to allow a client to taste several products and choose what seems most enjoyable. A client may also need variety in supplement flavors and textures, just as with conventional foods. Many commercial supplements taste best when chilled, rather than served at room temperature. It is also possible to combine commercial products with conventional foods. For example, a client who does not enjoy a liquid supplement may enjoy a milkshake made from the supplement plus ice cream. For clients who prefer it—or for certain dysphagia diets—specialized nutritional pudding products represent another choice. Pudding supplements that are nutritionally similar to liquid products are available. A garnish of whipped cream, chocolate shavings, or fruit may also make these products more appealing.

Incomplete or modular nutrition supplements offer another way to boost nutrition intake. For example, a product of carbohydrate powder with minimal flavor can be stirred into beverages, soups, applesauce, and other foods to add calories. This type of product does not provide protein. Therefore, it can be added to foods on a renal diet to boost calories without breaching a protein restriction. Yet another commercial product is a protein powder, which may be added to mashed potatoes, hot cereal, soup, or other products to boost protein content. If a client has developed an aversion or intolerance to meats and other high-protein foods, this can be a means of boosting protein content in the diet. As compared with a conventional dry milk powder, a commercial protein additive can be low in lactose.

A disadvantage of commercial nutritional supplements is that they tend to be more expensive than conventional foods. In many healthcare situations, third-party insurers reimburse for nutrition supplements if they are specified in physicians' diet orders. Another disadvantage may be how the commercial nutrition supplements are handled in your facility. In some facilities, the pharmacist or nursing staff orders them, and in others, they are ordered through nutrition services. Make sure the facility has a policy and procedure outlining who is responsible for these supplements, from ordering to serving.

The CDM, CFPP should monitor that the supplements are actually presented to the client in a timely manner and are consumed. Consider regular documentation so that actual consumption patterns may be gathered and utilized in the nutrition care plan and subsequent nutrition screening and assessments. The information/intake of the supplement and other documentation should be noted in the client's health record as part of the ongoing nutrition care plan. An audit of the acceptance may be initiated if problems with the delivery of the supplements arise. Maintain a list of formulas available, along with the Nutrition Facts label, so that the information is handy if needed. The Registered Dietitian Nutritionist and other members of the nutrition care team may assist the MD in recommending and choosing the correct product. The nutrition care team needs to monitor the client closely to be sure that they are tolerating the product. The CDM, CFPP may work directly with the client to identify and taste test some products to help with intake.

The nutrition care team may need to in-service direct care staff on the use and care of these products. Some clients may need assistance to open them and encouragement to consume them. Instruct the care staff to pour them into a glass and offer with a straw to increase intake and provide a nice presentation. The staff might also need instruction on how to record, monitor, and report poor intake to the nutrition care team. In addition, it may be necessary to conduct an audit of the acceptance of supplements and nourishments to assist with decision-making about the products and their consumption.

Tube Feeding

Enteral feeding refers to the provision of food directly via the gastrointestinal (GI) tract, bypassing the mouth. The GI tract is composed of the mouth, esophagus, stomach, and intestines. Enteral feeding is when nutritionally-complete formulas are given through a tube that goes directly to the stomach or small intestine. In the medical setting, the term enteral feeding is frequently called **tube feeding**. A person on enteral feedings usually has a condition or injury that prevents them from eating by mouth, however their GI tract is still able to function. Being fed through a tube allows a person to receive nutrition and keep their GI tract working. Enteral feeding may make up an individual's entire caloric intake, or in some situations, it may be used to supplement their intake.

GLOSSARY

Tube Feeding
Enteral feeding given through a feeding tube

Feeding tubes can be inserted, when necessary, through surgically-created openings in the stomach percutaneous endoscopic gastrostomy (PEG) or gastrostomy tube (g-tube), or jejunum (jejunostomy or j-tube). These types of tube feedings may be necessary for clients who will need to be fed enterally for long periods of time, such as three to six months. For shorter-term feedings, the tube can also be non-surgically inserted through the nose into the GI tract. This type of tube is called a nasogastric (NG) tube, or nasoduodenal (ND) tube. Figure 15.4 shows sites of feeding tubes and semi-permanent openings for tubes. Tube feedings may be used in clients:

- who are not able to swallow or take food by mouth, such as after head/neck surgery, stroke, trauma, or due to inflammation.
- whose caloric and protein needs are greater than can be ingested orally (such as with cancer or burns), and attempts to provide adequate nutrition through food and oral supplements have been unsuccessful.
- who have medical conditions that require modified diets the client can't tolerate orally (e.g., an elemental diet in which proteins are provided as amino acids, such as for treatment of Crohn's disease or pancreatitis).
- who will not eat (such as clients with anorexia nervosa).
- who are in a coma (nasogastric route is not used).

In cases where the gastrointestinal tract is not functioning, enteral nutrition is not an appropriate choice.

Tube feedings can be administered continuously or intermittently. A pump is often used to administer continuous drip feedings over a 12-24 hour period. This type of feeding allows more formula to be given and decreases the chances of diarrhea. Once tube feeding tolerance is well established, a feeding may be changed to an intermittent schedule. Intermittent feedings or bolus feedings are usually given four to six times each day by gravity drip for a period of 30 to 60 minutes. One advantage of intermittent feedings is that they give the client freedom of movement between feedings. For jejunal feedings, which enter low in the gastrointestinal tract, intermittent feedings usually aren't appropriate as they are quite likely to cause diarrhea. A typical

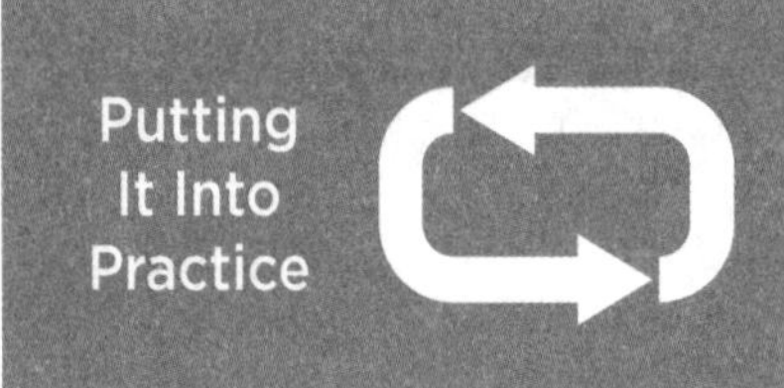

3. James is a 90 year-old client that was admitted one month ago. James is very thin and not eating well. The MD ordered 8 oz. Ensure® three times a day. The nurses report that James is not drinking the Ensure. James tells you the drinks are "too sweet" and he would rather have whole milk. You notice that James is on a low-fat, low-cholesterol diet due to a history of high cholesterol. What would you recommend to the MD?

jejunal feeding remains on a continuous drip regimen. In some cases, a client receiving feedings by gastrostomy tube may also be allowed to eat regular foods as desired.

Three types of complications can occur in tube fed clients: gastrointestinal disturbances, metabolic complications, and mechanical complications. The most common gastrointestinal disturbance is diarrhea, due to the fact that enteral products are concentrated. Concentrated components tend to pull water into the intestines. Sometimes this is a function of how quickly the feeding is administered. Fiber content of formulas may also play a role. To prevent diarrhea, it is usually necessary to begin a tube feeding at low concentrations (i.e., diluted with water) and a slow rate of administration, building up gradually as the feeding is tolerated. If diarrhea occurs, it may respond to drug therapy or a change in formula. Sanitation is essential during the preparation, storage, and administration of the enteral formula. This will prevent bacterial contamination that could cause foodborne illness. Feeding containers must be changed every 24-48 hours depending on manufacturer's recommendation and your facility's protocol.

Metabolic complications of tube feeding, such as electrolyte imbalance, frequently occur due to inadequate fluid intake, diarrhea, and/or vomiting. Tube feeding frequently serves as a client's sole source of fluid, so careful attention must be paid

Figure 15.4
Sites of Tube Feedings

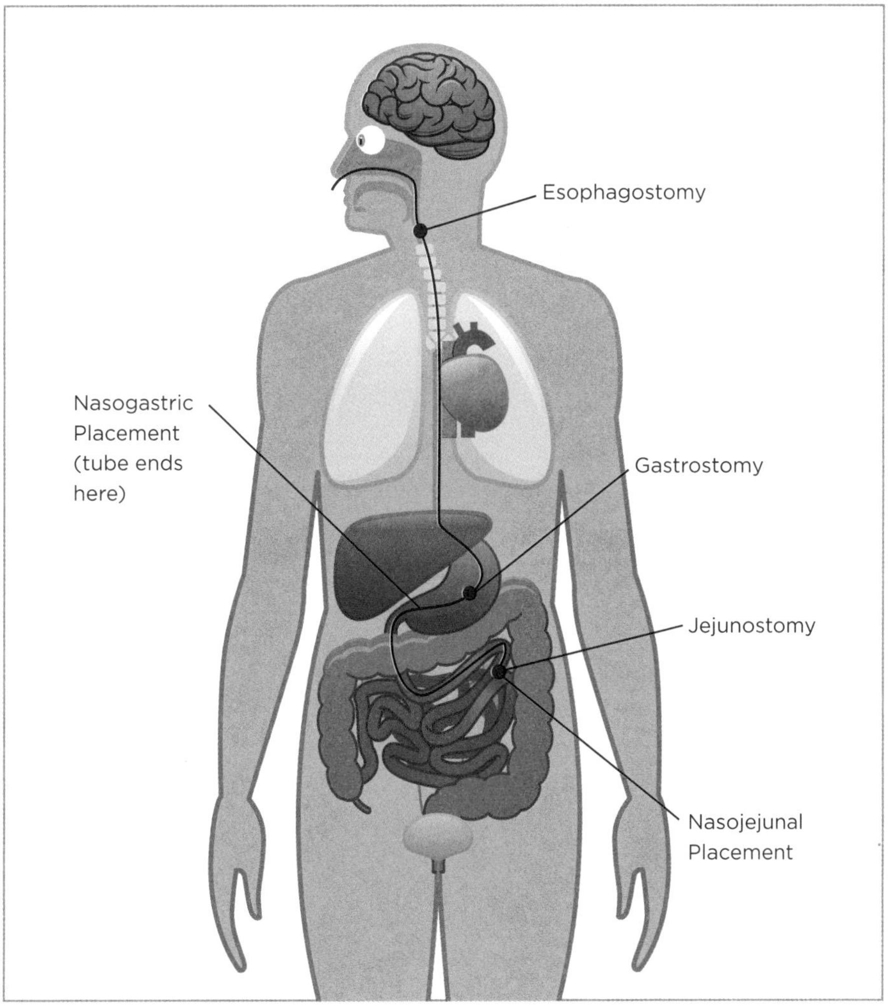

to fluid requirements. Fluid intake should be adequate to make up for normal losses. There is about a 500 ml difference between input and output over 24 hours. Fluid intake should accommodate unusual losses associated with increased body temperature, vomiting, and diarrhea.

Note that nursing personnel typically bear most of the responsibility for administering and managing tube feedings. The Registered Dietitian Nutritionist is involved in recommending a product, concentration, and rate of administration that will provide adequate nutrients. Like a menu, a tube-feeding regimen is a type of diet that must be matched to estimated nutrient needs and specific therapeutic needs. As a feeding progresses, a CDM, CFPP often assists in monitoring tolerance and administration while coordinating with the Registered Dietitian Nutritionist.

One type of enteral formula used for tube feeding but rarely for oral supplementation is a chemically defined formula. Whereas usual formulas require some digestion, chemically defined formulas (also called elemental or hydrolyzed formulas) are almost completely digested so they require only minimal digestion. These formulas are absorbed quickly and are useful for clients with severe digestive problems, such as pancreatitis. Chemically defined formulas generally cost more than other types of formulas and are less palatable.

In selecting an enteral product for oral or tube feeding, the nutrition professional should consider the product concentration; the need for a nutritionally-complete formulation; needs for modification in carbohydrate, fat, or protein composition; tolerance of lactose; location of the feeding tube; and whether or not to include fiber. A CDM, CFPP should be aware of taste, texture, and individual client acceptance as well.

Parenteral Nutrition

GLOSSARY

Parenteral Nutrition
Method of getting nutrition into your body through your veins

Parenteral nutrition, or intravenous feeding, is a method of getting nutrition into your body through your veins. Parenteral solutions may contain dextrose, lipids, amino acids, electrolytes, vitamins, and trace elements. They may be used in cases where the client's gastrointestinal tract is no longer able to digest and absorb food properly, or to maintain fluid and electrolyte balance both before and after surgery, or when a client is not receiving enough nourishment by other feeding methods. Other examples of situations that may require parenteral feedings include the following:

- severely malnourished clients with a nonfunctional gastrointestinal tract.
- clients with diseases of the small intestines who are not absorbing nutrients.
- clients with sepsis or burns who have very high nutrient needs.

When a client receives his or her total nutrient needs via parenteral nutrition, it is called total parenteral nutrition (TPN). Parenteral nutrition may use a central or peripheral vein. In central parenteral nutrition (CPN), a central vein near the heart is used because these veins are large in diameter. At other times, a peripheral vein (a vein in the arm or leg) is chosen, and this is called peripheral parenteral nutrition (PPN). PPN is used when only short-term support is needed and the client is not severely malnourished. PPN may be used to supplement ordinary eating. CPN is used in more severely malnourished clients who may also need more long-term nutrition support.

Although parenteral nutrition is very helpful to certain clients, it has its disadvantages. Inserting a catheter (tube) for parenteral nutrition is a surgical procedure, and once it is inserted, the catheter must be well cared for to prevent infection, a complication of parenteral nutrition. Also, when the gastrointestinal tract is not used for a long time, intestinal cells involved in absorption shrink in size, making a transition back to enteral feeding challenging. Furthermore, clients fed by vein have to forgo the usual satisfaction characteristic of eating, with all its social and emotional meanings. Lastly, parenteral solutions are very costly compared to enteral feedings.

In parenteral nutrition, an evaluation of nutritional status and an estimation of nutrient needs provide useful starting points for planning therapy, usually conducted by the Registered Dietitian Nutritionist. If a client is going to make a transition from parenteral feeding to conventional foods, the CDM, CFPP may be involved in the transition.

Chapter References

RESOURCES	
Academy of Nutrition and Dietetics: Position Paper. "Position of the Academy of Nutrition and Dietetics: Individualized Nutrition Approaches for Older Adults in Health Care Communities:" 2010' eatrightpro.org. Accessed March 30, 2020.	https://www.eatrightpro.org/news-center/nutrition-trends/foodservice-and-food-safety/individualized-nutrition-approaches-for-older-adults-in-health-care-communities
ANFP Comfort Foods and Comfort Care—5 hour CE course. Accessed March 30, 2020.	http://www.anfponline.org/marketplace
ANFP Fortification vs . Supplementation—5 hour CE Course. Accessed March 30, 2020.	http://www.anfponline.org/marketplace
California Coalition for Person-Centered Care. Accessed March 30, 2020.	https://www.cacpcc.org
Centers for Medicare & Medicaid Services (CMS). Accessed March 30, 2020.	http://www.cms.gov
Eden. Accessed March 30, 2020.	http://www.edenalt.org
The National Resource Center on Nutrition & Aging. Accessed March 30, 2020.	http://nutritionandaging.org
Pioneer Network-New Dining Practice Standards—Pioneer Network Food and Dining Clinical Standards Task Force. Accessed March 29, 2020.	https://www.pioneernetwork.net/wp-content/uploads/2016/10/The-New-Dining-Practice-Standards.pdf
The Food and Dining Side of the Culture Change Movement: Identifying Barriers and Potential Solutions to Furthering Innovations in Nursing Homes. Accessed March 30, 2020.	https://www.pioneernetwork.net/wp-content/uploads/2016/10/The-Food-and-Dining-Side-of-the-Culture-Change-Movement-Symposium-Background-Paper.pdf

Provide Nutrition Education

Overview and Objectives

Nutrition education enables clients to participate in caring for themselves. By developing basic skills in this area and adapting those skills to the educational needs of the client, a Certified Dietary Manager®, Certified Food Protection Professional® (CDM®, CFPP®) can be a valuable resource to clients. After completing this chapter, you should be able to:

- Develop a plan for nutrition education
- Select educational materials and resources
- Use resource materials and equipment for teaching
- Ascertain background and knowledge of clients
- Implement a teaching plan
- Suggest appropriate/available social resources
- Evaluate effectiveness of the teaching

A client takes part in the fine details of managing a diet. The client may choose particular foods from a selective menu. With knowledge, the client can choose foods that make meals enjoyable and support their own care by self-managing their diet. Providing appropriate nutrition education will enable the client to make better choices for him/herself. Using nutrition education principles, the CDM, CFPP begins to develop a plan for nutrition education.

The Academy of Nutrition and Dietetics defines nutrition education as "a process that assists the public in applying knowledge from nutrition science and the relationship between diet and health to their food practices. It is a deliberate effort to improve the nutritional well-being of people by assessing the multiple factors that affect food choices, tailoring educational methodologies and messages to the public being reached, and evaluating results. It can help individuals develop a knowledge base, make a commitment to good nutrition, select nutritionally adequate diets, and develop decision-making skills." According to this definition, nutrition educators can enhance knowledge, encourage skills to make decisions and select nutritious diets, and help clients develop a positive attitude toward nutrition. It can also help clients utilize the knowledge toward positive lifestyle behavioral changes. Nutrition education is one form of nutrition intervention, as defined by the Academy of Nutrition and Dietetics.

As was seen in the nutrition care process, the first step was screening and assessment. Similarly, the first step in the nutrition education process is an assessment of the learner (or client). The CDM, CFPP and/or the Registered Dietitian Nutritionist may have collected pertinent facts about the client, his/her preferences, previous diets that have been followed at home, likes/dislikes, and basic understanding of nutrition knowledge. In addition if this information is not available, nutrition screening and assessment can be conducted prior to the education, or as part of the nutrition education process.

Achieving Behavior Change: The Transtheoretical Model

The Transtheoretical Model of behavior change was originally developed by Prochaska and DiClemente to describe the process of behavior change for addictive behaviors. Over the past 30 years, it has been proven to be an effective model for nutrition behavior change as well.

The Transtheoretical Model assesses an individual's readiness to change or act on a new behavior. It helps the practitioner determine the readiness of change, and then provides strategies to move the individual through the five stages of change. The five stages of change include: pre-contemplation, contemplation, preparation, action, and maintenance. *Pre-contemplation* is when the individual is not ready or not thinking about making a change. Individuals in this stage may be characterized as resistant to change, unmotivated, or ambivalent. Those who are in the *contemplation* stage are getting ready to change— usually within six months. The next stage is *preparation* or change in the near future (within the next month). Individuals in this stage usually have a plan of action in place or are working on the steps. *Action* is the stage in which an individual takes action or makes a behavior change. *Maintenance* is the final stage in which individuals have made significant behavior change for a sustained period of time (usually six months or longer) and are working to prevent relapse back to old behavior patterns. (Prochaska, et al., 1984)

Developing Objectives

Before beginning any type of nutrition education, it is important to answer a few simple, direct questions: What does the client need to learn? What do they already know? What should the outcome be? The answers to these questions can be used to develop one or more learning objectives. A **learning objective** is a specific, measurable statement of the outcome of the education. To develop a learning objective, think about what the client will be able to do when he/she has successfully completed the nutrition education. An effective learning objective includes key elements, described in the acronym **S.M.A.R.T.**

Each learning objective should be relevant to the overall purpose of the instruction. For example, when educating a client about managing hypertension, there is no need to toss in nutrition information about diverticulitis. Focus on what the client needs and address this in an objective. Next, the objective needs to make sense, and be specific and meaningful to the client. An effective objective is also behavioral. This means it describes what a client will do. Needless to say, an objective must be attainable and realistic. It should also be specific and time sensitive. Why? So that an assessment can be made whether the education has been successful. Figure 16.2 lists examples of objectives that are and are not measurable.

GLOSSARY

Learning Objective
A specific, measurable statement of the outcome of a lesson, in-service, or nutrition education session

S.M.A.R.T. Objective
A learning objective that is **S**pecific, **M**easurable, **A**chievable, **R**easonable, and **T**imely

Figure 16.1
Criteria for Goals and Objectives

SMART GOALS
SPECIFIC: Answer questions such as: What precisely will happen? (Describe the outcome)
MEASURABLE: Answer questions such as: How will I determine if the goal is successful?
ACHIEVABLE: Answer questions such as: How can this be achieved with the resources available?
REASONABLE: Answer questions such as: What makes this possible to achieve?
TIMELY: Answer questions such as: When will this be accomplished?
EFFECTIVE OBJECTIVES
SPECIFIC: They describe what will be done, and by whom.
CHALLENGING: They represent growth rather than status quo, but are nevertheless practical.
OBSERVABLE: They describe a change that you as a CDM, CFPP can objectively observe.
MEASURABLE: They provide a form of a measure and time period you can use to evaluate achievement.
SIMPLE: They each cover one clear action item.

Source: https://www.smart-goals-guide.com

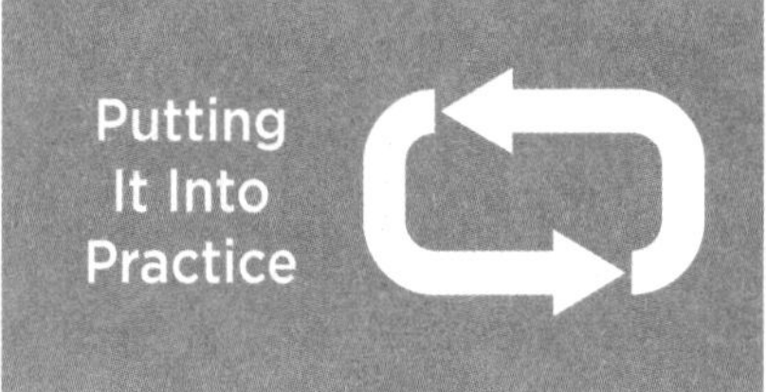

1. How could you rework the goal to "drink more water" to be a S.M.A.R.T. goal?

Figure 16.2
Measurable Objectives

MEASURABLE	NOT MEASURABLE
• Over the next 5 days, the client will choose foods on the daily menu that meet his 200-gram carbohydrate diet, within 10%.	• Client will do better with choosing foods on the daily menu.
• By December 1, the client will select foods that bring intake up to at least 1,600 calories.	• Client will eat more calories.

Group Instruction

Formal education of clients is most often accomplished through group instruction. An advantage of group instruction is that it allows clients to share experiences and develop a sense of group motivation. If the clients continue to have contact after an educational session, they can encourage and support each other. A group may include clients, as well as family members and others involved in care. In any facility where a group of clients has common educational needs, group instruction can be an excellent option. A CDM, CFPP may also combine group instruction with individual nutrition counseling (discussed later in this chapter). One of the most important things to remember for successful group education is to establish group rules that will help guide the sharing and discussion. In addition, it is important to maintain group control and not let one client/person dominate the conversation.

After developing learning objectives, a CDM, CFPP planning group instruction needs to develop a class outline that draws the learner into the topic. This includes: organized details of the lesson or comprehension, an opportunity for practice, and how to apply the material or application. Here are some tips for developing these sections of an outline.

Introduction

The introduction helps to pull the learner/client into the topic and serves to motivate changes. It orients learners to the subject. It gives the Registered Dietitian Nutritionist and/or CDM, CFPP an opportunity to learn more about the clients and establish rapport. It can also be used to create client involvement and interest, by, for example, tasting a new low-fat food. When beginning a class, pick an opening that will quickly engage participants' attention. It may be a question, such as: (or more open-ended) *Who finds some of the nutrition information you're supposed to follow confusing or annoying?* (This gets everyone paying attention, maybe nodding or smiling in agreement. Then you can look at some of the participants to engage more: *What do you find most confusing (or annoying) about your current diet?* Sometimes, a statistic can capture attention. An example is: *Did you know that 90 percent of people who go on weight loss diets end up heavier than when they started? Why do you think that is?* This introductory activity needs to feel non-threatening. For example, ask each participant to state a favorite food. Make the opening relevant to the group, and design it to put people at ease. As clients share information about themselves, avoid making judgments. Encourage open communication, which requires absolute acceptance of each person in the group. If the client is doing something undesirable, approach them in such a way to present information and help the client draw personal conclusions. During this section, also briefly describe the learning objectives. It may or may not be necessary to include every detail used in planning. Instead, provide a "general direction" for the session. Say something like: *When we are finished with this class, you will be able to determine the total amount of carbohydrates you need daily.*

Outline of the Lesson

This part of the class outline describes the content (what will be taught) and the teaching methods (how it will be taught). For each learning objective, sketch out what will be said and choose an appropriate teaching method. When choosing teaching material, pick information that is relevant and significant to the group. Be specific and use examples.

The learning objectives and subsequent material should be targeted toward the stage of change that has been identified for the learner. For example, if the client is planning to lose weight and is in the preparation stage, focusing on a menu and grocery list may be a better strategy than discussing ways of maintaining long-term weight loss. It is helpful to establish the short-term goals so that the client is not overwhelmed and can experience more immediate success.

Opportunity for Practice

When choosing the teaching methods, choose some that allow for participation and practice. By having clients actively participate in training, it can be expected that the clients will remember more of what they say and do than if you just tell them. Activities may include checking sample food labels and deciding how they fit into a diet, or marking a selective menu according to a meal plan. They may include practice in modifying recipes to fit special dietary needs, or even simple food preparation.

Application

Application is when the client is asked to apply the information learned to his/her own diet or situation. They make their own choices, work on their own, and correct their own work when possible. For some clients, the application may occur after leaving the facility and follow up with another meeting, an essential part of nutrition education. A follow-up meeting can help to reinforce the learning.

Figure 16.3 shows a sample outline for group instruction. Figure 16.4 lists some strategies for achieving effective communication.

Here are some additional ideas to enhance success in teaching groups to help motivate learning:

- Be prepared.
- Set up room or equipment in advance.
- Start on time.
- Use a seating arrangement such as a circle that enhances communication and vision.
- Make eye contact. Smile and nod to show positive reinforcement.
- Pay attention to the pace, volume, and tone of voice. Don't talk too fast, and be sure everyone can hear.
- It can be helpful, if you've just explained or said something, to ask someone in the group to help interpret what you just said, using their words.
- Ask clients what they already know about the topic to be discussed.
- Actively listen.

- Encourage and facilitate client participation.
- Ask open-ended questions.
- Praise and give encouragement.
- Use visual aids effectively.

Every person has a different preferred learning style. Some learn by seeing (visual), some by listening (auditory), and some learn more easily by touch (kinesthetic). Learning styles should be assessed and utilized for nutrition education.

Visual Aids

Visual aids can reinforce learning. Use simple handouts, posters, models, or slides. Visual aids keep clients' attention, reinforce main ideas, save time, and increase understanding and retention. Visual aids are also useful in making comparisons. Videos and slides (e.g., PowerPoint) may be useful, but do not use this to replace teaching. Make sure to use terms that the audience will know and understand. Avoid medical jargon. If medical jargon must be used, be sure to explain what is meant and ask for clarity before moving forward. What if everyone is not of the same ethnic background and can't all read the language on the visuals? Educational materials may need to be offered in various languages depending on the clientele or use pictures and models without words to assist in the education.

Make key points simple, and design handouts to be readable, especially for anyone with a vision impairment (14-point font or larger is recommended when working with senior citizens). The most effective visual aid is limited to one idea that can be communicated within three to five seconds. If using slides (e.g., PowerPoint) the font should be 24-point or larger; be careful not to put too many words per slide. Bullet points are helpful. If you do use slides to help you teach, be sure to keep your eyes on the audience. If there are more ideas, simply use more aids! Special visual aids for nutrition education include food models, which are synthetic replicas of food; measuring cups and spoons; food packages; and Nutrition Facts labels from foods. Compare the visual aids to the checklist in Figure 16.5 before using them.

Serving Sizes

It is important that the client understands what an appropriate amount of food is in a standard serving size. Many clients have no idea that a serving of bread is one ounce, nor can they state how much one ounce is. For example, one ounce of crackers or snack chips varies by the type of cracker or chip (e.g., 1 ounce of thin wheat crackers is 15 crackers; 1 ounce of soda crackers is 7 crackers).

In Chapters 1 and 6, there was a discussion regarding the serving sizes listed on MyPlate. The clients may be eating considerably more or less amounts of food than a standard serving size, depending on the food group. Visual aids are an appropriate way to help your clients see a standard serving. Sometimes, the palm of a person's hand is a good way to teach a client what 1/2 cup looks like when referring to cut-up fruits and vegetables, or grains; it can also be used to show what a 3-ounce size of chicken, meat, or fish looks like. It is also helpful for the clients to communicate to you how much they normally eat. Other diabetes-related topics may include complex carbohydrates vs. refined grains, and a discussion as to why clients may require different amounts of carbohydrates (gender, weight, medications, etc.).

Figure 16.3
Sample Education Session Outline: Carbohydrate Counting

TOPIC	ACTION
Introduction and Motivation	Ask clients if anyone has heard of diabetes. Then ask if anyone has any family members with diabetes. Ask them what type of diet they followed and what foods were restricted (It may be the exchange diet). Explain that the outcome today is for each client to be able to use a new eating plan where they have more choices and fewer restrictions. It is called carbohydrate counting.
Organized Detail of Lesson for Comprehension	Or you can begin by asking who's heard of a carbohydrate? Then ask if anyone can give an example of a food that is a carbohydrate. Once the audience is involved, give an explanation of what a carbohydrate is and why it is important for people with diabetes to know where carbohydrates are found. Keep it simple for now...only talk about starch, sugar, and fiber. Hand out nutrition labels and help them not only find the grams of carbohydrate, but also identify the sources of carbohydrate on the nutrition label. Explain how carbohydrates can be counted, and demonstrate that with a handout they can keep and refer to.
Opportunity for Practice	Divide the group into smaller groups or a sharing pair where they pair up with someone nearby to work on the activity. Give each group or pair some empty food packages and ask them to determine how many carbs each food would provide and the type of carbohydrate. Ask one person from each small group to report back to the full group.
Application	Each client should know how many carbohydrates (carbs) they have in one day and how carbs should be distributed. Ask them to select from the bin of food labels the foods they could have for one meal that would be equivalent to the number of carbs they are allowed. Ask a few of the groups to share their 'meals.'
Closing	Thank participants for their cooperation. Ask for questions and reactions. Summarize key points: What is a carbohydrate, why it is important, and where to find them. Briefly review how to count carbohydrates. Give session evaluation if you use a formal evaluation, or ask them to write one sentence about what they learned.

Source: Adapted from Nutrition411.com

Diet History

The diet history for each person is the foundation of personalized diet planning and education. For example, upon completion of the diet history, if it is discovered that a client frequently chooses fast foods, then help the client learn to choose foods from a fast food menu as part of the education process. If it is discovered that a client is a vegetarian, adapt the education and recommendations so that they are consistent with this dietary choice. To adapt teaching to client educational needs, use the communication tips in Figure 16.6.

Education Resources

While some facilities develop their own teaching materials, this is a time-consuming proposition. Many high-quality materials are available either free or at low cost from government agencies, industry groups, health organizations, food manufacturers, cooperative extension services, and education institutions. Of course the Internet has a multitude of resources; just make sure to abide by copyright laws if information is used from the Web. (See Figure 16.7 for a list of credible nutrition education resources.)

Figure 16.4
Keys to Effective Communication

Respect Personal Space	When sitting down to speak with clients, ask them to sit where they feel the most comfortable or let them tell you where to sit. This will allow people to choose the distance that feels right to them. Comfortable distance varies by culture and individual.
Learn the Cultural Rules About Touching	Find out the cultural rules regarding touch for the ethnic groups with whom you work, including differences based on gender. In some Asian cultures, the head should not be touched because it is the seat of wisdom. In many Hispanic cultures, the head of a child should be touched when you admire the child. A vigorous handshake may be considered a sign of aggression by Native Americans.
Establish Rapport	Take time to establish common ground through sharing experiences and exchanging information.
Ask Questions	Do not be afraid to ask someone about something with which you are unfamiliar or uncomfortable. Nutrition educators suggest open-ended, honest questions that show an interest in the person, a respect for his culture, and a willingness to learn. Have the client repeat back objectives or information in their own words to check for comprehension and understanding.
Listen to the Answers	Really listen. Do not interrupt the client or try to put words in his/her mouth. Let clients tell their own stories. Appreciate and use silence. Observe the client to get a feel for how he or she uses silence. Do not feel that silence has to be filled in with small talk. Give people a chance to formulate their thoughts, especially if they are trying to speak in a language that is not their native tongue. Cultures that value silence learn to distinguish varying qualities of silence, which may be hard for others to discern. "Pause time" is different for different cultures.
Notice Eye Contact	Notice the kind of eye contact your client is making with family members or your co-workers. Many cultures consider it impolite to look directly at the person speaking.
Pay Attention to Body Movements	Movements such as upturned palms of the hands, waving one's hand, and pointing with fingers or feet convey varying messages. Observe your clients for clues.
Note Client Responses	Note that a "yes" response does not necessarily indicate that a client has understood or is willing to do what is being discussed. It may simply be an offering of respect for the health professional's status. Some clients may not ask questions because this would indicate a lack of clear communication by the provider. In some cultures, smiling and laughing may mask other emotions or prevent conflict.

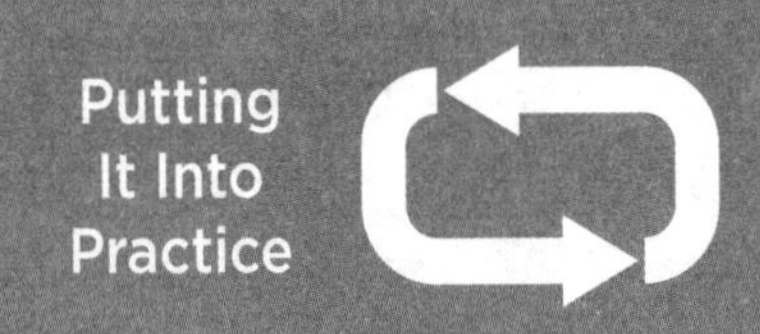

2. What are some common items that can demonstrate food portions if food models are unavailable?

Figure 16.5
Checklist for Evaluating Nutrition Education Materials (Handouts)

- The cover is attractive and clearly identifies the topic.
- The writing style is conversational and in active voice.
- Technical jargon is not used. In cases when a technical term must be used, it is defined.
- The text is at the appropriate reading level and is interesting and lively.
- The emphasis is on "what to do," or specific behavioral changes.
- The illustrations are simple and relevant to the content.
- The print size is large enough and the font is plain enough to be easily read.
- There is contrast between the color of the print and the color of the paper so the words are easily read.
- The pages are not cluttered with too much information.
- The material is appropriate for the intended audience (gender, culture, age, level of education).
- The publication invites reader thoughts and/or participation, e.g., through a questionnaire, a recipe, a worksheet, or other techniques.

Figure 16.6
Communication Techniques for Effective Instruction

Verbal Communication	• Describe behavior rather than judge it. • Treat clients with respect and trust. • Involve them in the problem-solving. • Empathize with the client. • Be receptive to other ideas.
Listening	• Listen to what the client has to say. • Maintain good eye contact with the client. • Restate, paraphrase, or clarify statements as a way to allow the client to elaborate on their feelings. Ask the client to share 1-2 things learned during the meeting.
Promote Effective Communication	• Use understandable language with few medical terms. • Allow for adequate time for the instruction. • Become aware of the client's concerns and limitations before they can interfere with communication. • Be genuine.

When teaching someone who will be preparing meals at home, help develop a plan for meal preparation. Consider developing a sample grocery list together or emphasize choices that meet dietary needs. If the client has any physical limitations, be sure that the food preparation facility can accommodate these, and that the food plan takes these into consideration. When working with a group, use the share/pair technique so the two can focus on what is practical for the client's abilities and lifestyle. Recommend additional resources as relevant, such as a local Meals on Wheels program.

Whether educating an individual or a group, effective communication is the foundation for success. Tailoring the education to meet the needs of the client is critical to achieving behavior change. Dietary instruction generally involves a client-driven change.

Figure 16.7
Sources for Credible Nutrition Education Resources

SOURCE	URL
Health Associations	
Association of Nutrition & Foodservice Professionals	www.anfponline.org
Academy of Nutrition and Dietetics	www.eatright.org
American Heart Association	www.heart.org
American Cancer Society	www.cancer.org
American Diabetes Association	www.diabetes.org
Federal Agencies	
Food and Drug Administration	www.fda.gov
National Institute of Diabetes and Digestive and Kidney Diseases	www.niddk.nih.gov
Centers for Disease Control and Prevention	www.cdc.gov
FDA Center for Food Safety and Applied Nutrition	www.fda.gov/food/foodsafety/default.htm
MyPlate	www.choosemyplate.gov
What's Cooking? USDA Mixing Bowl	www.whatscooking.fns.usda.gov
United Stated Department of Agriculture	www.usda.gov
Centers for Medicare & Medicaid Services	www.cms.gov
Others	
Nutrition411	Consultant360.com
Institute of Food Technologists	www.ift.org
Food & Health Communications	http://foodandhealth.com/
National Cooperative Extension System	www.extension.org

Note: This is a sample of highly-rated sources; your instructor may have others.

Evaluate the Effectiveness of the Education Session

The final, but very important, component of any nutrition education program is evaluation. The key purpose of evaluation is to determine whether or not learning objectives have been met. This is one of the main reasons learning objectives must be measurable. A description of how to measure behavior, as written in an objective, gives a solid gauge for evaluating the results of education. For example, if the objective says, *Client will consume at least 80 percent of the nutritional supplements provided*, the evaluation will include determining what percentage of nutritional supplements were consumed.

A second reason for evaluating nutrition education is to obtain feedback about the educational approach itself. Particularly for group education, good practice dictates that feedback is gathered from participants at the end. This information helps refine educational techniques and related materials. Sometimes, it provides feedback that helps to focus on how to work with a particular group or tackle a particular topic differently.

Following an educational session, three levels of evaluation may apply: client reaction, actual learning, and behavior change. Here is more information about each:

Client Reaction

Evaluation focused on client reaction answers the question: *How did the client(s) respond to the education sessions?* To evaluate client reaction for a group class, use a rating sheet such as a class evaluation, shown in Figure 16.8 in the Supplemental Materials. Client reaction often provides feedback to group leaders, too. For example, it may help determine which techniques worked best, or what questions may not have been addressed. This information can then be used to revise outlines for future classes. Following a one-on-one nutrition counseling session, it is also imperative to solicit the client's reaction. Usually, this is done informally by asking questions such as:

- Was this session helpful to you?
- What questions are left unanswered?
- Would you like to meet again to discuss your diet? If so, what would you like to talk about?

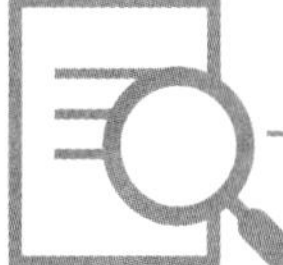

View the Supplemental Material to see Figure 16.8 Sample Class Evaluation Form.

Actual Learning

The second level of evaluation answers the question: *How much did clients learn?* To evaluate learning, use written and verbal questions, often given as a post-test. This is a test about facts and information presented. Some educational strategies require a pre-test before a session begins, and the same test at the end given as the post-test. This allows one to measure how much participants have learned.

Here are some examples of instructions/questions that could be used to evaluate how much a client learned:

- Divide the list of foods into two groups, those with ________ (e.g., high calories, the most vitamins, fat, sodium, etc.) or ________ (least vitamin C, low calories, low-fat, low-sodium).
- Write down one fact you learned that you will use.
- What is the difference between these food products? (e.g., sugar content, fat content, sodium content)
- Choose, from this group of foods, the best source of ________ (e.g., fiber, unsaturated fat, carbohydrate, calories, etc.).
- What would be a better way to increase ________ (e.g., calories, fiber, iron, vitamin A, etc.)?
- Create a menu you would eat that meets your fluid restrictions.

Behavior Change

The third level of evaluation answers the question: *Have dietary habits changed?* Refer to the learning objectives, and observe how behavior corresponds to the objectives themselves. In some cases, a food diary is useful. If clients are using a selective menu in a hospital or nursing facility, monitor how they make choices on menus. Likewise, if a client is choosing foods in a dining room, evaluate change by visiting the client at mealtime and making observations. There are many online self-tracking food diaries, which can help a client with immediate feedback.

Refining Plans

If the results of the evaluation show that education has not been as effective as planned, try to identify the reasons why that might be. A feedback tool such as the evaluation may help with this process. Since a rapport has already been established with the clients, it is easier to discover the reasons simply by asking the question(s) in a friendly, low-key manner. For example, three days after counseling a client about how to implement a high-calorie diet, say: *We are aiming to keep your daily calories up to 1500. Your calorie count for yesterday shows 900 calories. Why do you think that might be? (Or: Can you tell me a little bit about that?) Can you look at the meal plan and tell me what seems to be challenging?* Keeping the responses non-judgmental makes it easier for clients to trust the educator and allows the client to learn more effectively.

Consider all possible barriers to communication. These may include differences in language, ability to read (if relying on printed materials), use of terminology a client does not understand, state of alertness, and many others. If any of these barriers exists, re-evaluate how best to communicate with a client. Also keep in mind that individual learning styles vary. One person may learn best by reading words. Another may learn best by glancing at images and graphics. One needs to hear information. Another needs to do things (use hands-on activities). Each of these styles is valid, and each requires different educational techniques. If it is discovered that a client has not understood information, try using a different educational approach.

As the process and information is evaluated, it's important to be flexible. Do not expect perfection from clients, especially if they are striving to change long-standing dietary habits. Try to notice every positive step toward achieving objectives. Encouragement reassures a client about putting information into practice, and tends to bring about more of the same behaviors.

In addition, it's critical to recognize the distinction between knowledge and behavior. This distinction comes to the forefront continually when examining any type of health education. The client might know the information that will make them healthy. However, that doesn't mean they will automatically put it all into practice. Often, the challenge is not limited to explaining diets or relaying information. The real challenge is to help motivate and support an individual in making subtle improvements in habits. This may hinge on much more than nutrition knowledge. In fact, dietary habits have many cultural and psychological undertones. Values, emotional needs, and other life priorities may easily affect the final outcomes of nutrition counseling. As much as possible, try to understand these factors, and help clients address them. As needed, mold the suggestions to a client's preferences, customs, and concerns. It may be necessary to creatively weave nutrition ideas into specialized plans in order to match a client's needs.

Also consider the big picture. Nutrition education is only one component of a health plan. Consider the other components, and ask how these fit together for the client. Is the client overwhelmed? Is nutrition high or low on a priority list? If there are many

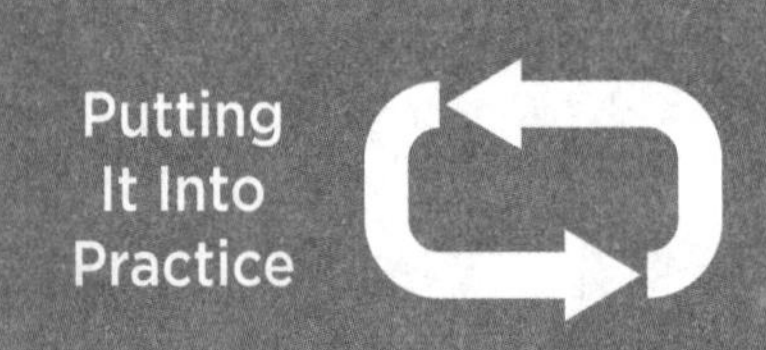

3. Your client is having trouble understanding nutrition education that was presented in a list form. What could be done to help?

health-related objectives and regimens, it may help to show the client how nutrition can support other needs. For example, a client who has hypertension and is also obese may appreciate discovering how weight loss will likely help reduce hypertension, too. The bottom line is to articulate a payoff for the client. Explain how the client will benefit, how he or she will feel, or what other desirable health effects could be expected from implementing dietary advice.

Furthermore, it is easy for a client to believe that sound nutrition is an all-or-nothing endeavor. This is key to the culture of dieting, and tends to affect our thinking when it comes to nutrition. Effective education depends on the ability to transform dietary advice into a series of small steps and to praise all positive changes. Any time a client experiences difficulty following a restrictive diet, we can provide reassurance and encouragement.

Sometimes, implementing dietary advice simply isn't practical for a client, due to one of various obstacles. As part of any reassessment, be alert to problems that may interfere with meeting nutrition-related objectives. Factors such as medications, dental changes, or changes in swallowing ability can easily affect how a person eats. If obstacles exist, try to help remove them. If that is not possible, refine the plan and the education to make them realistic for the client.

Documenting Evaluation

Like any aspect of a nutrition care plan, nutrition education requires evaluation and documentation. When providing nutrition counseling, be sure to document this information in the health record and sign and date it. Document who was involved (e.g., client and/or family members), what was covered, and what learning objectives were agreed upon. In addition, name/list any handouts that were provided. Document the assessment of a client's understanding of the educational content. As possible, state how the client has met or will meet behavioral objectives. For example: *Client accurately selected foods to total 160 grams of carbohydrates on tomorrow's menu.* Also, state the recommendation for follow-up. Upon reassessment of educational objectives, it is important to gather new information and continue to document progress in the medical record. If the plan for education is revised, be sure to indicate this in the progress note.

Reinforcing Education

Typically, one nutrition education session does not change a person's dietary habits. The most effective education is delivered in manageable chunks, over a period of time. Education of any type requires reinforcement. If there is opportunity to have ongoing contact with clients, as in a school, retirement community, or long-term care facility, this offers an excellent opportunity to provide intermittent education and reinforcement.

Reinforcement can be as simple as:

- Providing a nutrition tip on a menu
- Preparing a bulletin board in the facility to highlight a nutrition topic
- Labeling foods in a group dining area with nutrition facts
- Chatting with a client about daily food choices
- Noticing when a client implements a dietary change at any meal, and providing praise

- Giving a client an opportunity to ask a follow-up question a day or two after an educational session
- Highlighting a special item on a menu and noting how it meets particular needs

Summary

Nutrition education is the foundation of what helps clients participate in caring for themselves. The CDM, CFPP plays a critical role in helping the client develop basic skills in this area. It's important for the CDM, CFPP to understand all of the steps necessary that go into providing the most effective nutrition education.

Clearly, education is more than a one-shot endeavor. Quite often, CDM, CFPPs are in roles where they can have a tremendous impact on clients' individual dietary choices.

Chapter References

RESOURCES	
Academy of Nutrition and Dietetics. Accessed September 18, 2019.	https://www.eatright.org
Becky Dorner & Associates Inc. Accessed March 29, 2020.	https://www.beckydorner.com
How to Set & Achieve Your Goals. SMART Goals Guide. Accessed March 21, 2020.	https://www.smart-goals-guide.com
Metcalf, Tom. Listening to Your Clients. Life Association News. 1997;92(7):16	
Prochaska JO, Velicer WF, Rossi JS, et al. Stages of change and decisional balance for 12 problem behaviors. Health Psychol. 1994;13(1);39-46	
Pucket, RP, Lucas RA. *Food, Nutrition and Medical Nutrition Therapy Through the Life Cycle. 4th ed.* Dubuque, IA: Kendall Hunt Publishing; 2006.	
Smith B, Miller AW, Archer T, Hague C. Working with Diverse Cultures. Accessed March 29, 2020.	https://extension.usu.edu/diversity/ou-files/factsheet704.pdf

Participate in Regulatory Agency Surveys

Overview and Objectives

The last few chapters have addressed how critical it is to focus on clients and their quality of care. State and federal regulations also focus on clients and their quality of care. Learning the regulations, how to locate them, and some tips for following them will assist the Certified Dietary Manager®, Certified Food Protection Professional® (CDM®, CFPP®). After completing this chapter, you should be able to:

- Identify regulatory standards and recent revisions
- Develop an appropriate plan of correction
- Demonstrate professional interaction with surveyors
- Utilize regulatory agencies as professional resources
- Explain how regulations influence the quality management process

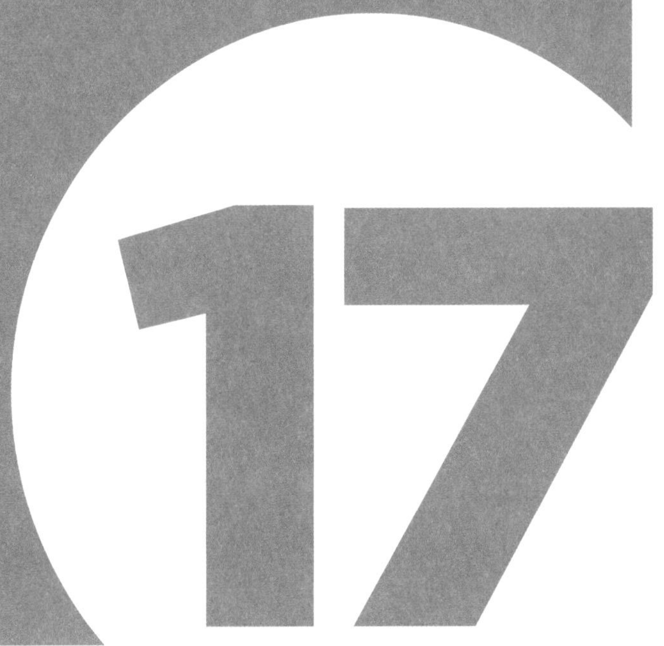

t is fitting that the last chapter in this textbook is about regulations. In many ways, regulations address everything that has been covered in this book. Let's look first at the regulatory agencies and the regulations that most impact the nutrition and foodservice department.

Regulatory/Accrediting Agencies

The **Centers for Medicare & Medicaid Services (CMS)** is a branch of the U.S. Department of Health & Human Services. CMS is the federal agency that administers the Medicare program and monitors the Medicaid programs offered in each state. All healthcare facilities have mandatory state licensing requirements according to their state law. The facility is held to the strictest regulatory requirements, either state or federal. It is important to know and follow the local state regulations. Once a facility has a state license to operate, it can voluntarily seek a federal CMS survey to determine if it is compliant with all the federal 'certification' requirements for federal funding. The long-term care initial and annual federal survey, required by the Omnibus Budget Reconciliation ACT (OBRA) 1987, is usually provided by state agency surveyors who wear the federal hat. Acute care hospital surveys may have a CMS deemed status and a survey process annually or every three years, and a skilled nursing facility or long-term care facility is surveyed about once a year (not later than 15 months after the last day of the previous standard survey). Since a CMS validation survey can be conducted at any time, it is important to be "survey ready" at all times. Any healthcare facility that offers services to clients who are funded by Medicare or Medicaid must follow CMS regulations. CMS also oversees HIPAA, the act that assures privacy for all healthcare client information.

GLOSSARY

Centers for Medicare & Medicaid Services (CMS)
A federal agency within the Department of Health & Human Services that administers the Medicare program. CMS works with state governments to administer Medicaid, Children's Health Insurance Program (CHIP), and Health Insurance Portability Standards

Regulations appear in a document called the CMS State Operations Manual (SOM). To access this information, go to www.cms.gov. Search for the CMS State Operations Manual. This is the document that will be used in the survey process. It is a large document and it is important for the CDM, CFPP and the Registered Dietitian Nutritionist to work together to address the nutrition components of the survey. The operations manual contains a great deal of helpful information besides the regulations. Regulations cover all areas of a healthcare facility including the following, that are specific to nutrition in:

483.25 Quality of Care

- 483.25(g) Tube Feeding Management
- 483.25(h) Parenteral/IV Fluids
- 483.25(c) Pressure Sores
- 483.25(i) Nutrition
- 483.25(j) Hydration

483.60 Food and Nutrition Services

- 483.60(a) Staffing
- 483.60(d) Food
- 483.60(e) Therapeutic Diets

For more information and specifics, refer back to Chapter 9. Other foodservice regulations are covered in the *Foodservice Management—By Design* textbook. Many other regulatory tags throughout the SOM overlap.

CMS Federal regulatory requirements for Nutrition in Long-Term Care and related tags for hospitals can be found on the CMS website (www.cms.gov). It is challenging to keep up with regulatory revisions, survey expectations, and changing evidence-based expectations in the industry. As interdisciplinary team members in a very demanding area of care, it is imperative to keep current and knowledgeable.

CMS provides investigative protocols that provide guidance for surveyors. The Investigative Protocol for Nutrition Status can be found on the CMS website. CMS guidelines use **F-Tag** numbers to identify specific guidance for long-term care; they use **A-Tag** numbers for hospitals. Changes to these documents are ongoing to improve quality of care. These changes make long-term care facilities more accountable for maintaining clients' nutrition status. CMS uses quality measures to assess the quality of care in healthcare facilities such as: Percent of Low-Risk Residents Who Have Pressure Sores (looks back seven days).

Small rural hospitals or critical access hospitals use **C-Tag** numbers. Some hospitals have a subacute or rehab unit on their license and must meet the regulatory requirements of both the acute and the long-term care regulations. Nutrition Services staff, including CDM, CFPPs in collaboration with Registered Dietitian Nutritionists, should study and know all the regulatory requirements for all levels of care that they provide. Work with the Registered Dietitian Nutritionist in the facility to review and educate the Nutrition Services staff regarding the CMS regulations.

Several for-profit agencies offer voluntary accreditation according to their established standards of care. They are not to be confused with the requirements of a state license or the requirement to certify for federal funds. The most well known is **The Joint Commission**, formerly The Joint Commission on Accreditation of Healthcare Organizations (JCAHO). Originally, The Joint Commission only accredited hospitals, but it has moved into other healthcare facilities such as long-term care. The Joint Commission is a nonprofit organization that accredits more than 22,000 U.S. health care organizations and programs. Most state governments recognize Joint Commission accreditation as a condition of licensure for the receipt of Medicaid and Medicare reimbursements. As of July 2010, The Joint Commission's hospital accreditation program is subject to Centers for Medicare & Medicaid Services (CMS) requirements for accrediting organizations. According to The Joint Commission, their mission is: *To continuously improve health care for the public, in collaboration with other stakeholders, by evaluating health care organizations and inspiring them to excel in providing safe and effective care of the highest quality and value.* The Joint Commission has established standards that each facility is measured against.

The Joint Commission accreditation for long-term care focuses on:

- Performance improvements
- The use of restraints
- Behavior management and treatment
- Quality control activities
- Medication errors
- Adverse drug indicators

GLOSSARY

F-Tag
An identification number of a CMS guideline for long-term care

A-Tag
An identification number of a CMS guideline for general acute care hospitals

C-Tag
An identification number of a CMS guideline for small rural or critical access hospitals

The Joint Commission
A non-profit organization that accredits healthcare organizations in the United States

The Survey Process

Both The Joint Commission and CMS use surveys as part of their accreditation or enforcement effort. As part of its enforcement effort, CMS and its contracted state agencies conduct on-site surveys of healthcare facilities. Each time a team of surveyors arrives to evaluate compliance of a healthcare facility with CMS regulations, all managers become involved. A survey is typically unannounced, and may occur on any day of the week. A standard LTC survey is designed to review compliance with CMS regulations, including all the detail of the various F-Tags.

A survey process for long-term care is called the **CMS Quality Indicator Survey (QIS)**. The QIS process provides for the review of larger samples of clients based on the MDS, observations, interviews, and clinical record reviews. Figure 17.1 shows an overview of the QIS process. This figure will help the CDM, CFPP follow the QIS survey process.

> **GLOSSARY**
>
> **CMS Quality Indicator Survey (QIS)**
> Survey process for long-term care facilities and provides for a broader review based on the MDS, observations, interviews, and review of clinical records

At the time of a survey, a CDM, CFPP may be asked to provide documentation and pertinent information (nutrition screening and assessment data, nutrition care plans, etc.). Surveyors will focus on interdisciplinary care with a resident-centered care focus, and increased continuity and timeliness of care. Part of the survey may include a detailed tour of dietary areas. A CDM, CFPP should accompany a surveyor and cooperate fully. When the survey concludes, the survey team will state any deficiencies noted and reference F-Tag numbers. Ask the Registered Dietitian Nutritionist in the facility to see the last forms from a survey and explain them, the deficiency noted, and discuss the corrective action taken. A deficiency is a finding that the facility is not in compliance with CMS Guidelines. The facility is cited and instructed to correct the deficiency. Deficiencies are categorized by the level of risk/harm that may occur. If problems are identified, the CDM, CFPP and other members of the interdisciplinary team need to follow up promptly and effectively to correct them. In all, a CDM, CFPP plays a critical role in assuring that the quality of dietary services meets the needs of clients, and that the end results of care are excellent. Use the State Operations Manual References found at www.cms.gov to prepare for the survey process.

Search the website for:

- State Operations Manual—Appendix P
- Guidance to Surveyors for LTC Facilities—Appendix PP
- Guidance to Surveyors for LTC Facilities—Appendix Q

Quality Assurance (QA)

Because a survey could occur at any time, a CDM, CFPP should always be prepared. In other words, a CDM, CFPP needs to manage the entire quality process day-to-day, and assure that standards are being met. Having a quality assurance program is a critical approach to quality management. Quality assurance is a process of evaluating and verifying whether your services meet or exceed the client's expectations.

In health care, there have been many names for quality assurance processes (e.g., CQI, QI, QA, PDCA, LEAN, QAPI). Today, health care is realizing that quality is an

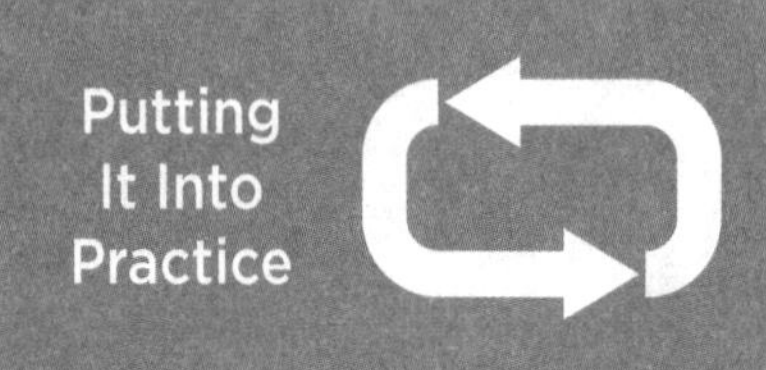

1. During last year's survey, a problem was identified with the timing of meals. Where can the CDM, CFPP go to find the regulations for timing of meals?

essential element of organizational strategy, not a single initiative. CMS calls it QAPI (Quality Assessment and Performance Improvement). The facility is required to have quality initiative(s). Whatever the facility calls the quality initiative, it should have these characteristics:

- Focus on clients and what they need, rather than on workers or departments and what they do.
- Be a team approach that is multidisciplinary.
- Use and evaluate the data. Make changes/improvements based on results.
- Is proactive and continuous. Don't wait for a problem to occur; continuously look at processes and ways to improve the processes.
- Contain a performance improvement segment.

Some states or corporate entities may have financial incentives for facilities that meet the annual QI goal(s).

Quality initiatives use some key terminology. One term is **outcome**. An outcome is the end result of work. In a healthcare environment, a health outcome describes the consequences of clinical interventions. For instance, if members of the healthcare team work together to improve a client's nutritional status, what happens to that client's nutritional status is the outcome of the clinical care plan. **Quality indicators (QIs)** are measures of outcomes. According to CMS, an indicator is "a key clinical value or quality characteristic used to measure, over time, the performance, processes, and outcomes of an organization or some component of healthcare delivery." As can be seen by this definition, indicators are designed to facilitate collection and analysis of data. They are objective and measurable.

GLOSSARY

Outcome
Outcome is the end result of work

Quality Indicators (QIs)
Quality indicators are measures of outcomes

A general process for implementing QA in health care uses two acronyms: FOCUS and PDCA. **FOCUS** means:

F—Find a process to improve.
O—Organize to improve a process.
C—Clarify what is known.
U—Understand variation.
S—Select a process improvement.

Once a process has been selected to improve, the next acronym relates to the plan itself. **PDCA** means:

P—Plan: Decide what will be done to improve the process. Decide what information to collect, and how to measure outcomes.

D—Do: Make the improvements.

C—Check: Collect and review data, and evaluate how the plan is working.

A—Act: Act on what has been learned. If successful improvement has been made, make sure it becomes part of the policies and procedures. If not, try an alternate plan.

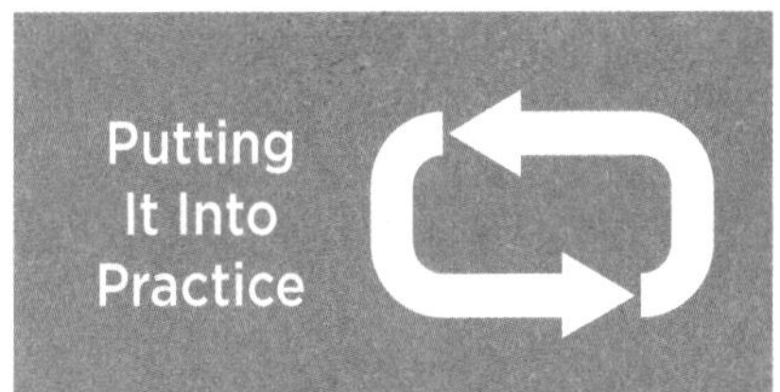

2. Residents are frequently complaining that they are not getting what they ordered. During the QAPI process, what measure might you track to audit for meal accuracy?

Figure 17.1
Overview of the QIS Process

Automation	• Each survey team member uses a tablet PC throughout the survey process to record findings that are synthesized and organized by the QIS software.
Offsite	• Review the OSCAR 3 Report and current complaints. • Download the MDS data to tablet PCs. • The production-grade software (ASE-Q) selects a random sample of residents for Stage I.
Tour	• No sample selection. • Initial overview of facility.
Sample Selection	• The production-grade software (ASE-Q) provides a randomly selected sample of residents for the following: > Admission sample is a review of 30 current or discharged resident records. > Census sample includes 40 current residents for observation, interview, and record review.
Survey Structure	• Stage I: Preliminary investigation of regulatory areas in the admission and census samples and mandatory facility-level tasks started. • Stage II: Completion of in-depth investigation of triggered care areas and/or facility-level tasks based on Stage I findings.
Group Interview	• Interview with Resident Council President or Representative.

Source: Centers for Medicare & Medicaid Services

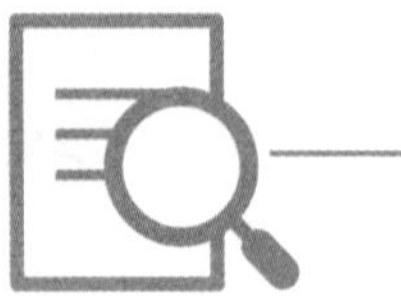

View the Supplemental Material to see Figure 17.3 Worksheet A: Identifying Areas for Improvement.

Quality Assessment and Performance Improvement (QAPI)

Not only are surveyors looking at what is done for quality assurance, they are also looking at how the data is used for performance improvement. CMS has language in both the hospital and long-term care regulations that facilities must:

- Develop, implement, and maintain an effective, ongoing, facility-wide, data-driven quality assessment and performance improvement program.
- Involve all departments and services.
- Focus on indicators related to improved health outcomes and prevention.

The Institute for Healthcare Improvement (www.ihi.org) has developed a worksheet that can help you with the Plan, Do, Check/Study, Act for performance improvement. Their tool is shown in Figure 17.2. The Medicare Quality Improvement Community (MedQIC) website is "a free online resource for quality improvement interventions and associated tools, toolkits, presentations, and links to other resources." The website is funded by CMS to provide a site to share resources based on the CMS scope of work. An example of a tool that is located there to help identify areas for improvement in the facility is shown in Figure 17.3, provided in the Supplemental Materials.

A CDM, CFPP is involved in many quality management issues. Remember that interdisciplinary effort is a strong focus of quality management and CMS regulations.

Thus, neither surveyors nor administrators divide up CMS regulations and hand a section to each manager. The CDM, CFPP is often the most accessible person during a survey and needs to understand the regulations, the facility's quality assessment process, and how the data supports the performance improvement.

The long-term care regulation F692 Nutrition/Hydration Maintenance & F808 Prescribed Therapeutic Diet requires that a therapeutic diet be provided based upon client needs and that client preferences and desires are honored as part of their quality of life. F550 Resident Rights/Exercise of Rights requires the facility to give the client a right of refusal of any therapeutic order. F561 Self Determination requires the facility to allow clients to make choices and self-determination. (This applies to hospital client rights as well.) The expectation is to ensure that the facility is aware of the client's preferences and desires. How will the client know that he/she has a choice? Review the nutrition screening and nutrition assessment information; does it document the client's preferences and desires? Interview questions should be specific to inform the client that this is his/her home and their right to make choices will be honored for increased quality of life. As can be seen, the CDM, CFPP plays a pivotal role in the lives of clients and in each facility.

Figure 17.2
PDSA Worksheet for Testing Change

Aim: (overall goal you wish to achieve)
Every goal will require multiple smaller tests of change

Describe the first (or next) test of change	Person responsible	When to be done	Where to be done

Plan:

List the tasks needed to set up this test of change	Person responsible	When to be done	Where to be done

Do: Describe what actually happened when the test was run.

Study: Describe the measured results and how they compared to the predictions.

Act: Describe what modifications to the plan will be made for the next cycle from what was learned.

Source: Institute for Healthcare Improvement

Chapter References

RESOURCES	
American Health Care Association.	http://www.ahcancal.org
Centers for Medicare & Medicaid Services (CMS).	http://www.cms.gov
Centers for Medicare & Medicaid Services (CMS) State Operations Manual Appendix Guide.	https://www.cms.gov/Regulations-and-Guidance/Guidance/Manuals/downloads/som107_appendicestoc.pdf
Centers for Medicare & Medicaid Services (CMS) State Operations Manual—Appendix PP.	https://www.cms.gov/Regulations-and-Guidance/Guidance/Manuals downloads/som107ap_pp_ guidelines_ltcf.pdf
Centers for Medicare & Medicaid Services (CMS) State Operations Manual—Appendix Q.	https://www.cms.gov
Centers for Medicare & Medicaid Services (CMS) Quality Measures.	https://www.cms.gov/Regulations-and-Guidance/Legislation/EHRIncentivePrograms/ClinicalQualityMeasures
Centers for Medicare & Medicaid Services (CMS) Survey Process.	https://www.cms.gov/Medicare/Provider-Enrollment-and-Certification/GuidanceforLawsAndRegulations/Downloads LTCSP-Procedure-Guide.pdf
Healthcentric Advisors.	http://healthcentricadvisors.org
Institute for Healthcare Improvement.	http://www.ihi.org
The Joint Commission.	https://www.jointcommission.org/

Accessed March 30, 2020.

APPENDIX A

Focus on Formulas

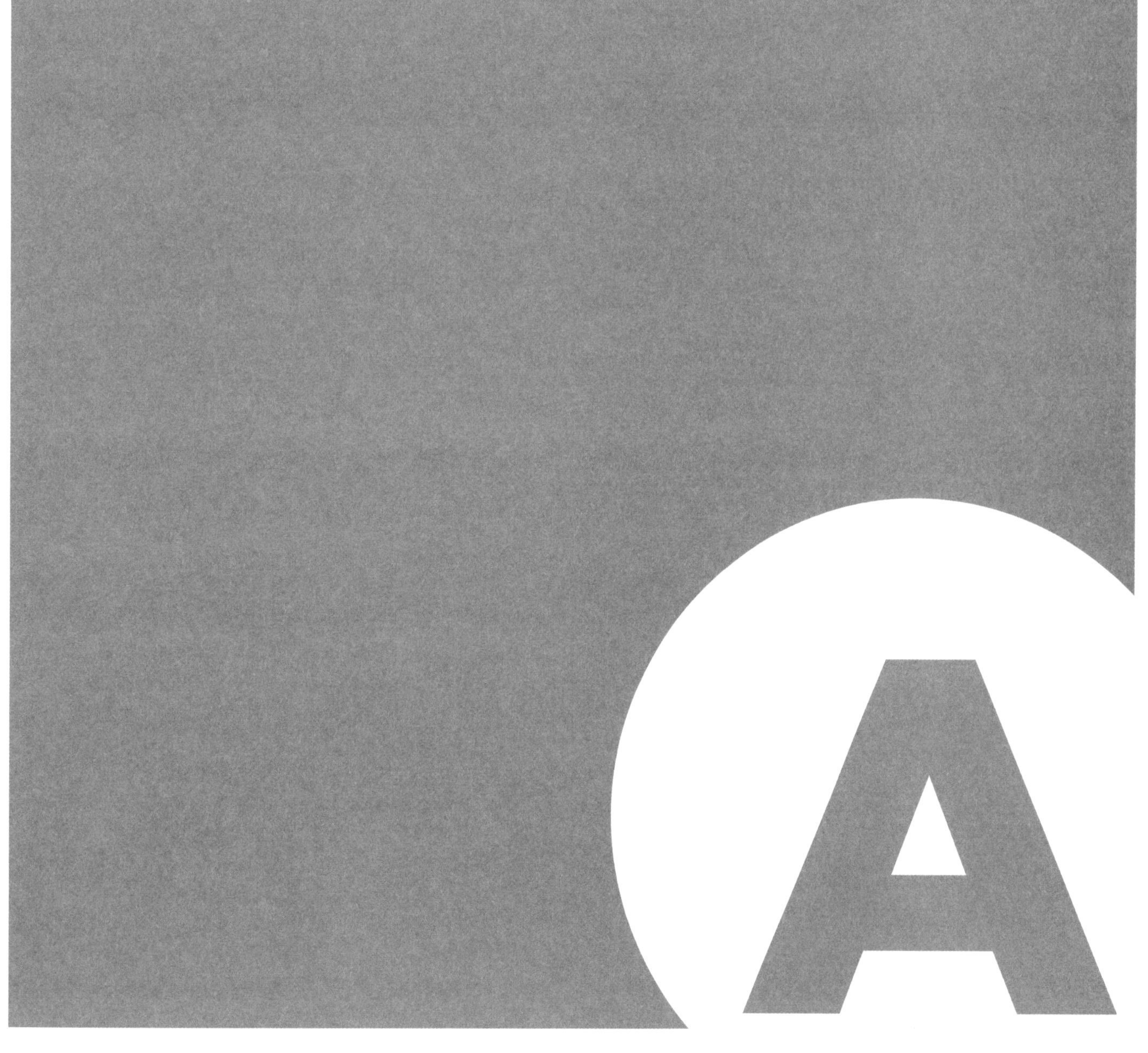

CALORIE EXCHANGE

COMPONENTS	FORMULA
1 gm of CHO = 4 calories 1 gm of protein = 4 calories 1 gm of fat = 9 calories	# of grams x # of calories
EXAMPLE	**RESULT**
If a diet order consists of 200 gm CHO, 45 gm protein, and 6 gm fat, how many calories does it have?	200 x 4 = 800 45 x 4 = 180 6 x 9 = 54 = 1,034 calories

View a step-by-step video of this formula on ANFPtv: https://videos.anfponline.org/calorie-exchange

FLUID INTAKE

COMPONENTS	FORMULA
Milliliters Cups Ounces	1 cup = 8 ounces = 240 mL
EXAMPLE	**RESULT**
A patient is on a restricted diet of 1200 mL per day. They are allowed 800 mL a day from meals and snacks. How many cups/day are they allowed?	1 cup = 240 mL Fluid Intake = 800/240 mL Fluid Intake = 5 cups per day

View a step-by-step video of this formula on ANFPtv: https://videos.anfponline.org/fluid-intake

FOCUS ON FORMULAS: NUTRITION

COMPONENTS	FORMULA
Healthy Adult: .8 grams x body weight in kg **Malnourished Adult:** 1.2 - 1.5 grams **Following Surgery:** 1-2 grams **Following Trauma, Severe Burns, or Multiple Fractures:** 2 grams	To determine the amount of grams of protein: • Determine the body weight in kg (# of lbs/2.2 kg per lb) • Identify protein needs
EXAMPLE	**RESULT**
Susan is a healthy female who weighs 144 pounds, what are her protein requirements?	144 / 2.2 = 65.45 kg 65.45 x .8 = 52.36 gm of protein per day

View a step-by-step video of this formula on ANFPtv: https://videos.anfponline.org/daily-protein-needs

IDEAL BODY WEIGHT

COMPONENTS	FORMULA
Height (H) **Weight (W)** **Frame Size (FS)**	**Women:** Ideal Body Weight (IBW) = 100 lbs. (W) for first 5 feet of height (H) plus 5 lbs. for each inch over 5 feet. If under 5 feet, subtract 5 lbs. for each inch under 5 feet. **Men:** Ideal Body Weight (IBW) = 106 lbs. (W) for first 5 feet of height (H) plus 6 lbs. for each inch over 5 feet. If under 5 feet, subtract 5 lbs. for each inch under 5 feet. **Frame Size:** • Small Frame = subtract 10% from the total • Medium Frame = no change • Large Frame = add 10% to the total
EXAMPLE	**RESULT**
John is a 6'2" male with a large frame BW = 106 lbs. + ((14 inches over 5 ft. x 6 lbs. per inch)) x 10% for large frame	BW = (106 + 84) x 1.1 BW = (190) x 1.1 BW = 209 or 209 lbs.

View a step-by-step video of this formula on ANFPtv: https://videos.anfponline.org/ideal-body-weight

PERCENTAGE OF IDEAL BODY WEIGHT

COMPONENTS	FORMULA
Body Weight **Ideal Body Weight (IBW)**	% of IBW = (Actual Weight/IBW) x 100
EXAMPLE	**RESULT**
Jose's Weight = 192 lbs. IBW = 175 lbs. What is his percentage of IBW?	192/175 x 100 = 109.7% (% of Jose's IBW)

View a step-by-step video of this formula on ANFPtv: https://videos.anfponline.org/percentage-of-ideal-body-weight

Index

A

B

E

F

G

L

M

N

O

P

W

Z